# Echocardiography in Acute Coronary Syndrome

Eyal Herzog, MD · Farooq Chaudhry, MD
Editors

# Echocardiography in Acute Coronary Syndrome

## Diagnosis, Treatment and Prevention

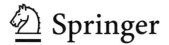 Springer

*Editors*
Eyal Herzog, MD
Division of Cardiology
St. Luke's Roosevelt Hospital Center
1111 Amsterdam Ave.
New York NY 10025
USA
EHerzog@chpnet.org

Farooq Chaudhry, MD
Division of Cardiology
St. Luke's Roosevelt Hospital Center
1111 Amsterdam Ave.
New York NY 10025
USA
FChaudhr@chpnet.org

ISBN 978-1-84882-026-5    e-ISBN 978-1-84882-027-2
DOI 10.1007/978-1-84882-027-2
Springer Dordrecht Heidelberg London New York

British Library Cataloguing in Publication Data
A catalogue record for this book is available from the British Library

Library of Congress Control Number: 2009921355

Printed on acid-free paper

Springer is part of Springer Science+Business Media (www.springer.com)

*To our late fathers, Abdul Din Chaudhry and Joseph Herzog, for their uncompromising commitments, principles and beliefs that guided our lives.*

*To our mothers, Safia B. Chaudhry and Ruth Gill, for their unconditional love and continuous and unrelenting support for their children.*

*To our wives, Sophia Zeb Chaudhry and Ronit Herzog, for their unwavering love, support, encouragement and complete devotion to our families.*

*To our children, Farhan, Fayzan, Faraz and Samia Chaudhry; Karin, Lee, and Jonathan Herzog for making everything worthwhile and in providing us with the greatest gift of all.*

# Preface

This is the first edition of Echocardiography in Acute Coronary Syndromes. There have been major advances and developments in both the field of Acute Coronary Syndrome and Echocardiography. This book is intended to address the important role echocardiography plays in diagnosing and evaluating patients with Acute Coronary Syndrome. It addresses current and new techniques in the field of echocardiography and how they can be applied in diagnosing and managing Acute Coronary Syndrome. All the contributing authors have been most gracious, dedicated, diligent and resourceful in their efforts to accomplish this.

The editors are thankful to Springer-London Company and its efficient staff for their overall professional handling and coordination of this book. The editors wish to express special appreciation to LaToya Selby and Jacqueline Wilkins whose spirit, efforts and hard work assured orderly and efficient manner to bring the book to fruition.

The editors are also especially thankful to their colleagues, past and present, especially fellows who have been an inspiration for constantly striving to keep abreast of the latest literature.

With deepest gratitude, we wish to express our thanks for the loyal support, understanding and encouragement during many hours required for preparation, reading and the reviewing for this book, to our families and in particular to our wives, Sophia Zeb Chaudhry and Ronit Herzog, and to our children, Farhan, Fayzan, Faraz and Samia Chaudhry, and Karin, Lee, and Jonathan Herzog; and a special thanks to our mothers Safia and Ruth.

Eyal Herzog and Farooq Chaudhry

# Contents

# Contributors

**Dr. Asimul Ansari, MD**  Department of Cardiology, Northwestern Memorial Hospital, Chicago, IL, USA

**Bilal Ayub, MD**  Resident Internal Medicine, Abington Memorial Hospital, Abington, Pennsylvania

**Emad Aziz, DO, MB, ChB**  Cardiology, St Luke's Roosevelt Hospital Center, New York, NY, USA

**Sripal Bangalore, MD, MHA**  Cardiology, Brigham and Women's Hospital, Harvard Medical School, Boston, MA, USA

**J. Todd Belcik, BS, RDCS, FASE**  Division of Cardiovascular Medicine, Oregon Health and Science University, Portland, OR, USA

**Farooq A. Chaudhry, MD**  Medicine, St. Luke's-Roosevelt Hospital Center, New York, NY, USA

**Mohamed Djelmami-Hani, MD**  Cardiology, Aurora Sinai Medical Center, Milwaukee, WI, USA

**Olivier Frankenberger, MD**  Cardiology, St. Luke's-Roosevelt Hospital, New York, NY, USA

**Kohei Fujimoto, MD, PhD**  Cardiology, Columbia University Medical Center, New York, NY, USA

**Linda D. Gillam, MD, FACC, FAHA, FASE**  Department of Medicine, Cardiology, Columbia University Medical Center, New York, NY, USA

**Eyal Herzog, MD**  St. Luke's Roosevelt Hospital Center, New York, NY, USA

**Shunichi Homma, MD**  Medicine, Colombia University, New York, NY, USA

**Mun K. Hong, MD**  Interventional Cardiology, St Luke's Roosevelt Hospital Center, New York, NY, USA

**Dr. Shao-Ling Huang, MD, PhD**  Department of Internal Medicine, University of Texas Health Science Center, Houston, TX, USA

**Gregory Janis, MD**  Cardiology, St Luke's-Roosevelt Hospital Center, New York, NY, USA

**Sandeep Joshi, MD**  Cardiology, St Luke's Roosevelt Hospital Center, 1111 Amsterdam Ave, New York, NY, USA

**Patrick Kee, MD, PhD**  Division of Cardiology, Department of Medicine, The University of Texas Health Science Center, Houston, TX, USA

**Sheila Khianey, MD**  St Luke's Roosevelt Hospital Center, New York, NY, USA

**Bette Kim, MD**  Division of Cardiology, St. Luke's-Roosevelt Hospital Center, New York, NY, USA

**Hyunggun Kim, PhD**  Department of Internal Medicine, University of Texas Health Science Center, Houston, TX, USA

**Melvin E. Klegerman, PhD**  Division of Cardiology, University of Texas Health Science Center-Houston, Houston, TX, USA

**Itzhak Kronzon, MD**  Department of Medicine (Cardiology), NYU Medical Center, New York, NY, USA

**Marrick Kukin, MD**  Cardiology, St Luke's-Roosevelt Hospital Centre, New York, NY, USA

**Jonathan R. Lindner, MD**  Cardiovascular Division, Oregan Health and Science University, Portland, OR, USA

**Kameswari Maganti, MD**  Cardiology, Northwestern University, Chicago, IL, USA

**David D. McPherson, MD**  Internal Medicine-Cardiology, UTHSC Houston, Houston, TX, USA

**Andrew P. Miller, MD**  Cardiovascular Disease/Medicine, University of Alabama at Birmingham, Birmingham, AL, USA

**Raaid Museitif, MD**  Cardiology, Aurora Sinai Medical Center, Milwaukee, Wisconsin, USA

**Merle Myerson, MD, EdD**  Director, Cardiovascular Disease Prevention Program, Division of Cardiology, St. Luke's-Roosevelt Hospital Center, New York, NY, USA

**Navin C. Nanda, MD**  University of Alabama at Birmingham, Birmingham, AL, USA

**Brian Nolan, DO**  Cardiovascular, Oregon Health and Science University, Portland, OR, USA

**Gurusher Singh Panjrath, MBBS**  The Johns Hopkins Hospital, Division of Cardiology, Baltimore, Maryland, USA

**Jyothy Puthumana, MD** Cardiology, Northwestern University Feinberg School of Medicine, Chicago, IL, USA

**Vera H. Rigolin, MD** Cardiology, Northwestern University Feinberg School of Medicine, Chicago, IL, USA

**Kiran B. Sagar, MD** Heart Care Associates, Milwaukee, WI, USA

**Rawa Sarji, MD** Resident Internal Medicine, St. Luke's Roosevelt Hospital, College of Physician and Surgeons, Columbia University, New York, NY, USA

**Muhamed Saric, MD, PhD** Department of Medicine, UMDNJ – New Jersey Medical School, Newark, NJ, USA

**Ajay S. Shah, MD** Cardiology, St Luke's-Roosevelt Hospital Center, New York, NY, USA

**Gregory S. Sherrid, MD** Mamaroneck, Westchester, NY, USA

**Mark V. Sherrid, MD** Cardiology, St Luke's-Roosevelt Hospital Center, 1000 10th Ave, New York, NY 10019, USA

**Dr. P. Tung, MD** Department of Internal Medicine, University of Texas Health Science Center, Houston, TX, USA

**Seth Uretsky, MD** Cardiology, St Luke's-Roosevelt Hospital Center, New York, NY, USA

**Dr. Kevin Wei, MD** Department of Internal Medicine/Cardiology, Oregon Health and Science University, Portland, OR, USA

**David Wild, MD** Cardiovascular Associates; Teaneck, NJ, USA

**Melana Yuzefpolsky, MD** Cardiology, St Luke's-Roosevelt Hospital Center, New York, NY, USA

# Chapter 1
# Introduction: Acute Coronary Syndrome and Echocardiography

Gurusher Singh Panjrath, Eyal Herzog, and Farooq A. Chaudhry

The last couple of decades have witnessed remarkable progress in the understanding of pathophysiology of acute coronary syndrome (ACS). This, in turn, has led to advances in imaging diagnosis and therapeutic options. Discovery of benefits of aspirin and thrombolytics was paralleled by the arrival of the coronary care units in the care of patients undergoing acute coronary syndromes and related arrhythmias. On the diagnostic front the development of noninvasive imaging modalities has achieved remarkable ground by assisting early diagnosis of an acute ischemic event. The hunger for technology was further fuelled by increasing options for invasive as well as medical revascularization. This furthered the need for availability of reliable and accessible modalities which could provide diagnostic as well as prognostic information to further risk stratify patients undergoing an ischemic event. Development of echocardiography paralleled the progress made in ACS. The initial use of echocardiography was to detect pericardial effusions and cardiac tumors. However, the current applications of various forms of echocardiography include an extended list of pathological and therapeutic indications. Advances in echocardiographic techniques and instrumentation have rivaled those in management of ACS.

This book is focused on the role of echocardiography in acute coronary syndrome. While plenty of books have examined the topics of echocardiography and acute coronary syndromes independently, the subsequent chapters in this book will discuss in detail the role of echocardiography pertaining specifically to acute coronary syndrome. Echocardiography today plays a quintessential role in the diagnosis of acute coronary syndrome and its related complications. Additionally, echocardiography plays an important role before and after ACS. The role of echocardiography in risk stratification and identifying subclinical disease is well established. Utility of echocardiography in cardiac resynchronization therapy in end-stage ischemic heart disease, as will be discussed later in this book, has been of increasing interest.

G.S. Panjrath (✉)
The Johns Hopkins Hospital, Division of Cardiology, Baltimore, Maryland, USA
e-mail: gpanjra1@jhmi.edu

E. Herzog, F.A. Chaudhry (eds.), *Echocardiography in Acute Coronary Syndrome*,
DOI 10.1007/978-1-84882-027-2_1, © Springer-Verlag London Limited 2009

## Echocardiography in the Emergency Room and Chest Pain Unit

Utility of echocardiography in the emergency room for diagnosis and management of chest pain has grown significantly over the years. Its utility has been noticed the most in patients with high clinical suspicion of ACS but a non-diagnostic ECG. Wall motion abnormalities, as a result of interrupted coronary blood flow, form the basis of this application. Reported sensitivity varies between 90 and 95% along with a negative predictive value of 90%.[1, 2] Echocardiography provides useful incremental prognostic data for identification of patients at risk of future cardiovascular events. Its use increases the sensitivity beyond that obtained from standard diagnostic criteria. Some authors, in an effort to evaluate its role in aggressive management and discharge of patients, demonstrated a negative predictive value of around 98%. This approach, however, would be considered too aggressive for most. A negative stress echocardiogram in patients with a negative electrocardiogram and biomarkers predicts excellent prognosis.[3] Pitfalls of such an aggressive approach include false negatives and undetected small infarctions in addition to concerns of dobutamine-induced platelet activation and myocardial injury.

## Risk Stratification in the Coronary Care Unit

Utility of echocardiography continues beyond diagnosis in the emergency room. Assessment of left ventricular function allows appropriate management and decision making regarding invasive versus conservative management. Event rate in patients with left ventricular dysfunction and mild to moderate wall motion abnormalities is greater than those with preserved ventricular function and wall motion abnormalities.[2] As will be discussed in detail later, additional information such as wall motion score index, left ventricular ejection fraction, end-systolic volume, and the presence of even mild mitral regurgitation are all early predictors of adverse outcome.

## Contrast Agents – Shadows with a Bright Future?

Since the first report in 1968 by Gramiak and Shah on the effect of contrast delineation of the aortic root during angiography,[4] contrast agents have traveled a long journey. Role of myocardial contrast echocardiography in noninvasive evaluation of myocardial perfusion and function awaits widespread clinical use in emergency departments and acute situations. Contrast agents can enhance the confidence to identify or exclude ischemia during stress echocardiography. However, even more exciting is the prospect to use micro bubbles for myocardial perfusion imaging.[5] Image quality and chamber opacification can be further improved by incorporating harmonic imaging.

Potential applications of micro bubbles vary from diagnosis of acute coronary syndromes to identifying the myocardial section at risk, myocardial viability,[6] collateral blood flow,[7] and outcomes of reperfusion intervention.[8] Furthermore, due to its ability to be destroyed by ultrasound, micro bubbles are under investigation as a vehicle for delivery of targeted agents including thrombolysis. Potential applications of micro bubbles have expanded to targeted imaging of inflammation,[9] apoptosis, gene[10] and liposomal drug delivery.[11]

However, the future of contrast agents and micro bubbles would depend on multiple factors, among them most important are safety and cost effectiveness.

## Future of Echocardiography in Acute Coronary Syndrome: Imaging and Beyond. . .

Despite technological challenges, its portability and ease of use is of utmost importance. Whether echocardiography is able to consolidate its position by overcoming safety issues pertaining to contrast agents and technological advancement in relation to instrumentation is of current experimental interest. Other areas of development will be targeted gene therapy or drug delivery systems (e.g., thrombolytics) and assessment of endothelial function and integrity using intravascular probes. Finally, techniques and instrumentation such as tissue Doppler imaging, strain rate imaging, and tissue characterization may be useful in assessment of ischemia and function.

## References

1. Peels CH, Visser CA, Kupper AJ, Visser FC, Roos JP. Usefulness of two-dimensional echocardiography for immediate detection of myocardial ischemia in the emergency room. *Am J Cardiol*. 1990 March 15;65(11):687–691.
2. Sabia P, Afrookteh A, Touchstone DA, Keller MW, Esquivel L, Kaul S. Value of regional wall motion abnormality in the emergency room diagnosis of acute myocardial infarction. A prospective study using two-dimensional echocardiography. *Circulation*. 1991 September;84(3 Suppl):I85–I92.
3. Colon PJ, 3rd, Guarisco JS, Murgo J, Cheirif J. Utility of stress echocardiography in the triage of patients with atypical chest pain from the emergency department. *Am J Cardiol*. 1998 November 15;82(10):1282–1284, A1210.
4. Gramiak R, Shah PM. Echocardiography of the aortic root. *Invest Radiol*. 1968 September–October;3(5):356–366.
5. Meza M, Greener Y, Hunt R, et al. Myocardial contrast echocardiography: reliable, safe, and efficacious myocardial perfusion assessment after intravenous injections of a new echocardiographic contrast agent. *Am Heart J*. 1996 October;132(4):871–881.
6. Shimoni S, Frangogiannis NG, Aggeli CJ, et al. Identification of hibernating myocardium with quantitative intravenous myocardial contrast echocardiography: comparison with dobutamine echocardiography and thallium-201 scintigraphy. *Circulation*. 2003 February 4;107(4):538–544.
7. Sabia PJ, Powers ER, Jayaweera AR, Ragosta M, Kaul S. Functional significance of collateral blood flow in patients with recent acute myocardial infarction. A study using myocardial contrast echocardiography. *Circulation*. 1992 June;85(6):2080–2089.

8. Ito H, Tomooka T, Sakai N, et al. Lack of myocardial perfusion immediately after successful thrombolysis. A predictor of poor recovery of left ventricular function in anterior myocardial infarction. *Circulation*. 1992 May;85(5):1699–1705.
9. Lindner JR, Dayton PA, Coggins MP, et al. Noninvasive imaging of inflammation by ultrasound detection of phagocytosed microbubbles. *Circulation*. 2000 August 1;102(5):531–538.
10. Shohet RV, Chen S, Zhou YT, et al. Echocardiographic destruction of albumin microbubbles directs gene delivery to the myocardium. *Circulation*. 2000 June 6;101(22):2554–2556.
11. Unger EC, Hersh E, Vannan M, Matsunaga TO, McCreery T. Local drug and gene delivery through microbubbles. *Prog Cardiovasc Dis*. 2001 July–August;44(1):45–54.

# Chapter 2
# A Novel Pathway for the Management of Acute Coronary Syndrome

Eyal Herzog, Emad Aziz, and Mun K. Hong

Acute coronary syndrome (ACS) subsumes a spectrum of clinical entities, ranging from unstable angina to ST elevation myocardial infarction.[1] The management of ACS is deservedly scrutinized, since it accounts for 2 million hospitalizations and a remarkable 30% of all deaths in the Unites States each year.[2] Clinical guidelines on the management of ACS, which are based on clinical trials, have been updated and published.[3, 4]

We have developed a novel pathway for the management of acute coronary syndrome at our institution, St. Luke's-Roosevelt Hospital Center (SLRHC), which is a university hospital of Columbia University College of Physicians and Surgeons.[5]

The pathway has been designated with the acronym of *PAIN* (*P*riority risk, *A*dvanced risk, *I*ntermediate risk and *N*egative/Low risk) that reflects patient's most immediate risk stratification upon admission (Fig. 2.1). This risk stratification reflects patient's 30 days risks for death and myocardial infarction following the initial ACS event.

The pathway is color-coded with "PAIN" acronym (P-red, A-yellow, I-yellow, N-green) that guides patient management according to patient's risk stratification. These colors – similar to the road traffic light code – have been chosen as an easy reference for the provider about the sequential risk level of patients with ACS.[6]

## The Goals of the Pain Pathway and a Road Map to the "Echocardiography in ACS" Book

### Initial Assessment of Patients with Chest Pain or Chest Pain Equivalent

Patients who present to emergency departments with chest pain or chest pain equivalent will be enrolled into this pathway.

E. Herzog (✉)
St. Luke's Roosevelt Hospital Center, New York, NY, USA
e-mail: EHerzog@chpnet.org

E. Herzog, F.A. Chaudhry (eds.), *Echocardiography in Acute Coronary Syndrome*,
DOI 10.1007/978-1-84882-027-2_2, © Springer-Verlag London Limited 2009

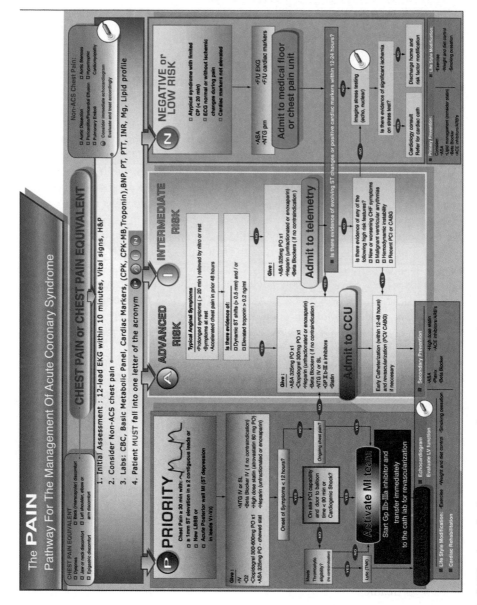

**Fig. 2.1** The PAIN pathway for the management of acute coronary syndrome

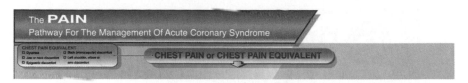

**Fig. 2.2** Chest pain and chest pain equivalent symptoms

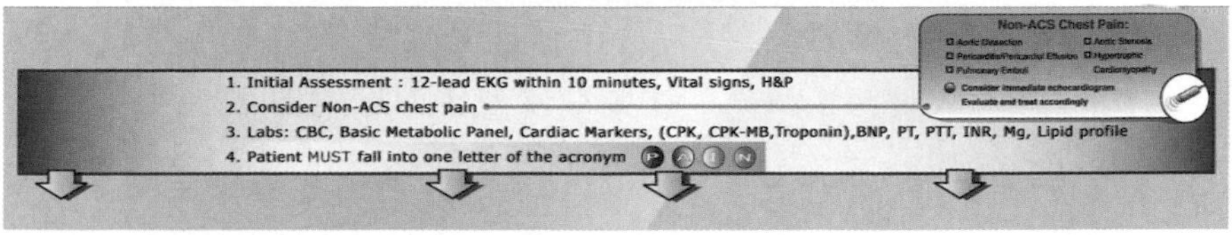

**Fig. 2.3** Initial assessment of patients with chest pain

Figure 2.2 shows the chest pain equivalent symptoms. The initial assessment is seen in Fig. 2.3. All patients should have an EKG performed within 10 min as well as detailed history and physical exam.

Non-ACS chest pain should be excluded urgently. These include aortic dissection, pericarditis and pericardial effusion, pulmonary emboli, aortic stenosis, and hypertrophic cardiomyopathy. If any of these emergency conditions is suspected, we recommend obtaining immediate echocardiogram or CT and to treat accordingly.

Our recommended initial laboratory tests include complete blood count, basic metabolic panel, cardiac markers (to include CPK, CPK-MB, and troponin), BNP, PT, PTT, INR, magnesium, and a lipid profile.

## Initial Management of PRIORITY Patients (Patients with ST Elevation Myocardial Infarction)

"PRIORITY" patients are those with symptoms of chest pain or chest pain equivalent lasting longer than 30 min with one of the following EKG criteria for acute myocardial infarction:

(1)  ≥1 mm ST elevation in two contiguous leads, or
(2)  New left bundle branch block, or
(3)  Acute posterior wall MI (ST segment depression in leads V1–V3)

The initial treatment of these patients includes obtaining an intravenous line, providing oxygen, treating patients with oral aspirin (chewable 325 mg stat), clopidogrel (300 or 600 mg loading dose), and intravenous beta blocker (if no contraindication), heparin (unfractionated or enoxaparin), nitroglycerin, and oral high-dose statin (Fig. 2.4).

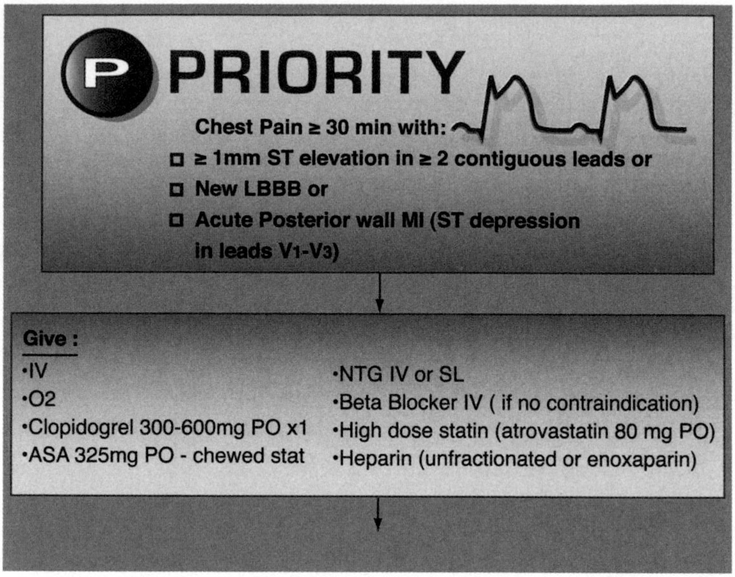

**Fig. 2.4** The initial management of PRIORITY patients (patients with ST elevation myocardial infarction)

The key question for further management of these patients is the duration of the patients' symptoms. For patients whose symptoms exceed 12 h, the presence of persistent or residual chest pain determines the next strategy. If there is no evidence of continued symptoms, these patients will be treated as if they had been risk stratified with the Advanced Risk group.

For patients whose symptoms are less than 12 h or with ongoing chest pain, the decision for further management is based on the availability of on-site angioplasty (PCI) capability with expected door to balloon time of less than 90 min or the presence of cardiogenic shock. Patients with expected door to balloon time of less than 90 min should be started on intravenous treatment of glycoprotein IIb–IIIa inhibitors and they should be transferred immediately to the cardiac catheterization lab for revascularization. The myocardial infarction (MI) team is activated for this group of patients (Fig. 2.5).

In our institution, a single call made by the Emergency Department physician to the page operator activates the MI team, which includes the following health-care providers:

(1) The interventional cardiologist on call
(2) The director of the CCU
(3) The cardiology fellow on call
(4) The interventional cardiology fellow on call
(5) The cath lab nurse on call
(6) The cath lab technologist on call

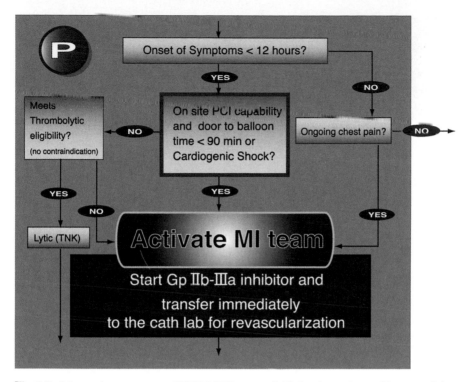

**Fig. 2.5** Advanced management of PRIORITY myocardial infarction patients with expected door to balloon time of less than 90 min

(7) The CCU nursing manager on call
(8) The senior internal medicine resident on call

Activating these groups of people have been extremely successful in our institution and have reduced markedly our door to balloon time. These strategies have been recently shown to decrease door to balloon time in the range of 8–19 min.[7]

For hospitals with no PCI capability or in situations when door to balloon time is expected to exceed 90 min, we recommend thrombolytic therapy if there are no contraindications.

## CCU Management and Secondary Prevention for Patients with PRIORITY Myocardial Infarction

Patients with "PRIORITY" myocardial infarction should be admitted to the CCU (Fig. 2.6). All patients should have an echocardiogram to evaluate left ventricle systolic and diastolic function and to exclude valvular abnormality and pericardial involvement. We recommend a minimum CCU stay of 24 h to exclude arrhythmia

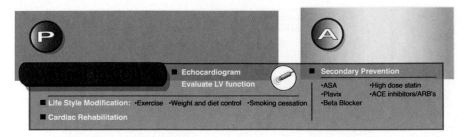

**Fig. 2.6** CCU management and secondary prevention for patients with PRIORITY myocardial infarction

complication or mechanical complication. For patients with no evidence of mechanical complications or significant arrhythmia, secondary prevention drugs should be started, including aspirin, clopidogrel, high-dose statin, beta blocker and ACE inhibitor, or angiotensin receptor blocker.

Most patients can be discharged within 48 h with recommendation for lifestyle modification including exercise, weight and diet control, smoking cessation, and cardiac rehabilitation. Secondary prevention drugs should be continued on discharge.

## Management of Advanced Risk Acute Coronary Syndrome

Typical anginal symptoms are required to be present in patients who will enroll into the Advanced or the Intermediate Risk groups.

These symptoms include the following:

1. prolonged chest pain ($>20$ min) relieved by nitroglycerine or rest;
2. chest pain at rest; or
3. accelerated chest pain within 48 h.

In order to qualify for the Advanced Risk group, patients must have either dynamic ST changes on the electrocardiogram ($>0.5$ mm) and/or elevated troponin ($>0.2$ ng/ml) (Fig. 2.7).

We recommend that patients be admitted to the CCU and be treated with aspirin, clopidogrel, heparin, glycoprotein IIb–IIIa inhibitor, beta blocker, statin, and nitroglycerin if there are no contraindications (Fig. 2.8).

These patients should have early cardiac catheterization within 12–48 h and revasularizaton by PCI or coronary artery bypass surgery (CABG) if necessary. All patients should have an echocardiogram to evaluate LV function. Recommendation for secondary prevention medication, lifestyle modification, and cardiac rehabilitation should be provided similar to the patients with PRIORITY risk group (Fig. 2.6).

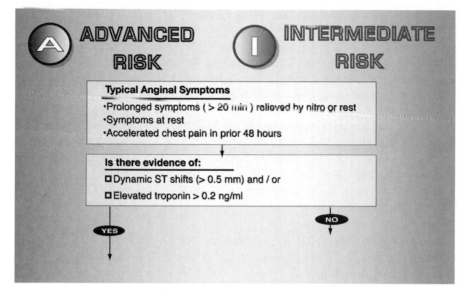

**Fig. 2.7**   Risk stratification as advanced risk acute coronary syndrome

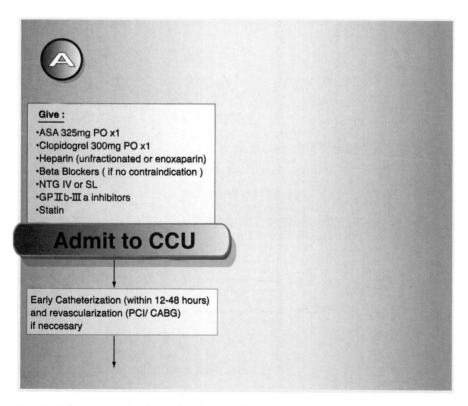

**Fig. 2.8**   Management of patients with advanced risk acute coronary syndrome

## Management of Intermediate Risk Group

Both Intermediate Risk group and Advanced Risk patients present to the hospital with typical anginal symptoms. Compared to the Advanced Risk patients, the Immediate Risk patients *do not* have evidence of dynamic ST changes on the electrocardiogram or evidence of positive cardiac markers. These patients should be admitted to the telemetry floor and be given aspirin, heparin, and beta blocker (Fig. 2.9). We recommend a minimum telemetry stay of 12–24 h. If during this period of time there is evidence of dynamic ST changes on the electrocardiogram or evidence for positive cardiac markers, the patients should be treated as if they had been stratified to the Advanced group.

The Intermediate Risk group patients are assessed again for the following high-risk features:

1. new or worsening heart failure symptoms;
2. malignant ventricular arrhythmias;
3. hemodynamic instability; or
4. recent (<6 months) PCI of CABG.

If there is an evidence of any of these high-risk features, we recommend transferring the patient for cardiac catheterization within 12–48 h and for revasculariza-

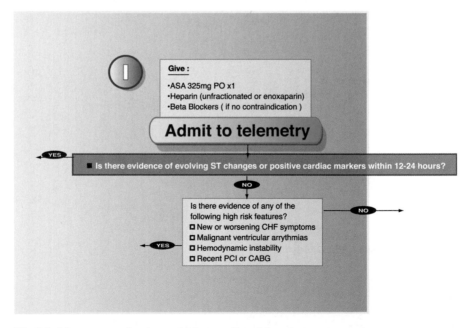

**Fig. 2.9** Management of patients with intermediate risk acute coronary syndrome

tion by PCI or CABG if necessary. Patients with no evidence of high-risk features should be referred for cardiac imaging stress testing (stress echocardiography or stress nuclear test).

## Management of Negative or Low-Risk Group Patients

These groups of patients have atypical symptoms and do not have significant ischemic EKG changes during pain and do not have elevated cardiac markers. These patients should be treated only with aspirin and given sublingual nitroglycerin if needed. If a decision was made to admit them to the hospital, they should be admitted to a chest pain unit or to a regular medical floor. They should be followed up for 12–24 h with repeated EKG and cardiac markers (Fig. 2.10). If there is evidence of evolving ST changes on the electrocardiogram or an evidence of positive cardiac markers, the patients would be treated aggressively as with the Advanced Risk group patients (Figs. 2.10, 2.11 and 2.12).

If there are no significant EKG changes and all cardiac markers are negative, we recommend a cardiac imaging stress testing by stress echocardiography or stress nuclear test (Fig. 2.11).

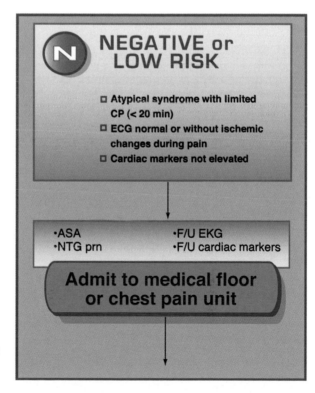

**Fig. 2.10** Initial management of patients with negative or low-risk acute coronary syndrome

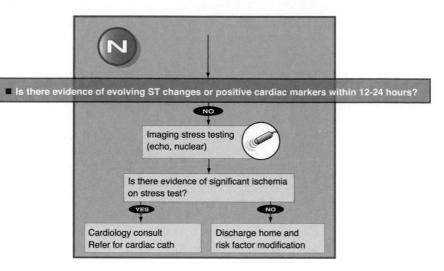

**Fig. 2.11** Risk stratification of low-risk patients by using cardiac imaging stress testing

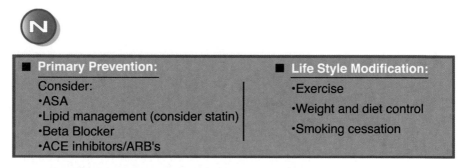

**Fig. 2.12** Primary prevention for low-risk patients

Evidence of significant ischemia on any of these stress imaging modalities will be followed by a referral for cardiac catheterization. If there is no evidence of signification ischemia on stress testing, the patients will be discharged home with a recommendation for risk factor modification to include primary prevention medication and lifestyle modification (Fig. 2.12).

# References

1. Herzog E, Saint-Jacques H, Rozanski A. The PAIN pathway as a tool to bridge the gap between evidence and management of acute coronary syndrome critical. *Pathw Cardiol*. 2004;3: 20–24.
2. Califf RM. *Acute Coronary Syndromes – ACS Essentials*. Royal Oak, MI: Pysicians' Press; 2003.

3. Braunwald E, Antman EM, Beasley JW, et al. ACC/AHA guidelines update for the management of patients with unstable angina non ST elevation myocardial infarction; a report of the American College of Cardiology/ American Heart Association Task Force on Practice Guidelines (Committee on the Management of Patients with Unstable Angina). *J AM Coll Cardiol.* 2000;36:970–1062.
4. Antman EM, Anbe DT, Armstrong PW, et al. ACC/AHA guidelines for the management of patients with ST-elevation myocardial infarction. *J Am Coll Cardiol.* 2004;44:671–719
5. Hong, MK, Herzog, F. *Multidisciplinary and Pathway-Based Approach.* New York: Springer; 2008.
6. Saint-Jacques H, Burroughs VJ, Watowska J, Valcarcel M, Moreno P, Maw M. Acute coronary syndrome critical pathway: chest PAIN caremap – a qualitative research study-provider-level intervention. *Crit Pathw Cardiol.* 2005;4:145–156.
7. Bradley EH, Herrin J, Yondfei Wang YF, et al. Strategies for reducing the door-to-balloon time in acute myocardial infarction. *N Engl J Med.* 2006;355:2308–2320.

# Chapter 3
# Echocardiography in Acute Coronary Syndrome: Anatomy, Essential Views and Imaging Plains

**Muhamed Saric**

## Introduction

A plentiful arterial circulation is required for an effective myocardial function during both systole and diastole. This supply/demand coupling is accomplished through regional matching of the arterial supply to a particular portion of the myocardium.

Arterial circulation of the heart consists of two parts: (1) large epicardial coronary arteries which serve as conduit vessels, and (2) medium-size and small intramyocardial coronary arterioles which serve as resistance vessels regulating the amount of coronary flow according to myocardial metabolic needs. Perturbation in any portion of this arterial tree will lead to a regional myocardial dysfunction. Acute coronary syndrome (ACS) is the clinical manifestation of a diminished coronary arterial blood supply in either conduit or resistance coronary vessels that is most commonly caused by atherosclerosis.

In this chapter, we will discuss the epicardial circulation; the anatomy and function of resistance vessels will be discussed in Chapter 5.

## Epicardial Conduit Vessels

In most humans, the entire epicardial circulation originates from the two initial branches of the aorta: the left coronary artery (LCA) and the right coronary artery (RCA). They originate from the left and the right sinus of Valsalva, respectively. The initial portion of the LCA is referred to as the left main coronary artery (LMCA); it branches into the left anterior descending artery (LAD) and the left circumflex artery (LCx). Although anatomically there are only two coronary arteries (LCA and RCA) in most individuals, in clinical parlance it is often said that there are three coronary vessels (RCA, LAD, and LCx).

---

M. Saric (✉)
Department of Medicine, UMDNJ – New Jersey Medical School, Newark, NJ, USA
e-mail: saricmu@umdnj.edu

E. Herzog, F.A. Chaudhry (eds.), *Echocardiography in Acute Coronary Syndrome*,
DOI 10.1007/978-1-84882-027-2_3, © Springer-Verlag London Limited 2009

In a few individuals, there may be anomalies in the origin of the coronary arteries pertaining to the number and location of coronary ostia within the aortic root as well as anomalies in the initial course of the vessels. A more detailed discussion on the anomalous origin of the coronary arteries is beyond the scope of this textbook.

The LAD supplies the largest portion of the left ventricles; the size of the LAD territory tends to be relatively constant among individuals and encompasses about 50% of the left ventricle. The LAD initially runs in the anterior interventricular groove parallel to the long axis of the heart, then turns over the left ventricular apex and terminates in most individuals in the apical region of the posterior interventricular groove. The LAD gives off septal branches that penetrate into the anterior two-thirds of the interventricular septum and diagonal branches which supply large areas of the anterior wall of the left ventricle and much smaller area of the anterior wall of the right ventricle (Fig. 3.1A).

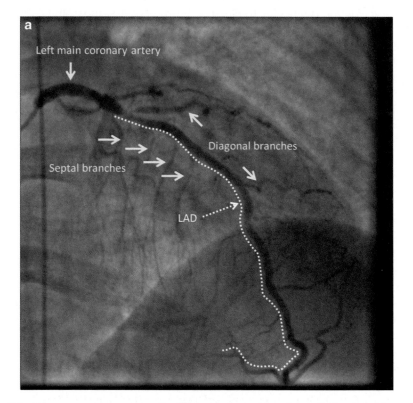

**Fig. 3.1** Coronary anatomy as visualized by coronary angiography. **A**: Left anterior descending artery (LAD) and its major branches visualized in a cranially and a slightly rightward angulated view [right anterior oblique (RAO) −9°; cranial +36°]. **B**: Dominant right coronary artery (RCA) and its major branches visualized in a slightly cranially angulated left anterior oblique (LAO) view (LAO +28°; cranial +3°). **C**: Nondominant left circumflex (LCx) artery and its major branches visualized in a caudally and a slightly rightward angulated view [right anterior oblique (RAO) −6°; caudal −21°)

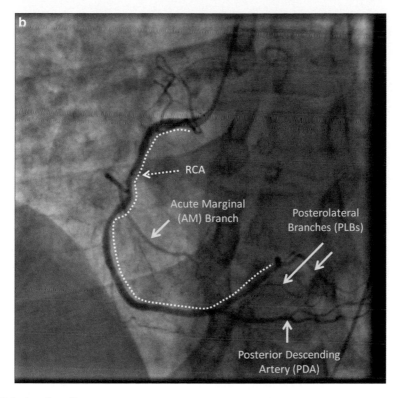

**Fig. 3.1** (continued)

The other half of the left ventricle is supplied by both the RCA and the LCx in proportions that vary between individuals. In about 70% of humans, the RCA subtends a larger section of the left ventricle than the LCx (the so-called right-dominant circulation); in about 20% of individuals the contribution of the two arteries is equal (codominant or balanced circulation), and in the remaining 10% the LCx is larger than the RCA (left-dominant circulation).[1] The dominance type does not affect the initial course of either the RCA or the LCx; it arises from the pattern of terminal branching in the two vessels.

In all individuals, the initial course of the RCA is within the right atrioventricular groove and thus perpendicular to the long axis of the heart. During this initial course, the RCA gives off acute marginal (AM) branches which run roughly parallel to the long axis of the right ventricle to supply the acute margin of the heart made up by the right ventricle. The RCA is the principal source of arterial blood supply to the right ventricle; when there is a right ventricular dysfunction during ACS, it is almost invariably caused by abnormalities in the RCA tree (Fig. 3.1B).

In a roughly mirror-image pattern, the LCx initially runs in the left atrioventricular groove perpendicular to the long axis of the heart and gives off obtuse marginal

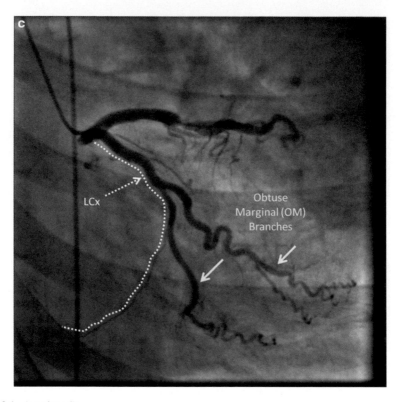

**Fig. 3.1** (continued)

(OM) branches. They run parallel to the long axis of the heart and supply the obtuse margin of the heart made up by the lateral wall of the left ventricle (Fig. 3.1C).

The inferoposterior aspects of the interventricular septum and the left ventricle are supplied by the posterior descending artery (PDA) and one or more posterolateral branches (PLBs). The PDA usually runs along the proximal two-thirds of the posterior interventricular groove and its course is parallel to that of the LAD in the anterior interventricular groove. Along its interventricular course, the PDA gives off septal branches to the inferior aspect of the interventricular septum and then meets the LAD in the apical portion of the posterior interventricular septum. PLBs are arterial branches that run along the long axis of the left ventricle and roughly parallel to the course of the PDA and the OMs. PLBs supply the inferior and posterior walls of the left ventricle.

It is the origin of the PDA and the PLBs that determines whether the coronary circulation is right-dominant, left-dominant, or balanced (codominant). In the right-dominant circulation, the PDA and PLBs are branches of the RCA; in the left-dominant circulation, the PDA and PLBs are terminal branches of LCx; in balanced (codominant) circulation, both the RCA and the LCx supply the PDA and/or PLBs.

# Imaging of Epicardial Coronary Arteries

Invasive coronary angiography using selective iodinated contrast dye injection into the RCA or the LCA has traditionally been the gold standard for imaging of epicardial coronary circulation. It is now being supplanted by high-resolution noninvasive computed tomographic (CT) angiography. The role of echocardiography in imaging epicardial coronary vessels in ACS remains limited. In adult, the origins of the RCA and the LCA can be visualized occasionally by transthoracic echocardiography and almost always by transesophageal echocardiography.[2] However, such information is rarely valuable in ACS unless an anomalous origin of the coronary arteries or dissection in the proximal coronary arteries is suspected as the cause of the patient's chest pain.

Two-dimensional gray-scale and color Doppler echocardiographic imaging beyond the origins of the coronary arteries is rarely feasible or clinically useful in ACS unless coronary fistulas are suspected. In such instances, coronary arteries are enlarged (often markedly so) and thus detectable by standard gray-scale and color Doppler techniques.

Transthoracic and transesophageal spectral Doppler recordings are feasible and are routinely used for measuring coronary flow reserve in research protocols involving the LAD,[3] the RCA,[4] and the LCx.[5] However, the utility of such recordings in routine clinical evaluation of ACS patients remains limited.

# Segmental Anatomy of the Left Ventricle

In order to correlate coronary arterial circulation to the myocardial function, the left ventricle is commonly divided into 17 segments according to a standardized American Heart Association consensus model adopted for all forms of modern cardiac imaging including echocardiography, nuclear cardiology, computed tomography, and magnetic resonance imaging.[6]

In this model, the left ventricle is first cut perpendicular to its long axis to create three myocardial rings: basal, mid-cavity, and apical. The basal and the mid-cavity ring each accounts for about 35% of the left ventricular mass, while the apical segments comprise the remaining 30%. This is in general agreement with autopsy studies of human hearts.[7]

The basal and the mid-cavity rings are then cut into six circumferential segments each; every segment accounts for 60° of the left ventricular circumference. These circumferential segments in the basal and the mid-cavity rings are referred to as anterior, anteroseptal, inferoseptal, inferior, inferolateral, and anterolateral in the consensus model. Note, however, that inferolateral and anterolateral segments have traditionally been referred to by echocardiographers as the posterior and the lateral wall, respectively.

The apical ring is subdivided into five segments: an apical cap which does not subtend the left ventricular cavity and four circumferential cuts of 90° each: anterior, septal, inferior, and lateral.

Each segment is given a unique number according to the following three principles:

1. Sequential numbering starts in the basal myocardial ring and ends in the apical portion of the left ventricle.
2. In each myocardial ring, the numbering starts with the anterior segment and proceeds counterclockwise.
3. Segment 17 refers to the apical cap.

Note that the traditional echocardiography model differs slightly from the consensus model; the apical cap is not counted as a separate segment giving rise to a 16-segment model of conventional echocardiography.[8]

In the 2005 guidelines for chamber quantification jointly sponsored by the American Society for Echocardiography and the European Association for Echocardiography,[8, 9] it is stated that:

1. Both the 17- and the 16-segment models can still be used.
2. The 17-segment model should be used for myocardial perfusion studies or when a comparison between echocardiography and other cardiac imaging modalities is necessary.
3. The 16-segment model is appropriate for studies assessing wall motion abnormalities since the apical cap (segment 17) does not move.

The nomenclature of the 17-segment consensus model is summarized in Table 3.1. To represent all 17 segments simultaneously the so-called "bull's eye" plot is used (Fig. 3.2).

**Table 3.1**  17-Segment left ventricular model

|                          | Basal | Mid-cavity | Apical |                 |
| ------------------------ | ----- | ---------- | ------ | --------------- |
| Anterior                 | 1     | 7          | 13     | Anterior        |
| Anteroseptal             | 2     | 8          | 14     | Septal          |
| Inferoseptal             | 3     | 9          | 15     | Inferior        |
| Inferior                 | 4     | 10         | 16     | Lateral         |
| Inferolateral (posterior)| 5     | 11         | 17     | Apical cap      |
| Anterolateral (lateral)  | 6     | 12         |        |                 |
| Total number of segments | 6     | 6          | 5      | Grand total = 17|

Based on data from Cerqueira et al.[6]

A major shortcoming of either the 16-segment or the 17-segment model is their failure to include any right ventricular (RV) segments. The right ventricle is supplied primarily by the RCA branches; only a small portion of the anterior right ventricle may be supplied by the LAD. Since RV dysfunction in ACS has major prognostic implications, echocardiographers should always comment on RV function in ACS patients.

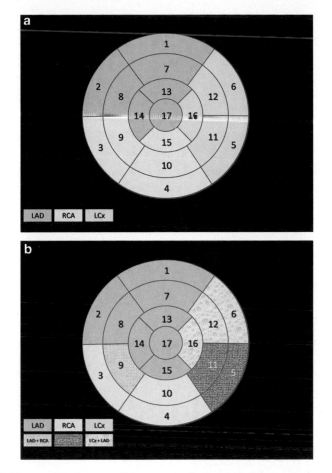

**Fig. 3.2** Bull's eye plot of myocardial segments. **A** represents left ventricular assignments to coronary territory based on data from the 2002 American Heart Association consensus statement.[6] **B** represents left ventricular assignments to coronary territory based on data from the 2005 consensus statement by the American Society for Echocardiography and the European Association for Echocardiography[9]

## Relating Standard Echocardiographic Views to Segmental Left Ventricular Model

The left ventricle is commonly visualized echocardiographically in three short-axis and three long-axis views. The three short-axis views are obtained at the cardiac base, mid-papillary level, and the cardiac apex. The short-axis views correspond to the three myocardial rings of the consensus model.

In echocardiography, the long-axis views are termed apical four-chamber view, apical two-chamber view, and apical three-chamber view (which is roughly equivalent to the parasternal long-axis views). In radiology, however, different terminology is used; the American Heart Association consensus statement encourages

**Table 3.2** Correlation between echocardiographic and radiologic views

| Echocardiography | Radiology |
|---|---|
| Apical four-chamber view | Horizontal long-axis view |
| Apical two-chamber view | Vertical long-axis view |
| Apical three-chamber view | No equivalent standard view |
| (parasternal long-axis view) | |
| Short-axis view | Short-axis view |

Based on data from Cerqueira et al.[6]

adoption of the radiologic nomenclature by echocardiographers. The relationship between echocardiographic and radiologic views is summarized in Table 3.2.

The apical four-chamber view (horizontal long-axis view) and the apical two-chamber view (vertical long-axis view) are roughly 90° apart. The apical three-chamber view (roughly equivalent to the parasternal long-axis view) is wedged in between the apical four- and the two-chamber views.

On standard tomographic views of transthoracic echocardiography, only a subset of the 17-segment model is visualized in each view. Segmental analysis of all standard 2D transthoracic views is given in Fig. 3.3. With the advent of real-time 3D

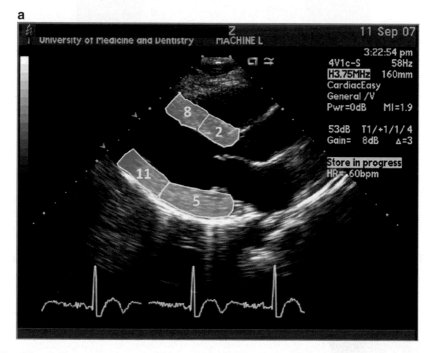

**Fig. 3.3** Left ventricular segments on standard 2D echocardiographic views. **A**: Parasternal long-axis view. **B**: Apical four-chamber view (horizontal long-axis view). **C**: Apical two-chamber view (vertical long-axis view). **D**: Parasternal short-axis view at the basal left ventricular level. **E**: Parasternal short-axis view at the mid-papillary level. **F**: Apical short-axis view. Coronary angiograms are courtesy of Drs. Marc Klapholz and Edo Kaluski, New Jersey Medical School, Newark, NJ

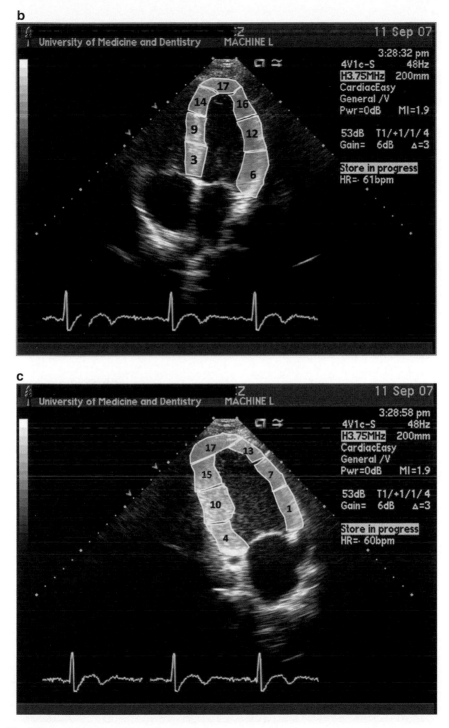

**Fig. 3.3** (continued)

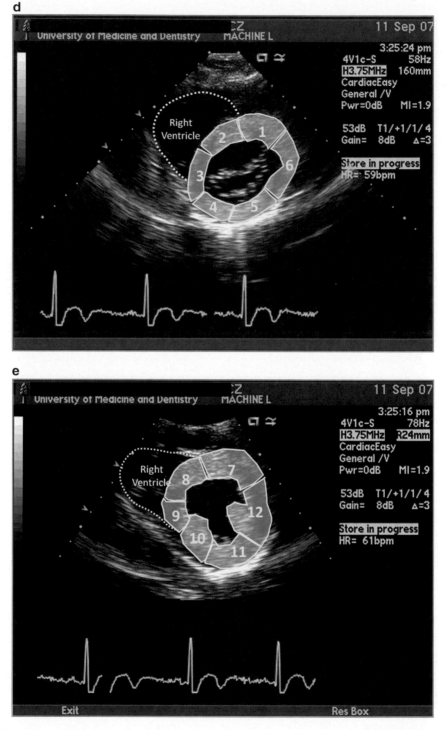

**Fig. 3.3** (continued)

f

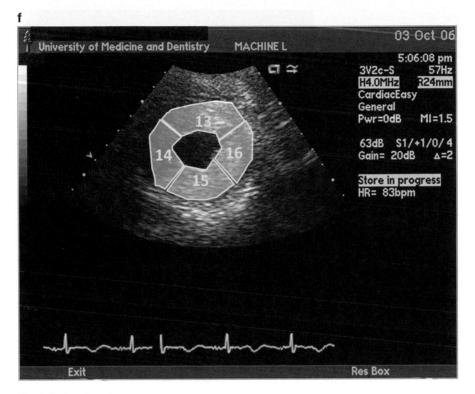

**Fig. 3.3**  (continued)

transthoracic echocardiography, the entire left ventricle can be reconstructed which allows for visualization of the 17-segment model in a 3D space (Fig. 3.4).

## Relating Coronary Circulation to Segmental Left Ventricular Model

Because there is a great variability in human coronary arterial circulation, a precise correlation between myocardial segments and coronary arterial branches cannot be established in a way that would be applicable for every individual. However, it is generally agreed upon that it is appropriate to assign individual left ventricular segments to specific coronary territories.[10] Below we will discuss the left ventricular assignments to coronary territories based on the 2002 American Heart Association consensus statement.[6] Note, however, that the 2005 consensus statement by the American Society for Echocardiography and the European Association[9] for Echocardiography provides a more complex view which emphasizes significant overlap in border zones between different coronary territories. The difference between the two schemes is summarized in Fig. 3.2 and in Table 3.3.

**Fig. 3.4** Left ventricular segments on 3D echocardiography. With real-time 3D transthoracic echocardiography, the entire 17-segment model can be visualized in a 3D space

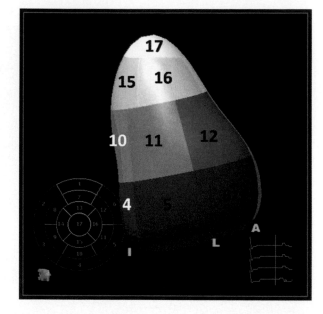

Of the three coronary arteries, the LAD probably exhibits the least amount of variability. It supplies the entire anterior wall (segments 1, 7, and 13), the entire anterior septum (segments 2, 8, and 14), and most often the apical cap (segment 17). However, one has to bear in mind that the segment 17 exhibits the greatest variability in blood supplies compared to all other left ventricular segments and that it can be supplied by any of the three coronary arteries.

Given the variability of the PDA origin, there is a great variability in the supply of the segments in the RCA and the LCx territories. Since the PDA is the branch of the RCA in the majority of humans, the RCA territory generally covers more left ventricular segments than the LCx. In most individuals, the RCA territory supplies the entire inferior wall (segments 4, 10, and 15) as well as the basal and the mid segment of the inferior septum (segments 2 and 9). In a left-dominant or codominant circulation, many of these segments may be supplied by the LCx.

Since the majority of humans have right-dominant coronary circulation, the LCx territory is restricted to the anterolateral wall (lateral wall in traditional echocardiography parlance; segments 6, 12, and 16) as well as the basal to mid portion of the inferolateral wall (posterior wall in traditional echocardiography parlance; segments 5 and 11).

Since in acute coronary syndrome echocardiographic imaging is often done before coronary angiography, echocardiographers cannot a priori determine whether the coronary circulation is right-dominant, left-dominant, or codominant. Without this information, an inevitable misassignment of myocardial segments in the RCA vs. the LCx territory will occasionally arise. In order to avoid misunderstandings with coronary angiographers, it is customary in our echocardiography laboratory to

**Table 3.3** Correlation between left ventricular segments and coronary artery territories

| Coronary artery | Left ventricular region | Basel segments | Mid-cavity segments | Apical segments | Apical cap | Total number of segments | Percentage of all left ventricular segments |
|---|---|---|---|---|---|---|---|
| Left anterior descending (LAD) | Anterior | 1 | 7 | 13 | 17 | | |
| | Anteroseptal or septal | 2 | 8 | 14 | | | |
| | Total LAD segments | | | | | 7 | 41 |
| Right coronary artery (RCA) | Inferoseptal | 3 | 9 | 15 | | | |
| | Inferior | 4 | 10 | | | | |
| | Total RCA segments | | | | | 5 | 29 |
| Left circumflex artery (LCx) | Inferolateral (posterior) | 5 | 11 | 16 | | | |
| | Anterolateral (lateral) | 6 | 12 | | | | |
| | Total LCx segments | | | | | 5 | 29 |
| | Grand total | | | | | 17 | 100 |

Based on data from the 2002 American Heart Association consensus statement.[6] Please note that the 2005 consensus statement by the American Society for Echocardiography and the European Association for Echocardiography[9] assigns segments somewhat differently: segment 15 (apical inferior wall) is assigned to the LAD territory; segment 9 (mid inferior septum) is shared between the LAD and the RCA; segments 5 and 11 [basal and mid inferolateral (posterior) wall] are shared between the RCA and the LCx; segments 6, 12, and 16 [anterolateral (lateral) wall] are shared between the LAD and the LCx. Interestingly, the 2005 statement assigns no left ventricular segments exclusively to the LCx.

refer to segments supplied by the PDA as being in the non-LAD territory without specifying whether such segments are in the RCA or in the LCx territory.

It is also important to emphasize that the above assignments of LV segments to particular coronary artery assume the absence of significant native collateral circulation or surgical bypass grafting.

## Overlap Zones Between Coronary Territories

The RCA/LCx dominance pattern is not the only cause of significant variability among humans in coronary arterial supply to individual LV segments. The variability is particularly pronounced in border zones where one coronary territory meets another.

ALL THREE TERRITORIES: The three coronary territories converge at the LV apex. The apical cap (segment 17 seen in all apical long-axis views) thus may be supplied by any of the three arteries although most commonly is supplied by the LAD.

LAD MEETS PDA TERRITORY: The distal LAD usually wraps around the LV apex to meet the PDA in the distal portion of the posterior interventricular groove. Since the magnitude of the LAD wraparound is variable, the border zone segments of the apical to mid inferior wall (segments 15 and 10 seen on the apical two-chamber view) and the inferior septum (segments 14 and 9 seen on the apical four-chamber view) may be supplied by either the LAD or the RCA. Most commonly, the mid segments (9 and 10) are in the PDA territory, while the apical segments (14 and 15) are in the LAD territory.

LAD MEETS LCx TERRITORY: The two territories meet around the segment 16 (apical lateral wall seen on the apical four-chamber view) and thus both LAD and LCx can contribute to its arterial supply. The overlap may even extend to the mid and basal segments of the lateral wall (segments 12 and 6).

RCA MEETS LCx TERRITORY: The two territories converge at the basal to mid inferolateral (posterior) left ventricular wall (segments 5 and 11 seen on the apical three-chamber view or the parasternal long-axis view). These segments are supplied by the posterolateral branches (PLBs), which may come from either RCA or LCx depending on the coronary dominance pattern.

Overlap zones are illustrated in Fig. 3.2B.

## Conclusion

Regional myocardial systolic and diastolic function is dependent on regional arterial blood supply. Although there is a significant variability in coronary arterial anatomy, it is generally agreed that individual left ventricular segments can be paired with branches of one of the three major coronary arteries (LAD, LCx, and RCA). If on an echocardiogram of a person suspected of having ACS one observes regional left ventricular dysfunction in a segmental pattern consistent with expected coronary artery distribution, one may conclude that the dysfunction is indeed ischemic in origin, thus confirming the diagnosis of ACS.

## Clinical Case

Gerard Oghlakian, MD, and Yuliya Kats, MD have contributed to the following clinical case.

## *Subjective*

An 87-year-old man with history of systemic hypertension and benign prostatic hypertrophy was brought in to our tertiary hospital by Emergency Medical Service (EMS) after sustaining multiple bruises and a forehead laceration in a car accident. According to the bystanders, the patient was involved in a single, unprovoked car accident where his car drove off the road and into a street-side pole. He had no recollection of the car accident itself; however, he did recall having lightheadedness just prior to the crash. There were no other symptoms such chest pain, shortness of breath, or palpitations. He had no prior established cardiovascular disease aside from systemic hypertension for which he was taking doxazosin. He denied any use of tobacco, alcohol, or illicit drugs.

## *Objective*

In the emergency department, his physical exam showed a blood pressure of 180/50 mmHg and a heart rate of 105 beats per minute. His respiratory rate was 20 respirations per minute and his oxygen saturation was 99% on a 100% nonrebreather mask. On a physician exam he had a normal jugular venous pressure. Lung auscultation revealed diffuse rhonchi in the right lung fields. Cardiac exam demonstrated normal S1 and S2; no murmurs or gallops were appreciated. There was no lower extremity edema.

Electrocardiogram performed in the emergency department revealed sinus tachycardia with frequent premature ventricular complexes and mild ST depressions in inferior and lateral leads (Fig. 3.5). On laboratory exam, complete blood count and basic chemistries were unremarkable. With respect to cardiac markers, the troponin I level at time of presentation was 2.06 ng/mL (normal <0.4 ng/mL); creatine phosphokinase at 365 units per liter (normal <200 units per liter), and MB isoenzyme at 23 ng/mL with an MB index of 6.3%. Computed tomography (CT) of the head revealed no intracranial pathology. CT of the chest showed right-sided lung contusion and multiple right and left rib fractures.

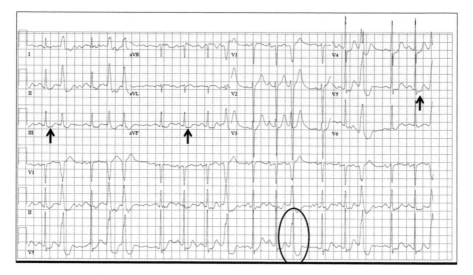

**Fig. 3.5** Electrocardiogram (EKG) performed in the emergency department. EKG revealed sinus tachycardia with frequent premature ventricular complexes (*oval*) and mild ST depressions in inferior and lateral leads (*arrows*)

## Assessment and Plan

Patient was suspected of having a non-ST elevation myocardial infarction that likely led to ventricular arrhythmia, syncope, and the car accident. An alternative explanation for his preadmission course was syncope of a noncardiac etiology leading to a car accident, traumatic cardiac contusion, and subsequent release of cardiac markers.

## Indication for the Echo

A transthoracic echocardiogram was ordered to determine the presence, the location, and the extent of regional left ventricular wall motion abnormalities that would support or refute the clinical diagnosis of a non-ST elevation myocardial infarction.

## Echo Imaging

Transthoracic echocardiogram (Fig. 3.6) performed in the emergency department revealed hypokinesis of the basal to mid segments of the inferior wall (segments 4 and 10; Fig. 3.6A) and the posterior (inferolateral) wall (segments 5 and 11; Fig. 3.6B). The pattern of left ventricular wall motion abnormalities was consistent with an ischemic damage in the distribution of either the right coronary artery

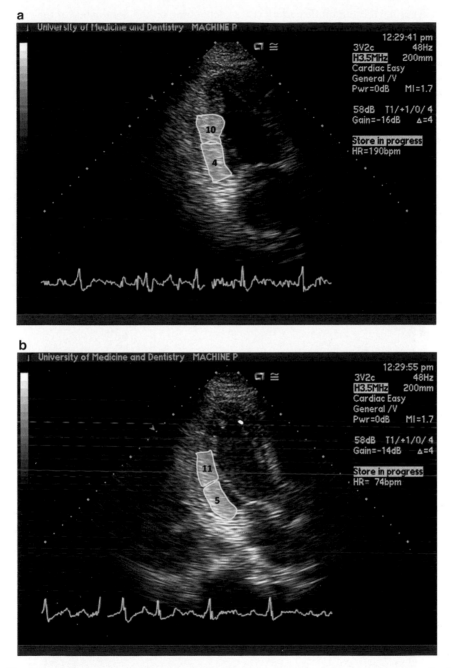

**Fig. 3.6**  Transthoracic echocardiogram. **A:** Apical two-chamber view revealed hypokinesis of the basal and the mid segment of the inferior wall (segments 4 and 10). **B:** Apical three-chamber view revealed hypokinesis of the basal and the mid segment of the posterior (inferolateral) wall (segments 5 and 11)

(RCA) or the left circumflex artery (LCx) depending on the dominance of the coronary circulation.

Other left ventricular segments were hyperkinetic and the global left ventricular ejection fraction was preserved. The size and function of the right ventricle – the chamber that is most likely to suffer contusion in a car accident – was normal. The study demonstrated neither pericardial effusion nor a significant valvular disease.

## *Management*

Given the combination of elevated cardiac serum markers and the echocardiographic findings of regional wall motion abnormalities in the distribution of the PDA, patient was referred for prompt coronary angiography. His coronary circulation revealed a left-dominant pattern with the PDA being a branch of the left circumflex artery. LCx had a critical 98% stenosis in its mid course just at the bifurcation of the $OM_2$ branch (Fig. 3.7). There were no left-to-left or right-to-left collaterals, suggesting that the LCx stenosis was acute.

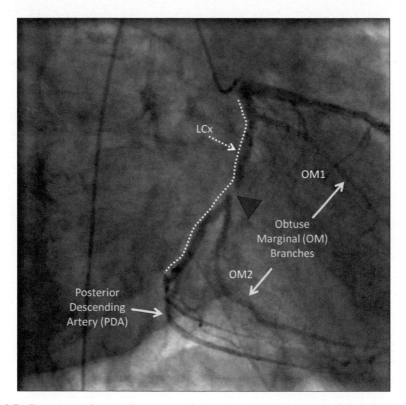

**Fig. 3.7** Coronary angiogram. Coronary angiogram reveals severe stenosis of the left circumflex (LCx) artery (*arrow head*) just prior to the origin of the second obtuse marginal branch (OM2)

## Outcome

LCx stenosis was successfully treated with a percutaneous placement of a bare-metal stent. After stenting, he underwent an electrophysiologic study which revealed no arrhythmia. His subsequent hospital course was uneventful. He was sent home in good condition and was free of symptoms on follow-up.

# References

1. Sos TA, Sniderman KW. A simple method of teaching three-dimensional coronary artery anatomy. *Radiology*. 1980;134:605–606.
2. Biederman RW, Sorrell VL, Nanda NC, Voros S, Thakur AC. Transesophageal echocardiographic assessment of coronary stenosis: a decade of experience. *Echocardiography*. 2001 January;18(1):49–57.
3. Chammas E, Dib C, Rahhal M, Helou T, Ghanem G, Tarcha W. Noninvasive assessment of coronary flow reserve in the left anterior descending artery by transthoracic echocardiography before and after stenting. *Echocardiography*. 2007 September;24(8):789–794.
4. Murata E, Hozumi T, Matsumura Y, Fujimoto K, Sugioka K, Takemoto Y, Watanabe H, et al. Coronary flow velocity reserve measurement in three major coronary arteries using transthoracic Doppler echocardiography. *Echocardiography*. 2006 April;23(4):279–286.
5. Auriti A, Pristipino C, Cianfrocca C, Granatelli A, Guido V, Pelliccia F, Greco S, et al. Distal left circumflex coronary artery flow reserve recorded by transthoracic Doppler echocardiography: a comparison with Doppler-wire. *Cardiovasc Ultrasound*. 2007 June 16;5:22.
6. Cerqueira MD, Weissman, NJ, Dilsizian V, et al. Standardized myocardial segmentation and nomenclature for tomographic imaging of the heart: a statement for healthcare professionals from the Cardiac Imaging Committee of the Council on Clinical Cardiology of the American Heart Association. *Circulation*. 2002;105;539–542.
7. Edwards WD, Tajik AJ, Seward JB. Standardized nomenclature and anatomic basis for regional tomographic analysis of the heart. *Mayo Clin Proc*. 1981;56:479–497.
8. Schiller NB, Shah PM, Crawford M, et al. Recommendations for quantitation of the left ventricle by two-dimensional echocardiography: American Society of Echocardiography Committee on Standards, Subcommittee on Quantitation of Two-Dimensional Echocardiograms. *J Am Soc Echocardiogr*. 1989;2:358–367.
9. Lang RM, Bierig M, Devereux RB, et al. Recommendations for chamber quantification: a report from the American Society of Echocardiography's Guidelines and Standards Committee and the Chamber Quantification Writing Group, developed in conjunction with the European Association of Echocardiography, a branch of the European Society of Cardiology. *J Am Soc Echocardiogr*. 2005 December;18(12):1440–1463.
10. Gallik DM, Obermueller SD, Swarna US, Guidry GW, Mahmarian JJ, Verani MS. Simultaneous assessment of myocardial perfusion and left ventricular function during transient coronary occlusion. *J Am Coll Cardiol*. 1995;25:1529–1538.

# Chapter 4
# Echo Assessment of Systolic and Diastolic Function in Acute Coronary Syndrome

Muhamed Saric

## Introduction

The human heart, being almost exclusively dependent on aerobic metabolism, requires a constant supply of oxygen to avoid tissue injury. Even at rest, the human myocardium extracts almost the entire oxygen content of the passing blood. This results in extremely low resting oxygen saturation in the coronary sinus, the final repository of the coronary blood (35% at rest; 25% at peak exercise). Therefore, the primary means of increasing oxygen delivery to the myocardium is through augmentation of coronary blood flow. From rest to maximal physical exertion, coronary flow increases up to fivefold.[1]

Although the pressure in the epicardial coronary arteries may vary significantly, the precapillary pressure in the myocardium is held almost constant at 45 mmHg thanks to autoregulation accomplished through dynamic changes in the arteriolar resistance.[2] Due to this autoregulation, a narrowing in an epicardial coronary artery has to be very severe (about 90% diameter loss) for the stenosis to become clinically evident at rest; blood supply limitation with exercise become evident when the stenosis reaches 70%.

Once the epicardial stenosis reaches a critical level, the loss of myocardial function and the development of clinical signs and symptoms proceed in an orderly fashion. This stepwise process is referred to as ischemic cascade.[3] It starts with an intramyocardial perfusion defect and progresses through a diminished left ventricular diastolic function, a decreased myocardial contractility, an increased left ventricular end-diastolic pressure, ST-segment changes, and ends, occasionally, with angina pectoris (Fig. 4.1).

Intramyocardial perfusion defects are the earliest sign of limitations in the coronary blood supply and can be detected by either myocardial contrast echocardiography (MCE) or nuclear imaging. MCE is discussed elsewhere in this textbook. In this

M. Saric (✉)
Department of Medicine, UMDNJ – New Jersey Medical School, Newark, NJ, USA
e-mail: saricmu@umdnj.edu

E. Herzog, F.A. Chaudhry (eds.), *Echocardiography in Acute Coronary Syndrome*,
DOI 10.1007/978-1-84882-027-2_4, © Springer-Verlag London Limited 2009

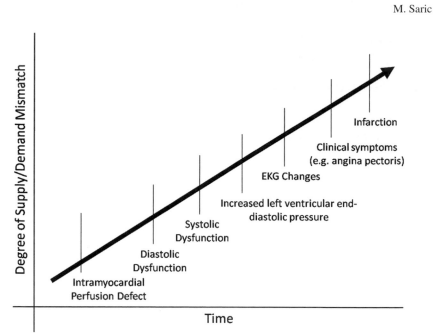

**Fig. 4.1** Ischemic cascade. The loss of myocardial function and the development of clinical signs and symptoms proceed in a stepwise fashion as the cardiac demand increases

chapter, we will concentrate on the next two steps in the ischemic cascade, namely the loss of diastolic and systolic function during acute coronary syndromes.

## Regional vs. Global Parameters of Dysfunction

Once the coronary supply/demand mismatch reaches a certain threshold level, there is a loss of normal myocardial function. The fundamental characteristic of ischemic dysfunction (either diastolic or systolic) is that it occurs regionally and that its distribution pattern conforms to the expected coronary blood supply of the 17-segment model discussed in Chapter 3. Conversely, when regional dysfunction is due to non-ischemic causes its distribution tends to be patchy and often spread over two or more coronary territories.

In the absence of extensive collaterals or surgical bypass grafting, the loss of myocardial function usually occurs first in the distal segments and spreads gradually toward the cardiac base. For instance, in a case of a proximal left anterior descending (LAD) artery stenosis, the first segments to lose function tend to be the apical ones followed by mid-cavity and basal segments.

When assessing myocardial systolic or diastolic dysfunction in acute coronary syndrome, one may evaluate regional abnormalities directly or measure their impact on the global ventricular function. Although diastolic dysfunction precedes the systolic one in the ischemic cascade, we will discuss systolic dysfunction first since in routine clinical practice it is assessed in almost all patients. This is in contrast to diastolic dysfunction for which there is a much smaller body of echocardiographic evidence to guide the diagnosis, treatment, and prognosis.

## Assessment of Regional Systolic Function in Acute Coronary Syndrome

Occlusion of an epicardial coronary artery at the time of acute coronary syndrome may lead to a loss of contractile function in the myocardial segments subtended by that artery. The magnitude and duration of such a contractile loss is dependent on both the severity and the duration of the coronary occlusion (Fig. 4.2).

In unstable angina, left and right ventricular wall motion is usually normal unless resting transthoracic echocardiography happens to be performed fortuitously during an episode of chest pain.

Non-ST elevation myocardial infarction (NSTEMI) usually results from an occlusion of a coronary branch vessel often in an elderly patient with preexisting collateral coronary circulation. Typically the loss of contractile function is restricted to the subendocardial layer which is most vulnerable to ischemia. However, on standard echocardiography the contractility loss will be observed in the entire thickness of the affected myocardial segment. This overestimation of contractile loss is attributed to tethering (an apparent passive loss of contractility in normal segments due to contractile loss in an adjacent area).

ST elevation myocardial infarction (STEMI) often results from an occlusion of a major coronary vessel and tends to occur in a younger age group compared to

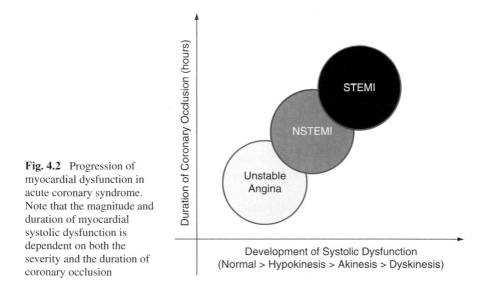

**Fig. 4.2** Progression of myocardial dysfunction in acute coronary syndrome. Note that the magnitude and duration of myocardial systolic dysfunction is dependent on both the severity and the duration of coronary occlusion

NSTEMI. If the total session of coronary flow lasts for more than 6 h, myocardial necrosis will occur and the myocardium in the affected segments will be replaced with a fibrous scar over the ensuing weeks.

The magnitude of regional contractile loss in acute coronary syndrome is usually assessed semiquantitatively; one reports descriptively on the following three parameters:

1. Magnitude of contractile loss in each affected segment

   NORMAL          Contractility preserved
   HYPOKINESIS     Partial loss of contractility
   AKINESIS        Complete loss of contractility
   DYSKINESIS      Paradoxical movement of the affected segment away from
                   The center of the ventricle during systole
   ANEURYSMAL      Outward movement of the affected segment during both
                   Systole and diastole

2. Number and location of affected segments
3. Suspected coronary artery distribution (left anterior descending artery vs. right coronary artery vs. left circumflex artery)

Wall scoring provides a more rigorous quantitative approach to assessing wall motion abnormalities in acute coronary syndrome. However, the wall scoring method assesses the contractility of all ventricular segments and is thus described in the next section.

## Assessment of Global Systolic Function in Acute Coronary Syndrome

Global ventricular systolic function in acute coronary syndrome may be assessed through either wall motion scoring or calculation of global ventricular ejection fraction.

### *Wall Motion Scoring*

Wall motion scoring analysis assigns a numeric value to the degree of contractile dysfunction in each segment. The actual numeric values given to particular forms of contractile (dys)function vary in the published literature; the most common scheme is given in Table 4.1.

Once all segments are given individual scores, a total score is calculated as a sum of individual scores. A wall motion score index (WMSI) in then calculated as a ratio between the total score and the number of evaluated segments. The WMSI is a dimensionless number; its range of values depends on the scoring scheme used. For the scoring scheme shown in Table 4.1, the WMSI would range between 1 and 5.

**Table 4.1** Left ventricular wall motion scoring

|            | Score |
| ---------- | ----- |
| Normal     | 1     |
| Hypokinesis | 2     |
| Akinesis   | 3     |
| Dyskinesis | 4     |
| Aneurysmal | 5     |

$$\text{Wall motion score index} = \frac{\text{Sum of individual segment scores}}{\text{Number of evaluated segments}}$$

For a fully visualized normal ventricle, the total score is 17 (all segments have normal contractility). Since all 17 segments are evaluated, the wall score index of a normal heart is 17/17 = 1. For abnormal ventricles, the higher the WMSI, the more the contractile dysfunction. The theoretical maximum for a WMSI is 5 in the scoring scheme depicted in Table 4.1; such a score would assume that all left ventricular segments are aneurysmal, a condition incompatible with life. Between the extremes of 1 and 5 are the values obtained in patients with acute coronary syndrome.

Using the same methodology, one can use the 16-segment model instead of the 17-segment one. The underlying notions will not change: the higher the WMSI, the worse the systolic dysfunction. For example, in a patient with acute coronary syndrome who had a total occlusion of the proximal LAD, akinesis was observed in the entire apical region (segments 13, 14, 15, and 16), while hypokinesis was observed in the remaining LAD territory (segments 1, 2, 7, and 8). Segments in the territories of other coronaries were normal. This patient's global WMSI was calculated as [4(3) + 4(2) + 8(1)]/16 = 1.75 (Fig. 4.3).

Instead of a global WMSI, one can also calculate a regional WMSI taking into account only segments supplied by a particular artery. For the patient above, the regional LAD score would be [4(3) + 4(2)]/8 = 2.5 (Fig. 4.3). Because of tremendous variability in the size of RCA and LCx territories between patients, it is often more prudent to provide a regional score for the entire non-LAD (RCA + LCx) territory rather than individual scores for RCA and LCx when there is no prior knowledge of a coronary dominance pattern in an individual patient.

A major shortcoming of the above WMSI analysis is that it does not include right ventricular wall segments despite the fact that the presence of right ventricular systolic dysfunction may portend a worse prognosis in patients with acute coronary syndrome.[4]

## Assessment of Ventricular Ejection Fraction

Numerous studies have shown that the left ventricular ejection fraction (LVEF) is one of the most powerful predictors of future mortality and morbidity in patients

**Fig. 4.3** Wall motion score index (WMSI) calculations using a 16-segment left ventricular model. This patient with acute coronary syndrome had a total occlusion of his proximal left anterior descending (LAD) artery leading to akinesis of the four apical segments and hypokinesis in the basal and mid segments of the anterior wall and the anterior septum. Other left ventricular segments were normal. Note the global WMSI (WS Index) of 1.75, and the regional LAD score (LAD Index) of 2.50. Note also that the regional scores were normal (1.00) for both the right coronary artery (RCA) and the left circumflex (LCx) artery; this indicates that the wall motion abnormalities in this patient were confined to the LAD territory

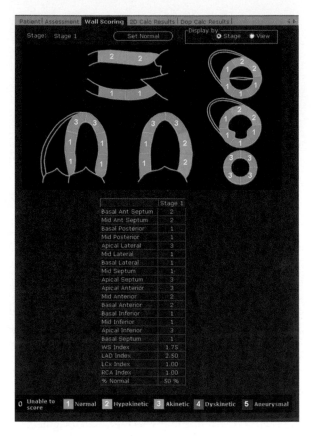

with left ventricular systolic dysfunction of any cause including ischemic heart disease.[5] For instance, LVEF is the single most powerful predictor of mortality and the risk for life-threatening ventricular arrhythmias after myocardial infarction.[6] Furthermore, once the acute coronary syndrome resolves, the residual LVEF is important for treatment as LVEF cutoff values are built into recommendations for both medical and electrical device therapies. Even with treatment and clinical stabilization of heart failure, there is an inverse, almost linear, relationship between LVEF and survival in patient whose LVEF is less than 45% (Fig. 4.4).[7]

By definition, LVEF is the percentage of the end-diastolic volume that is ejected with each systole as the stroke volume. Thus, to calculate the LVEF one needs to estimate the end-systolic and end-diastolic volume of the left ventricle.

Current recommendations of the American Society for Echocardiography and the European Association for Echocardiography discourage the use of M mode-derived methods such as the cube rule for calculation of left ventricular volumes.[8] M mode is particularly ill-suited for estimating LVEF in patients with ischemic heart disease involving the apical regions of the left ventricle because M mode measurements are made at the base of the heart; the calculated regional LVEF at the mid-papillary level

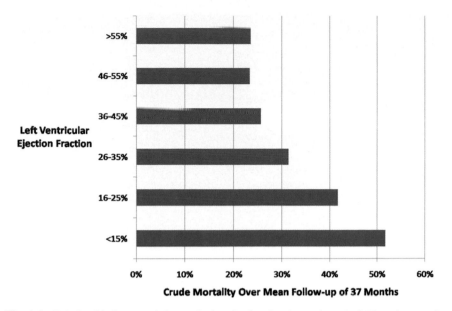

**Fig. 4.4** Relationship between left ventricular ejection fraction and survival. Note the negative almost linear relationship between survival and left ejection fractions <45%. Based on numeric data from Curtis et al.[7]

is clearly not representative of the global LVEF in patients with apical wall motion abnormalities.

For two-dimensional echocardiography, biplane Simpson's rule is the gold standard for estimation of the LVEF[9] Most modern ultrasound systems provide a semi-automated software package for the Simpson's rule analysis. Operators are usually required only to trace the left ventricular border of an end-diastolic and an end-systolic frame in the apical four-chamber and two-chamber views; the software package then automatically calculates the left ventricular end-diastolic volume, end-systolic volume, and LVEF (Fig. 4.5). One should be aware, however, that when mitral or aortic regurgitation is present, Simpson's rule calculates the total stroke volume which is the sum of the regurgitant volume and the true antegrade stroke volume; therefore, the calculated LVEF, although technically correct, may not be a good measure of left ventricular systolic performance.

With the advent of real-time three-dimensional (RT3D) transthoracic techniques, left ventricular volumes and LVEF can now be calculated with even greater accuracy than is possible with the biplane Simpson's rule (Fig. 4.6). RT3D-derived left ventricular volume data are now comparable to those obtained by cardiac magnetic resonance imaging, the prior gold standard for such calculations.[10]

In conclusion, whenever available, left ventricular volumes and LVEF in acute coronary syndrome should be calculated from an RT3D system; the biplane Simpson's rule should be the next best method for such calculations when only a two-dimensional ultrasound system is available.

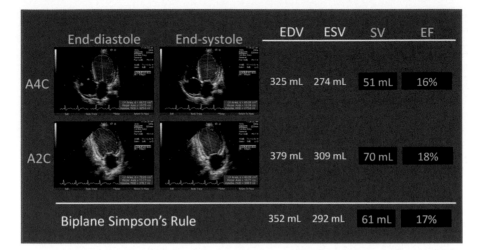

**Fig. 4.5** Calculation of left ventricular ejection fraction (LVEF) by biplane Simpson's rule. The operator of an ultrasound system is required to trace the endocardial border of an end-diastolic and an end-systolic frame in the apical four-chamber (A4C) and two-chamber (A2C) views. The system then calculates the end-diastolic volume (EDV), end-systolic volume (ESV), stroke volume (SV), and LVEF

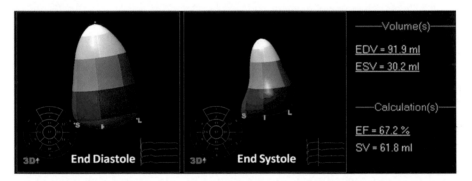

**Fig. 4.6** Calculation of left ventricular volumes and ejection fraction (EF) by three-dimensional echocardiography. A 3D ultrasound system calculates the end-diastolic volume (EDV), end-systolic volume (ESV), stroke volume (SV), and LVEF automatically from a 3D data set after an operator manually enters key reference points of the left ventricle

## Comparing Wall Motion Scoring to Left Ventricular Ejection Fraction

A major feature of the wall scoring system is that it does not differentiate between normal and hyperdynamic left ventricular segments. This may be viewed as either an advantage or a shortcoming of the wall scoring method.

Let us take an example of two patients with acute coronary syndrome both of which have hypokinesis in all LAD segments. In one patient, however, the left ventricular segments in the non-LAD territory are hyperdynamic, while in the other patient they move normally. According to the wall scoring method described above, both would have the same wall motion score index yet their LVEF would be different (LVEF is expected to be higher in the first patient). WMSI in this case accurately reflects the extent of wall motion abnormalities due to acute coronary syndrome in the two patients but is unable to take into account the compensatory hyperkinesis in the second patient the way global LVEF can.

## Strain Imaging in Acute Coronary Syndrome

Wall motion scoring described above relies on subjective 'eyeballing' of left ventricular thickening and wall motion during the cardiac cycle and thus requires a large degree of experience and expertise. Strain imaging has recently entered the armamentarium of echocardiography and promises to provide a more objective and quantitative basis for wall motion analysis.

Strain imaging is based on the fact that each of the 17 segments in the left ventricular model changes its length throughout the cardiac cycle. In the longitudinal direction, each segment *shortens* from end diastole to peak systole; this can be observed in apical four-chamber, two-chamber, and three-chamber views. In the radial direction, each segment *lengthens* (*thickens*) from end diastole to peak systole; this can be observed in any of the short-axis views of the left ventricle. From peak systole to end diastole, the process reverses: each ventricular segment *lengthens* in the longitudinal direction and *shortens* (*thins*) in the radial direction.

Strain is a unitless ratio between the segment length at any point in the cardiac cycle and the reference length at end diastole. In other words, strain is a fractional change in the segment length during the cardiac cycle. Because left ventricular segments *shorten* in the longitudinal direction during systole, their longitudinal systolic strain has a negative value. This is in contrast to radial strain which has a positive value in systole due to wall thickening. The opposite is true for both longitudinal and radial strain during diastole. Echocardiographically, strain data are obtained from either tissue Doppler velocity data or speckle tracking.[11]

In a normally contracting left ventricular segment, peak strain value is achieved just prior to aortic valve closure. In patients with unstable angina or non-ST elevation (nontransmural) infarction, two changes occur: the magnitude of systolic strain diminishes and the peak strain occurs progressively later well past the aortic valve closure. The latter phenomenon is referred to as 'postsystolic thickening' and is still poorly understood despite decades of experimental work in animal models. It is important to emphasize that postsystolic thickening is a sensitive but not a specific sign of ischemia; it may also be observed in other disorders such as myocardial storage diseases and in states of high left ventricular afterload (such as aortic stenosis and elevated systemic blood pressure).[11]

In ST elevation (transmural) infarction with nonviable myocardium, no active strain is present and may be replaced with outward bulging (dyskinesis). Strain pattern in normal and ischemic myocardium is summarized diagrammatically in Fig. 4.7.

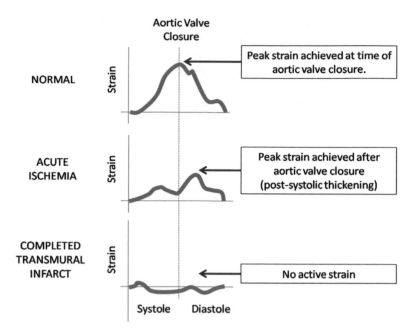

**Fig. 4.7** Patterns of left ventricular strain in normal and ischemic myocardium. Schematic representation of radial strain recordings. Note that in the normal myocardium, peak systolic strain occurs at the time of aortic valve closure. During ischemia, the magnitude of systolic strain diminishes and the peak strain occurs past the aortic valve closure (postsystolic thickening). In the fully infracted myocardium, there is no active systolic or postsystolic strain. Drawn based on data from Bijnens et al.[11]

## Assessment of Diastolic Function in Acute Coronary Syndrome

In patients with acute syndrome, assessment of left ventricular diastolic function should follow the general guidelines of echocardiographic analysis of diastolic parameters. The analysis should include at least the following three aspects:

1. Evaluation of the pattern of mitral and pulmonary venous blood flow velocity determined by pulsed wave Doppler.
2. Measurement of diastolic mitral annular tissue excursion using tissue Doppler techniques.
3. Calculation of the left atrial volume.

It is important to emphasize that the diastolic changes described in this chapter are not specific to acute coronary syndrome and occur in a wide variety of cardiac and extra-cardiac disorders (renal failure, anemia, high afterload due to stiff aortic tree, etc.).

## *Mitral and Pulmonary Venous Blood Flow Velocity Pattern*

In young individuals, left ventricular filling occurs primarily during the early (E) phase of diastole with only a minor contribution from atrial contraction in late diastole (A phase). Furthermore, the filling of the left atrium from the pulmonary veins is more prominent during ventricular diastole (D wave) and during ventricular systole (S wave) and the atrial reversal of flow (AR wave) from the left atrium into the valveless pulmonary veins during atrial contractions is small. In summary, in a young individual the diastolic pattern is characterized by mitral E wave dominance, pulmonary vein D wave dominance, and a small AR (Fig. 4.8).

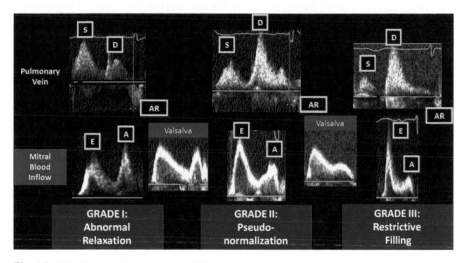

**Fig. 4.8** Mitral and pulmonary venous filling patterns. *Top panel* shows pulmonary vein tracings; S, systolic wave; D, diastolic wave; AR, atrial reversal wave. *Bottom panel* shows mitral blood inflow tracings; E, early diastolic wave; A, atrial kick

The amplitude (peak velocity) of the mitral E wave is governed by the pressure gradient between the left atrium and the left ventricle in early diastole; similarly the magnitude of the pulmonary D wave is determined by the pressure gradient between the pulmonary veins and the left ventricle during the early period of ventricular diastole.

In young individuals, these gradients are characterized by very low ventricular pressures and flow from the pulmonary veins and the left atrium driven by ventricular suction.

In humans, the 'normal' aging process is characterized by a loss of relaxing properties in the left ventricle during diastole. Due to slowed relaxation, the left ventricular pressure remains relatively high during early diastole which in turn diminishes the left atrial-to-left ventricular and pulmonary venous-to-left ventricular gradients during early diastole. As a consequence, the amplitude of the E wave and the pulmonary venous D wave diminishes progressively, while the deceleration of the E wave prolongs. In an elderly person, the pattern of diastolic flow thus becomes A dominant, S dominant, and with a prominent AR wave (both in amplitude and duration). This pattern has been termed abnormal relaxation or grade I (mild) left ventricular dysfunction.

Left ventricular relaxation during early diastole is an active, energy-consuming process requiring a continuous supply of oxygen. It can therefore be expected that in acute coronary syndrome left ventricular relaxation is impaired; indeed such impairment precedes systolic dysfunction in the ischemic cascade (Fig. 4.1). Using the pulsed wave Doppler mitral inflow velocity pattern, one can easily show transition from an E dominant pattern at baseline to an A dominant pattern with prolonged E wave deceleration time within seconds of acute coronary occlusion. In humans, this is infrequently observed because most acute coronary syndromes occur in late middle-age and elderly patients who have the pattern of abnormal relaxation at baseline due to 'normal' aging.

When relaxing properties are severely impaired in moderate and severe left ventricular dysfunction, there is a compensatory increase in the left atrial pressure (preload) in an attempt to normalize the filling pressure gradient. As a result, the magnitude of the E and D waves rises in proportion to the rise in the left atrial pressure. In moderate diastolic dysfunction, the combination of abnormal left ventricular relaxation and moderately elevated left atrial pressure gives rise to the so-called pseudonormal filling pattern (E dominant, D dominant with an E wave deceleration time >150 ms; grade II diastolic dysfunction). Severe diastolic dysfunction is characterized by ever taller E and D waves but with an E wave deceleration time <150 ms and is referred to as restrictive filling (grade III diastolic dysfunction).

Pseudonormal and restrictive filling patterns are combinations of diminished left ventricular relaxing properties (left ventricular dysfunction) and elevated preload (elevated left atrial pressures). The Valsalva maneuver diminishes preload and unmasks the underlying left ventricular relaxation abnormalities. After the Valsalva maneuver the pseudonormal pattern will become the abnormal relaxation pattern; this is important in distinguishing a normal from a pseudonormal pattern.

Pseudonormal and restrictive filling patterns are frequently encountered in patients with acute coronary syndrome, especially when there is concomitant systolic dysfunction and diminished left ventricular ejection fraction. When such patterns are observed, they are indicative of elevated left atrial pressures and should alert a clinician to actively pursue the diagnosis and treatment of pulmonary edema. This is further discussed in the section on mitral annular tissue Doppler.

After a Valsalva maneuver, restrictive filling pattern will often revert to a pseudonormal pattern (reversible restrictive filling pattern). When this fails to occur (irreversible restrictive filling pattern), the prognosis is very poor.[12]

In summary, grade I left ventricular dysfunction is indicative primarily of left ventricular dysfunction, while grades II and III (pseudonormal and restrictive filling patterns) are primarily indicative of elevated left atrial pressures.

## Mitral Annular Tissue Doppler Analysis

After placing a pulsed Doppler sample volume at the level of either septal or lateral mitral annulus in the apical four-chamber transthoracic view, one obtains E and A waves similar to the mitral blood velocity pattern described above except that the mitral annular tissue Doppler waves move in the direction opposite to the blood flow. These annular waves are often labeled E′ and A′ to distinguish them from the equivalent mitral blood velocity waves (Fig. 4.9).

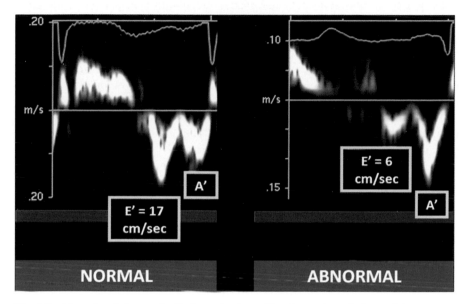

**Fig. 4.9**   Normal and abnormal mitral annular tissue Doppler tracings. *Left panel* shows a normal pattern; *right panel* reveals diminished E′ velocity consistent with abnormal left ventricular relaxation

The amplitude (peak velocity) of E′ is inversely related to left ventricular relaxing properties (the lower the E′ velocity, the greater the left ventricular dysfunction). In the elderly, peak E′ velocities of less than 8 cm/s is abnormal; in young individuals the cutoff value of 10 cm/s is used. Mitral tissue Doppler E′ measures primarily the diastolic properties of the left ventricle and is relatively preload independent (unaffected by left atrial filling pressures); this is in contrast with mitral and pulmonary venous blood velocities, which simultaneously reflect both the left ventricular diastolic properties and the left atrial filling pressures.

Clinically, the most useful application of the mitral annular tissue Doppler analysis is the ratio of the mitral blood velocity E wave and the mitral annular E′ velocity. When the E′ sampling is performed at the *medial* annulus, an E/E′ ratio of <8 is indicative of normal filling pressures. An E/E′ ratio >15 implies elevated filling pressures. When one observes an E/E′ >15 in a patient with acute coronary syndrome, there is a strong possibility that the patient is in pulmonary edema. When

E/E′ values range between 8 and 15, left atrial pressure may be either normal or elevated.[13] In addition, estimation of left ventricular filling pressures by E/E′ ratio is a powerful predictor of survival after acute myocardial infarction; the higher the E/E′ ratio, the lower the survival.[14]

## *Left Atrial Volume*

Usually, left atrial volume does not change precipitously in patients with acute coronary syndrome. However, chronic remodeling over weeks and months after completed myocardial infarction leads to progressive left atrial enlargement due to chronically elevated left atrial pressures. Conversely, in the absence of significant mitral and aortic valve disease, the mere finding of increased left atrial volume is indicative of abnormal left ventricular filling characterized by chronically elevated left atrial pressures.

Left atrial volumes are usually calculated using the area-length method and indexed for body surface area (Table 4.2). The same reference values are used for both women and men.

**Table 4.2**   Normal and abnormal left atrial volumes

| Left atrial size | Left atrial volume indexed to body surface area (mL/m$^2$) |
| --- | --- |
| Normal | $22 \pm 6$ |
| Mildly enlarged | 29–33 |
| Moderately enlarged | 34–39 |
| Severely enlarged | $\geq 40$ |

Based on data from Lang et al.[8]

## Conclusion

In patients with acute coronary syndrome, assessment of left ventricular function should be based on the 17-segment model for both standard wall motion analysis and strain imaging. Assessment of left ventricular diastolic function should include mitral inflow and pulmonary vein blood velocity pulsed Doppler recordings, mitral annular tissue Doppler tracings, E/E′ ratio, and calculation of the left atrial volume indexed to patient's body surface area.

## Clinical Cases

Gerard Oghlakian, MD, Ramzan Zakir, MD, and Christine Gerula, MD of New Jersey Medical School in Newark, NJ have contributed to the following cases.

## Clinical Case #1

### Subjective

A 72-year-old man with history of hypertension, diabetes mellitus, and coronary artery disease (CAD) presented to the emergency room complaining of intermittent chest pain of 5 days duration. He described the chest pain as being left-sided, nonexertional, waxing and weaning, and lasting few minutes at a time. He denied concomitant shortness of breath, nausea, or vomiting. There was no diaphoresis, lightheadedness, or syncope.

His past medical history of CAD consisted of a previous myocardial infarction and stent placement in the distal left anterior descending (LAD) artery 1 year ago. He also had history of mechanical aortic valve replacement 10 years prior. He denied any tobacco, alcohol, or drug abuse. He was compliant with all his medications including an angiotensin-converting inhibitor, a beta blocker, a statin, and aspirin.

### Objective

In the emergency room, his physical exam revealed a blood pressure of 110/73 mmHg and a heart rate of 89 beats per minute. His respiratory rate was 22 respirations per minute and his oxygen saturation was 99% on room air. He did not appear to be in any distress. He had a normal jugular venous pressure. His lungs were clear to auscultation. His cardiac auscultatory findings were normal. There was no peripheral edema.

The electrocardiogram obtained in the emergency department showed normal sinus rhythm, inferior Q waves, and lateral T wave abnormalities consisting of a slight ST depression in the precordial lead $V_6$ and T wave inversions in leads I and $aV_L$ (Fig. 4.10).

### Assessment and Plan

A presumptive diagnosis of cardiac biomarker-negative unstable angina was established.

### Indication for the Echo

While still in the emergency department, the patient had another episode of chest pain. His electrocardiogram obtained during the chest episode remained unchanged from the baseline. A stat echocardiogram was performed in the emergency department while the patient was still having chest pain.

### Echo Imaging

Transthoracic echocardiography at the time of chest pain revealed hypokinesis of the basal and mid segments of the inferior and posterior (inferolateral) walls (segments

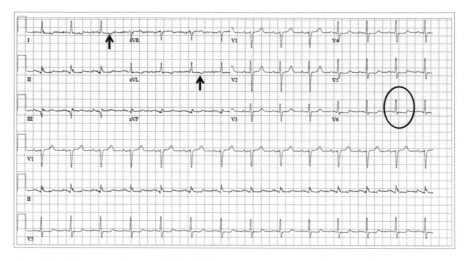

**Fig. 4.10** Electrocardiogram (EKG). EKG reveals normal sinus rhythm, inferior Q waves, and lateral T wave abnormalities consisting of a slight ST depression in the precordial lead $V_6$ (*circles*) and T wave inversions in leads I and $aV_L$ (*arrows*)

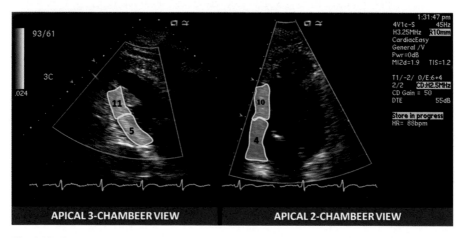

**Fig. 4.11** Transthoracic echocardiogram. Transthoracic echocardiography at the time of chest pain revealed hypokinesis of the basal and mid segments of the inferior and posterior (inferolateral) walls (segments 4, 5, 10, and 11). There were no other left ventricular wall motion abnormalities including the regions supplied by the distal LAD (segments 13–17) where in-stent restenosis had occurred

4, 5, 10, and 11). There were no other left ventricular wall motion abnormalities including the distal anterior wall and the apex (segments 13–17). Left ventricular ejection fraction was diminished and was calculated at 40% (Fig. 4.11).

## Management

Patient was taken to the cardiac catheterization laboratory. His coronary angiogram revealed that the right coronary artery was dominant and that it had no significant stenosis. In the distal left anterior descending (LAD) artery, there was in-stent restenosis. Just proximal to the takeoff of the first obtuse marginal branch, there was a 95% diameter stenosis of the left circumflex (LCx) artery (Fig. 4.12).

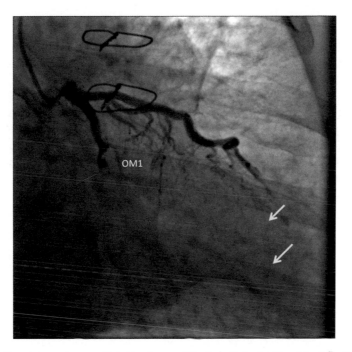

**Fig. 4.12** Coronary angiogram. Note the abnormalities in both the LAD and the LCx. In the distal LAD, there is in-stent restenosis (*arrows*). Just proximal to the takeoff of the first obtuse marginal branch (OM$_1$), there is a 95% diameter stenosis of the LCx (*arrow head*). The image is obtained in the right anterior oblique (RAO) view (−27°) with caudal angulation (−30°). Coronary angiogram is courtesy of Drs. Marc Klapholz and Edo Kaluski, New Jersey Medical School, Newark, NJ

Given the echocardiographic findings, the LCx was deemed to be the culprit vessel and the stenosis was successfully treated with the deployment of a drug-eluting stent. Despite restenosis of the stent in the distal LAD, there were no wall motion abnormalities in the LAD distribution likely due to natural collaterals.

## Outcome

Following the percutaneous intervention, his chest pain resolved and he was discharged home. He remained chest pain free on subsequent follow-up.

## Clinical Case #2

### Subjective

A 69-year-old man with history of hypertension was found unresponsive in a local park. Emergency medical service was called and patient was transported to the hospital. No details of his past medical history could be obtained as the patient was unresponsive and no relative or friend could be contacted.

### Objective

In the emergency department, his blood pressure was 185/65 mmHg and a heart rate of 55 beats per minute. His respiratory rate was 10 respirations per minute and his oxygen saturation was 99% on a 100% nonrebreather mask. There was no evidence of trauma. He had a normal jugular venous pressure. Patient was intubated for airway protection and auscultatory exam of the lungs was difficult. His cardiac exam revealed no murmurs, rubs, or gallop. He did not have any peripheral edema.

An electrocardiogram performed in the emergency department revealed sinus bradycardia, left atrial enlargement, and lateral T wave inversions (Fig. 4.13). Basic laboratory exam was remarkably for elevated serum glucose level (239 mg/dL; normal <109 mg/dL).

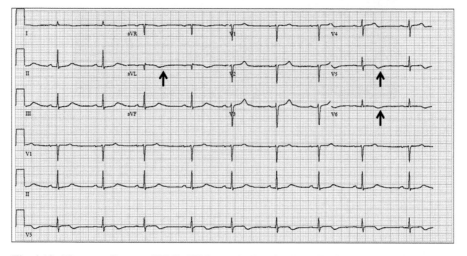

**Fig. 4.13** Electrocardiogram (EKG). EKG reveals sinus bradycardia, left atrial enlargement, and lateral T wave inversions (*arrows*)

Serum troponin I peaked at 20.8 ng/mL (normal <0.4 ng/mL). Brain natriuretic peptide (BNP) was elevated at 1550 pg/mL (normal <100 pg/mL). Chest radiograph revealed pulmonary vascular congestion (Fig. 4.14).

**Fig. 4.14** Chest radiograph.
Pulmonary vascular
congestion is present in both
lungs. Radiograph is courtesy
of Dr. Pierre Maldjian, New
Jersey Medical School,
Newark, NJ

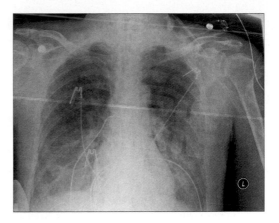

## Indication for the Echo

A presumptive diagnosis of acute coronary syndrome complicated by an acute pulmonary edema was established and transthoracic echocardiogram was ordered to assess left ventricular systolic and diastolic function.

## Echo Imaging

Transthoracic echocardiogram revealed severe global LV systolic dysfunction. Assessment of left ventricular diastolic dysfunction revealed a restrictive filling pattern (grade III left ventricular diastolic dysfunction) based on mitral and pulmonary venous flow velocity recordings. Peak velocity of the mitral annular tissue Doppler E′ wave was low (6 cm/s) indicative of diminished left ventricular relaxation. E/E′ ratio was greater than 15 indicative of elevated left atrial pressures (Fig. 4.15). In summary, echocardiographic findings were consistent with the clinical diagnosis of

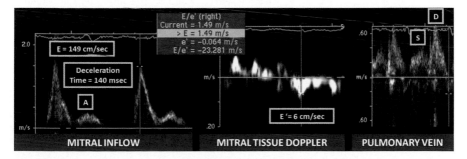

**Fig. 4.15** Echocardiogram. Mitral inflow blood velocity pattern reveals restrictive filling pattern. Pulmonary venous flow with S < D is consistent with such a pattern. Peak velocity of the mitral annular tissue Doppler E′ is low. E/E′ ratio is greater than 15 indicative of elevated left atrial pressures and consistent with the clinical diagnosis of congestive heart failure

congestive heart failure (pulmonary vascular congestion on chest radiograph; highly elevated BNP).

## Management

Patient was treated with an angiotensin-converting enzyme, a beta blocker, a statin, and an intravenous diuretic. His oxygenation improved and pulmonary vascular congestion resolved.

## Outcome

The patient's neurologic status did not improve significantly and he continued to be in a persistent vegetative state and ventilator dependent. He had a tracheostomy and gastrostomy tube placed and was transferred to a long-term facility. He had no further cardiac evaluation or intervention in view of his poor neurologic outcome.

## References

1. Kaijser L, Berglund B. Myocardial lactate extraction and release at rest and during heavy exercise in healthy men. *Acta Physiol Scand*. 1992;144(1):39–45.
2. Kaul S, Ito H. Microvasculature in acute myocardial ischemia: part I: evolving concepts in pathophysiology, diagnosis, and treatment. *Circulation*. 2004;109(2):146–149.
3. Nesto RW, Kowalchuk GJ. The ischemic cascade: temporal sequence of hemodynamic, electrocardiographic and symptomatic expressions of ischemia. *Am J Cardiol*. 1987;59(7): C23–C30.
4. Zehender M, Kasper W, Kauder E, et al. Right ventricular infarction as an independent predictor of prognosis after acute inferior myocardial infarction. *N Engl J Med*. 1993;328:981–988.
5. Multicenter Postinfarction Research Group. Risk stratification and survival after myocardial infarction. *N Engl J Med*. 1983 August 11 ;309(6):331–336.
6. Carlson MD, Krishen A. Risk assessment for ventricular arrhythmias after extensive myocardial infarction: what should I do? *ACC Curr J Rev*. 2003;12(2):90–93.
7. Curtis JP, Sokol SI, Wang Y, et al. The association of left ventricular ejection fraction, mortality, and cause of death in stable outpatients with heart failure. *J Am Coll Cardiol*. 2003;42(4):736–742.
8. Lang RM, Bierig M, Devereux RB, et al. Recommendations for chamber quantification: a report from the American Society of Echocardiography's Guidelines and Standards Committee and the Chamber Quantification Writing Group, developed in conjunction with the European Association of Echocardiography, a branch of the European Society of Cardiology. *J Am Soc Echocardiogr*. 2005 December;18(12):1440–1463.
9. Otterstad JE. Measuring left ventricular volume and ejection fraction with the biplane Simpson's method. *Heart*. 2002 December;88(6):559–560.
10. Jenkins C, Bricknell K, Hanekom L, Marwick TH. Reproducibility and accuracy of echocardiographic measurements of left ventricular parameters using real-time three-dimensional echocardiography. *J Am Coll Cardiol*. 2004;44:878–886.
11. Bijnens B, Claus P, Weidemann F, Strotmann J, Sutherland GR. Investigating cardiac function using motion and deformation analysis in the setting of coronary artery disease. *Circulation*. 2007;116:2453–2464.
12. Kirkpatrick JN, Vannan MA, Narula J, Lang RM. Echocardiography in heart failure. *J Am Coll Caardiol*. 2007;50:381–396.

13. Ommen SR, Nishimura RA, Appleton CP, Miller TA, Oh JK, Redfield MM, Tajik AJ. Clinical utility of Doppler echocardiography and tissue doppler imaging in the estimation of left ventricular filling pressures: A comparative simultaneous Doppler-catheterization study. *Circulation*. 2000;102:1788–1794.
14. Hillis G, Moller J, Pellikka P, et al. Noninvasive estimation of left ventricular filling pressure by E/e' is a powerful predictor of survival after acute myocardial infarction. *J Am Coll Cardiol*. 2004;43:360–367.

# Chapter 5
# Echocardiography Assessment of the Right Ventricle in Acute Coronary Syndrome

Linda D. Gillam

## Introduction

When echocardiographers evaluate patients with cardiac decompensation following acute myocardial infarction, the abnormalities sought are typically left-sided problems such as profound left ventricular systolic dysfunction and/or mechanical complications of infarction. However, right ventricular infarction, which may also present as cardiogenic shock, is often overlooked. Although echocardiography is ideally suited to make this diagnosis, echocardiographic imaging protocols frequently include only limited images of the right ventricle and rarely include regional or quantitative assessment of function. As a consequence, the diagnosis of myocardial infarction may be missed.

This chapter will first provide an overview of the clinical features of right ventricular infarction to help the echocardiographer identify clinical scenarios in which this diagnosis should be suspected. Subsequent sections will provide a road map for the global and regional assessment of right ventricular function using echocardiography. Both qualitative and quantitative approaches will be discussed. The chapter will conclude with a review of complications of right ventricular infarction and the role that echocardiography can play in their detection and management.

## Blood Supply of the Right Ventricle

The right ventricle receives virtually all of its blood supply from the right coronary artery. The left anterior descending coronary artery supplies small proximal branches to the right ventricular outflow tract; when it wraps around the left ventricular apex, it perfuses the right ventricular apex as well.

In the majority of people (60%),[1] the right coronary artery also supplies the inferior septum and the inferoposterior wall of the left ventricle through the posterior

L.D. Gillam (✉)
Department of Medicine, Cardiology, Columbia University Medical Center, New York, NY, USA
e-mail: gillam@cvus.columbia.edu

E. Herzog, F.A. Chaudhry (eds.), *Echocardiography in Acute Coronary Syndrome*, DOI 10.1007/978-1-84882-027-2_5, © Springer-Verlag London Limited 2009

descending artery and posterolateral left ventricular branches. This is termed a right dominant coronary circulation. In approximately 25% of cases,[1] these regions are perfused by the left circumflex coronary artery (left dominant circulation). In the remaining 15%,[1] the circulation is codominant with both the right and the left circumflex coronary arteries contributing blood supply to these segments.

Thus, right ventricular infarction, which occurs when the right coronary artery is occluded, is typically accompanied by left ventricular inferior wall infarction. Isolated occlusion of a nondominant right coronary almost certainly occurs and is presumably associated with isolated right ventricular infarction. However, this phenomenon is rarely recognized clinically, perhaps because right-sided EKG leads are not routinely recorded and the small muscle mass of the infarcted right ventricle results in small enzyme leaks that may be overlooked or attributed to other causes of chest pain. Moreover, as discussed more fully below, echocardiography may either fail to detect right ventricular systolic dysfunction or attribute such dysfunction to other etiologies. Therefore, the true frequency of isolated right ventricular infarction is unknown. With occlusion of the left anterior descending coronary artery, right ventricular involvement (apex and/or outflow tract) may occur but is rarely clinically significant. Inferior wall infarction attributable to left circumflex occlusion does not involve the right ventricle.

The overall incidence of right ventricular infarction varies widely. Autopsy series[2,3] report RV involvement in 24–90% of patients with inferior wall myocardial infarction. Clinically evident right ventricular infarction is reported to occur in 15–20%[4] with severe involvement in 3–8%. Echocardiographic studies[5] have reported that up to 40% of patients with inferior wall myocardial infarction have right-sided involvement. It is hypothesized that right ventricular hypertrophy with resulting increased oxygen demand renders the right ventricle more vulnerable to ischemic insult.

## Clinical Manifestations and Significance of Right Ventricular Infarction

Right ventricular infarction should be suspected and sought echocardiographically in any patient with inferior wall myocardial infarction. More specific clinical findings include manifestations of acute right ventricular decompensation such as hypotension and jugular venous distention, particularly if associated with clear lung fields. The clinical differential diagnosis of right ventricular infarction includes left ventricular myocardial infarction with pump failure (in patients presenting with cardiogenic shock), cardiac tamponade, pulmonary embolus, and cor pulmonale. Right-sided precordial EKG leads should be routinely performed and will show ST-T changes and Q waves.[6]

In many patients, right ventricular infarction may be associated with no or minimal signs and symptoms. However, even in such individuals it may be clinically important since, in aggregate, right ventricular infarction has been shown to be an independent predictor of morbidity and mortality.[7-9] It is notable, however, that right ventricular infarction may cause cardiogenic shock. In the SHOCK (SHould we emergently revascularize Occluded coronaries for Cardiogenic shocK) study,[10] right ventricular infarction accounted for 5.3% of patients with MI-associated shock. Importantly, in this series, adverse outcomes defined as recurrent infarction (8.8%), recurrent ischemia (12.1%), and death (53.1%) occurred just as frequently when shock was on the basis of predominant right versus left ventricular infarction. The pathophysiologic basis for cardiogenic shock in right ventricular infarction may be multifactorial. Importantly, a right ventricle that is unable to pump blood through the pulmonary vascular bed will result in left ventricular underfilling. Moreover, due to pericardial constraint, an acutely dilated right ventricle will result in deviation of the interventricular septum toward the left with a tendency to distort and impede filling of the left ventricle.[11]

# Echocardiographic Diagnosis of Right Ventricular Infarction

## *Qualitative Assessment*

Echocardiographers have, for many years, used a qualitative (visual) assessment as the initial approach to evaluate left ventricular global and regional function. While it has its limitations, this approach has permitted the reliable diagnosis of left ventricular infarction. Moreover, there is a well-established correlation between regional wall motion abnormalities and the site of coronary occlusion. This is the basis of the 17-segment model of the left ventricle that has been adopted for all imaging modalities.[12]

The qualitative assessment of the left ventricle emphasizes the use of multiple echocardiographic windows that collectively demonstrate all 17 segments in a manner that is intrinsically redundant, i.e., each segment is shown in more than one window. Seeing a regional wall motion abnormality in more than one echocardiographic view increases the confidence with which the diagnosis of regional dysfunction is made. While the assessment of regional left ventricular function is arguably one of the most difficult echocardiographic skills, it is well established that it can be acquired with formal training and practice.

A similar approach can be applied to the right ventricle. Thus the right ventricle should be evaluated in multiple views, and it behooves the echocardiographer to fully evaluate the right ventricle in all patients so that the spectrum of normal right ventricular function is learned. Only with this approach will the qualitative assessment of RV function be robust.

Unfortunately in many echocardiographic studies, the assessment of the right ventricle is limited to the apical four-chamber view. However, the routine two-dimensional echocardiographic examination of the right ventricle should include multiple views as follows (Fig. 5.1):

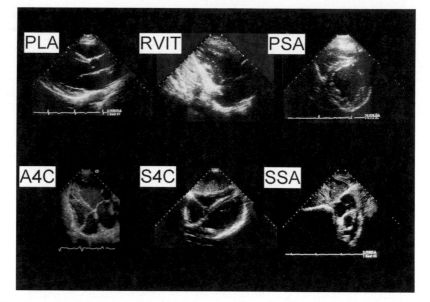

**Fig. 5.1** Standard imaging planes for the two-dimensional echocardiographic evaluation of the right ventricle. PLA = parasternal long axis; RVIT = right ventricular inflow tract; PSA = parasternal short axis (the image obtained is at the level of the ventricles); A4C = apical four-chamber; S4C = subcostal four-chamber; SSA = subcostal short axis (in the image, the plane is at the level of the great vessels). However, with transducer angulation, a series of short-axis views at the level of the ventricles that is analogous to those obtained parasternally may be recorded

1) Parasternal right ventricular inflow tract view.
2) Parasternal short-axis views at multiple levels. (Note: In order to see the right ventricle optimally, it may be necessary to widen the sector and/or sacrifice a complete simultaneous display of the left ventricular short axis. In this situation a series of RV-optimized and LV-optimized short-axis views should be recorded.)
3) Apical four-chamber view. (Note: While this view is routinely optimized for the left ventricle, a second RV-optimized four-chamber view should also be recorded.) This typically requires medial transducer angulation and a degree of foreshortening of the left ventricle.
4) Subcostal four-chamber view.
5) Subcostal short–axis view.

## The Utility of Echocardiographic Contrast Agents in Assessing the Right Ventricle

When RV endocardial definition is poor, echocardiographic contrast agents may be enormously helpful in improving image quality although RV endocardial border enhancement is an off-label indication. On occasion, satisfactory right ventricular opacification may be achieved with saline contrast. While contrast perfusion imaging of the right ventricle has been reported in a canine model,[13] it is technically challenging given the thin right ventricular wall. There has been no published study of this technique in humans.

## *A Segmental Approach to the Right Ventricle*

As is discussed in greater detail below, a segmental approach to the right ventricle is also important since regional rather than global RV dysfunction may occur in a number of clinically important scenarios including both right ventricular infarction and arrhythmogenic RV dysplasia. One such approach and the relationship between echocardiographic views and segments visualized are shown in Fig. 5.2. This recognizes four right ventricular segments: the right ventricular outflow tract (typically supplied by branches of the left anterior descending coronary artery), and the anterior, lateral, and inferior (diaphragmatic) free walls, all supplied by the right coronary. While the anterior and lateral walls are supplied by the acute marginal branches, the inferior wall is perfused by the posterior descending artery. While this system has value, particularly in the setting of right ventricular ischemia/infarction, it should be noted that there has not yet been agreement within the echocardiographic or larger imaging community on this or any other system. Moreover, it is limited by the fact that it does not provide a standardized nomenclature for differentiating between basal and apical segments.

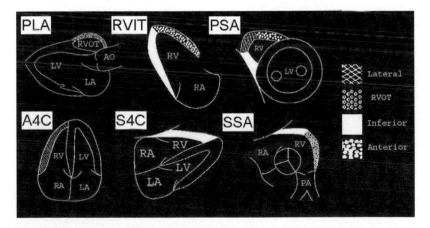

**Fig. 5.2** The segmental approach to the right ventricle recognizes four segments: the right ventricular outflow tract (RVOT) as well as the anterior, lateral, and inferior (diaphragmatic) walls. As shown schematically, the parasternal long-axis view displays the right ventricular outflow tract; the right ventricular inflow tract demonstrates the anterior and inferior walls; parasternal short-axis views at the level of the ventricles show the anterior, lateral, and inferior walls; the apical four-chamber view reveals the lateral wall; the subcostal view shows the inferior wall, and the subcostal short axis at the level of the great vessels reveals the inferior wall and the right ventricular outflow tract

When properly displayed, the right ventricular inflow tract view displays the right ventricular anterior and inferior walls and attached anterior and posterior leaflets of the tricuspid valve. However, there is a frequent variation on this view in which the interventricular septum rather than the right ventricular inferior wall is imaged (Fig. 5.3). In this case, the anterior and septal leaflets of the tricuspid valve are displayed. The parasternal long-axis view shows the right ventricular outflow tract, while short-axis views from either a parasternal or a subcostal view reveal the right ventricular anterior, lateral, and inferior walls. The apical four-chamber view demonstrates the right ventricular lateral wall, while the subcostal four-chamber view shows its inferior wall. Thus, the subcostal four-chamber view is not identical to the apical four-chamber view.

The importance of a segmental approach to the right ventricle is underscored by the fact that right ventricular infarction will vary in extent with the site of occlusion as reported in a study of 40 patients with inferior wall infarction due to right coronary artery occlusion and EKG-defined right ventricular infarction.[14] In this study, using the segmental scoring system described above, 90% of patients with the most extensive RV dysfunction (wall motion abnormalities involving the anterior, inferior, and lateral segments) had obstruction proximal to the first acute marginal branch. In 83% of patients with dysfunction involving the anterior and

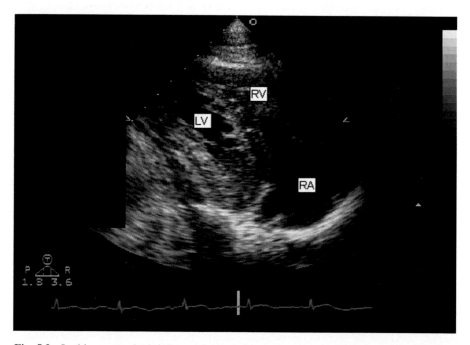

**Fig. 5.3** In this nonstandard right ventricular inflow tract view, the transducer has been rotated to reveal the interventricular septum and adjacent left and right ventricles. This view shows only the anterior wall of the right ventricle and typically does not show it well. The inferior wall is no longer visible

inferior segments, occlusion was proximal to the second marginal branch while wall motion abnormalities limited to the inferior segment correlated with obstruction either immediately proximal to the third marginal branch (50%) or distal to this vessel (50%). In all patients in whom there was no detectable right ventricular dysfunction, obstruction was distal to the third marginal branch. No patient had right ventricular outflow tract dysfunction or dysfunction isolated to the anterior or lateral walls. This study supports the concept that the right ventricular inferior wall is in the distal perfusion bed of the right coronary artery and, as such, will be at risk with both proximal and distal occlusion. In contrast, the anterior wall will be affected only with proximal occlusions.

This fact has important ramifications when one considers the echocardiographic views of the right ventricle. Views such as the apical four-chamber view that image only the lateral wall may fail to detect infarction when the culprit lesion is distal and the resultant wall motion abnormality is limited to the inferior wall. Since the inferior wall may be difficult to see in short-axis views, the subcostal four-chamber and properly aligned right ventricular inflow tract views are essential to the echocardiographic detection of right ventricular infarction. Figure 5.4 demonstrates severe hypokinesis to akinesis of the RV as evidenced by nearly identical right ventricular size at both end-diastole and end-systole. This patient had a proximal RCA occlusion.

It should be noted that all patients in this study have undergone successful primary angioplasty prior to echocardiographic imaging and that it has previously been reported that, in the setting of acute right coronary artery occlusion, early reperfusion improves right ventricular as well as left ventricular function.[15]

## Additional Studies of Right Ventricular Infarction Using Qualitative Two-dimensional Echocardiography

Using a semiquantitative segmental scoring system (normal, hypokinesis, kinesis/dyskinesis), Ketikoglu and colleagues reported abnormal right ventricular function at baseline with improvement at 3 months in patients with LV inferior wall infarction and EKG-defined RV involvement.[16] In the RV infarct group, they also noted abnormal diastolic function (increased tricuspid A wave, E deceleration time, and RV isovolumic relaxation time as well as decreased E/A ratio).

Dobutamine stress echocardiography has been used to demonstrate viability in patients with right ventricular infarction who had undergone successful acute reperfusion. Contractile reserve demonstrated at day 5 correlated with recovery of function at the time of 3 month follow-up.[17]

## Three-Dimensional Echocardiography

Three-dimensional echocardiography is ideally suited to the assessment of the right ventricle given the geometric complexity of this chamber. However, there has not yet been a report of the utility of this technique in right ventricular infarction.

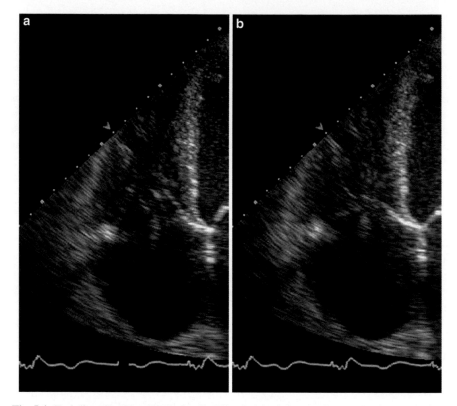

**Fig. 5.4** End-diastolic (**A**) and end-systolic (**B**) apical four-chamber images of a patient with right ventricular infarction due to proximal right coronary artery occlusion. Although it is difficult to convey wall motion with static images, it should be apparent that there has been little change in the size or the contour of the right ventricle. In real time, the RV lateral wall is seen to be severely hypokinetic to akinetic

## Quantitative Assessment of the Right Ventricle

A number of methods have been proposed for the quantitative echocardiographic assessment of global right ventricular function although none has achieved widespread clinical use. A major obstacle to the development and adoption of such tools has been the unusual shape of the right ventricle that handicaps its assessment with planar two-dimensional imaging. Moreover, there has been a relative lack of interest in abnormalities of the right heart with the result that few gold standards exist. The advent of three-dimensional echocardiography has spurred interest in developing quantitative three-dimensional analytic techniques which have, to date, been applied to right ventricular volumes. Additional applications will likely be forthcoming.

Validated two-dimensional methods for assessing the right ventricle include the following:

1. *Fractional area change.* This measure is easily obtained using the apical four-chamber view in which the end-diastolic and end-systolic areas are simply planimetered. The fractional area change is expressed as:

$$\frac{(\text{Area at end-diastole}) - (\text{Area at end-systole})}{\text{End-diastolic area}}$$

   Normal values are greater than 35%.
2. Tricuspid annular plane systolic excursion has also been widely used. This measure (TAPSE) is easily obtained using either two-dimensional or M-mode measurements using the apical four-chamber view.
3. Tricuspid regurgitant jets may be used to derive right ventricular dP/dt. The tricuspid regurgitant jet is displayed at high sweep speeds. Using analysis systems that have been developed for the assessment of left ventricular dP/dt, two calipers are placed on the ascending limb of the tricuspid regurgitation jet typically at 1 and 2 m/sec. Based on the Bernoulli equation, the velocity spectrum can be used to calculate the rate of rise of pressure (dp/dt).
4. The myocardial performance (Tei) index originally described for the left ventricle has also been adapted to the right ventricle. This index is expressed as follows:

$$\frac{(\text{Isovolumic contraction time}) + (\text{Isovolumic relaxation time})}{\text{Ejection time}}$$

   Since it is usually difficult to simultaneously record tricuspid inflow and pulmonary outflow given the relative positions of the tricuspid and pulmonic valves, sequential inflow and outflow recordings are usually employed.
5. Doppler tissue imaging has also been used to look at the right ventricle and more recently, strain and strain rate have been derived using both Doppler tissue imaging and speckled tracking approaches. Using Doppler tissue imaging, the acceleration rate of isovolumic contraction has been suggested to be a load-independent index of right ventricular contractility.

## Studies of Right Ventricular Infarction Using Quantitative Methods

Using right ventricular free wall Doppler tissue imaging, Dokainish et al.[18] reported that a reduced S wave correlated with right ventricular infarction as defined by proximal right coronary occlusion. Moreover, it was prognostically important, predictive of cardiac death and rehospitalization at 1 year. In a small series of patients with ECG-defined right ventricular infarction,[19] right ventricular tissue velocity strain and strain rate were noted to be abnormal in the basal and midventricular segments. However, apical values were not statistically different from those in patients with isolated left ventricular inferior wall infarction.

The myocardial performance index has also been reported to be abnormal in the setting of right ventricular infarction.[20] Using an EKG gold standard, a right ventricular performance index of >30 had a sensitivity of 82% and specificity of 95% for RV infarction in the setting of left ventricular inferior wall infarction. In the study group, the mean performance index for those with RV myocardial infarction was $0.53 \pm 0.22$.

In a group of patients with acute EKG-defined RV myocardial infarction, abnormal tricuspid annular plane excursion (17 mm) and Doppler tissue imaging S wave (10.3 cm/s) were noted when they were compared to those with inferior wall infarction without RV involvement.[21] In a later study of patients with both anterior and inferior infarction[22] reduced tricuspid annular plane excursion was noted to be a marker of poor prognosis, particularly in patients with anterior wall infarction. This study did not report the number of patients with EKG evidence of right ventricular involvement.

## Echocardiography in the Differential Diagnosis of Right Ventricular Infarction

In addition to being able to make a positive diagnosis of right ventricular infarction, echocardiography can also easily confirm or exclude some alternative clinical diagnoses such as tamponade or left heart abnormalities. The key features of right ventricular infarction are regional or global right ventricular systolic dysfunction accompanied by left ventricular inferior wall and inferoseptal regional wall motion abnormalities. Dysfunction of the inferior wall and the inferior septum will help exclude cor pulmonale or pulmonary embolus where left ventricular function is typically normal. However, the septal distortion associated with pulmonary hypertension in these conditions may distort the left ventricular inferior wall making it more difficult to assess inferoseptal and inferior wall regional function.

Apical sparing with otherwise global RV systolic dysfunction[23] has been reported as a marker of pulmonary embolus but is neither specific nor sensitive for this diagnosis. Since the RV apex may be supplied by the left anterior descending coronary artery, a similar pattern is theoretically possible with right ventricular infarction. Finally, it is possible that in patients with nondominant RCA occlusion and right ventricular infarction, echocardiography alone may fail to reach the correct diagnosis since there will be no left-sided involvement in these patients. Clinical correlation and right ventricular ECGs are always helpful.

## Complications

### Tricuspid Regurgitation

Ischemic mitral regurgitation as a complication of left ventricular infarction has been extensively studied and is recognized to occur as a result of an imbalance between tethering and closure forces. As first described by Gibson et al.,[24] apical tethering, the hallmark of functional/ischemic mitral regurgitation, is also observed in cases of functional tricuspid regurgitation (Fig. 5.5). However, functional tricuspid regurgitation in the context of acute or chronic right ventricular infarction has not been extensively studied although one small reported series suggested that significant functional tricuspid regurgitation was rare in the setting of acute right ventricular infarction unless there was pulmonary hypertension.[25] Further study, ideally with three-dimensional technique, is warranted.

## *Ventricular Septal Defect*

Ventricular septal rupture is a recognized complication of acute myocardial infarction (Fig. 5.6). Of relevance to this discussion is the fact that reduced right ventricular function is a strong predictor of poor outcome. Thus a full assessment of the right ventricle is essential in all such patients.[26]

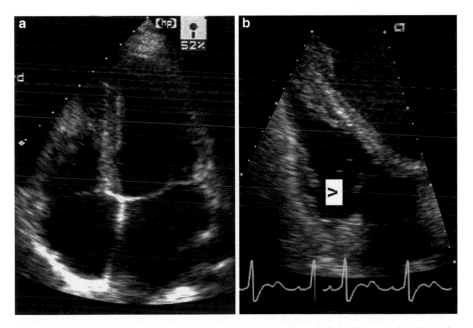

**Fig. 5.5** Normal closure of the tricuspid valve is shown in **panel A**. The septal and anterior leaflets close in the plane of the annulus. In contrast, in the setting of functional (ischemic) tricuspid regurgitation (**panel B**), the leaflets are apically tethered with a point of coaptation that is apically displaced from the plane of the annulus. Apical tethering is best appreciated in the apical four-chamber view

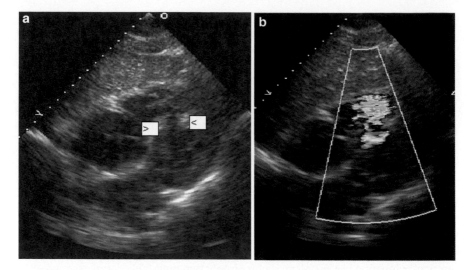

**Fig. 5.6**  Subcostal four-chamber view (**panel A**) of a patient with a ventricular septal defect (*arrows*). Color flow mapping (**panel B**) shows a large left to right shunt. In real-time, the right ventricle is noted to be severely hypokinetic, a poor prognostic sign

## *Intraventricular Thrombus ± Pulmonary Embolus*

The development of intracardiac thrombi with the potential for pulmonary embolism is another complication that has been the subject of isolated case reports.[27] While echocardiography, particularly with contrast enhancement, might facilitate the identification of this complication, it is frequently confounded by normal prominent right ventricular trabeculation.

## *Right to Left Shunting*

An additional complication that may be detectable by echocardiography is the development of right to left shunt across a patent foramen ovale.[28] As a consequence of elevated right-sided pressures and right atrial dilatation, the foramen may be stretched open and a significant right to left shunt with systemic hypoxia may ensue. Saline contrast echocardiography may establish the diagnosis and intracardiac or transesophageal echocardiography may help guide device closure.

## *Free Wall Rupture*

Right ventricular free wall rupture is a rare complication of right ventricular infarction.[29] As with left ventricular rupture, the echocardiographic manifestations typically consist of hemopericardium with echocardiographic features of tamponade. The rupture site is rarely demonstrable since the right ventricle is dramatically underfilled (Fig. 5.7).

**Fig. 5.7** Subcostal view from a patient with right ventricular free wall rupture following myocardial infarction. A large hematoma as well as free blood is seen in the pericardial space. The heart is compressed and the right ventricle is virtually empty. The suspected site of rupture is identified by the *arrow* although no color flow signal was detectable. Autopsy confirmed this to be the site of rupture

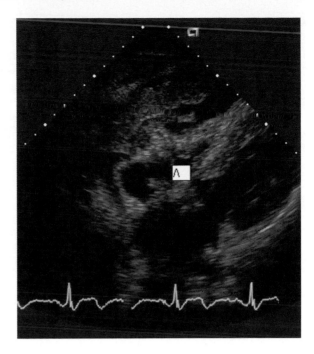

## Treatment and Outcomes

A full discussion of the treatment of right ventricular infarction is beyond the scope of this chapter. However, elements of treatment include volume repletion, inotropic support with dobutamine, antiarrhythmic support for the maintenance of sinus mechanism, reperfusion, and, in patients who are acutely decompensated, temporary right ventricular assist device placement. Nitrates and morphine are typically avoided. Since such treatment differs in many respects from that of left-sided myocardial infarction, the ability to make the correct diagnosis with echocardiography is obviously of extreme importance.

The prognosis in right ventricular infarction is generally favorable if the acute event is survived and if appropriate treatment is provided. There is typically variable residual dysfunction but this is often clinically inapparent. Patients with right ventricular infarction may recover RV systolic function over a period of weeks, perhaps attributable to a favorable oxygen supply–demand ratio as well as a greater capacity for quickly developing a functional collateral vascular supply. These results suggest that in many cases RV myocardial stunning takes place during ischemia instead of irreversible damage.

# Conclusion

Right ventricular myocardial infarction is a clinically important and frequently over-looked complication of acute occlusion of the right coronary artery. While it may easily be detected by careful echocardiographic evaluation, current echo protocols frequently fail to systematically evaluate the right ventricle. Suboptimal apical views are particularly problematic. To date, the cornerstone of echocardiographic evaluation of the right ventricle is a qualitative approach. However, quantitative methods for assessing the right ventricle exist and will continue to evolve.

# References

1. Gorlin R. Coronary anatomy. *Major Probl Intern Med.* 1976;11;40–58.
2. Isner JM, Roberts WC. Right ventricular infarction complicating left ventricular infarction secondary to coronary artery disease. Frequency, location, associated findings and significance from analysis of 236 necropsy patients with acute or healed myocardial infarction. *Am J Cardiol.* 1978;42(6):885–894.
3. Anderson HR, Falk E, Nielsen D. Right ventricular infarction: frequency, size, and topography in coronary heart disease: a prospective study comprising 107 consecutive autopsies from a coronary care unit. *J Am Coll Cardiol.* 1987;10(6):1223–1232.
4. Kinch JW, Ryan TJ. Right ventricular infarction. *N Engl J Med.* 1994;330(17):1211–1217.
5. D'Arcy B, Nanda NC. Two-dimensional echocardiographic features of right ventricular infarction. *Circulation.* 1982;65:167–173.
6. Braat SH, Brugada P, den Dulk K, van Ommen V, Wellens HJ. Value of lead V4R for recognition of the infarct coronary artery in acute inferior myocardial infarction. *Am J Cardiol.* 1984;53(11):1538–1541.
7. Zehender M, Kasper W, Kauder E, et al. Right ventricular infarction as an independent predictor of prognosis after acute inferior myocardial infarction. *N Engl J Med.* 1993;328(14): 981–989.
8. Serrano CV, Jr., Ramires JA, Cesar LA, et al. Prognostic significance of right ventricular dysfunction in patients with acute inferior myocardial infarction and right ventricular involvement. *Clin Cardiol.* 1995;18(4):199–205.
9. Bueno H, Lopez-Palop R, Bermejo J, Lopez-Sendon JL, Delcan JL. In-house outcomes of elderly patients with acute myocardial infarction and right ventricular infarction. *Circulation.* 1997;96(2):436–441.
10. Jacobs AK, Leopold JA, Bates E, et al. Cardiogenic shock caused by right ventricular infarction: a report from the SHOCK registry. *J Am Coll Cardiol.* 2003;41:1273–1279.
11. Dell'Italia LJ, Starling MR, Crawford MH, Boros BL, Chaudhuri TK, O'Rourke RA. Right ventricular infarction: identification by hemodynamic measurements before and after volume loading and correlation with noninvasive techniques. *J Am Coll Cardiol.* 1984;4(5): 931–939.
12. Cerqueira MD, Weissman NJ, Dilsizian V, et al. Standardized myocardial segmentation and nomenclature for tomographic imaging of the heart: a statement for healthcare professionals from the Cardiac Imaging Committee of the Council on Clinical Cardiology of the American Heart Association. *Circulation.* 2002;105(4):539–542.
13. Masugata H, Senda S, Fujita N, Mizushige K, Ohmori K, Kohno M. Spatial distribution of right ventricular perfusion abnormalities following acute right coronary artery occlusion: a study by myocardial contrast echocardiography and blue dye staining. *Int J Cardiovasc Imaging.* 2005;21:599–607.
14. Gemayel CY, Fram DB, Fowler LA, Kiernan FJ, Gillam LD. In vivo correlation of the site of

right coronary artery occlusion and echocardiographically defined right ventricular infarction. *Circulation*. 2000;102:II-542.

15. Bowers TR, O'Neill WW GC, Pica MC, Safian RD, Goldstein JA. Effect of reperfusion on biventricular function and survival after right ventricular infarction. *N Engl J Med*. 1998;338(14):933–940.

16. Ketikoglou DG, Karvounis HI, Papadopoulos CE, et al. Echocardiographic evaluation of spontaneous recovery of right ventricular systolic and diastolic function in patients with acute right ventricular infarction associated with posterior wall left ventricular infarction. *Am J Cardiol*. 2004;93(7):911–913.

17. Karvounis HI, Ketikoglou DG, Zaglavara TA, Parharides GE, Louridas GE. Usefulness of low-dose dobutamine stress echocardiography for the evaluation of spontaneous recovery of stunned myocardium in patients with acute right ventricular infarction. *J Am Soc Echocardiogr*. 2005;18:351–356.

18. Dokainish H, Abbey H, Gin K, Ramanathan K, Lee PK, Jue J. Usefulness of tissue Doppler imaging in the diagnosis and prognosis of acute right ventricular infarction with inferior wall acute left ventricular infarction. *Am J Cardio*. 2005;95(9):1039–1042.

19. Sevimli S, Gundogdu F, Aksakal E, et al. Right ventricular strain and strain rate properties in patients with right ventricular myocardial infarction. *Echocardiography*. 2007;24:732–738.

20. Chockalingam A, Gnanavelu G, Alagesan R, Subramanian T. Myocardial performance index in evaluation of acute right ventricular myocardial infarction. *Echocardiography*. 2004;21:487–494.

21. Alam M, Wardell J, Andersson E, Samad BA, Nordlander R. Right ventricular function in patients with first inferior myocardial infarction: assessment by tricuspid annular motion and tricuspid annular velocity. *Am Heart J*. 2000;139:710–715.

22. Samad BA, Alam M, Jensen-Urstad K. Prognostic impact of right ventricular involvement as assessed by tricuspid annular motion in patients with acute myocardial infarction. *Am J Cardiol*. 2002;90(7):778–781.

23. McConnell JV, Solomon SD, Rayan ME, Goldhaber SZ, Lee RT. Regional right ventricular dysfunction detected by echocardiography in acute pulmonary embolism. *Am J Cardiol*. 1996; 78: 469–472.

24. Gibson TC, Foale RA, Guyer DE, Weyman AE. Clinical significance of incomplete tricuspid valve closure seen on two-dimensional echocardiography. *J Am Coll Cardiol*. 1984;4: 1052–1057.

25. Gemayel CY, Fram DB, Kiernan FJ, Gillam LD. Tricuspid regurgitation complication right ventricular infarction: a prospective echocardiographic study. *J Am Soc Echocardiogr*. 2001;14:455A.

26. Radford MJ, Johnson RA, Daggett WM, Jr., et al. Ventricular septal rupture: a review of clinical and physiologic features and an analysis of survival. *Circulation*. 1981;64(3): 545–553.

27. Mittal SR, Arora H. Pulmonary embolism with isolated right ventricular infarction. *Indian Heart J*. 2001;53:218–220.

28. Cox D, Taylor J, Nanda NC. Refractory hypoxemia in right ventricular infarction from right-to-left shunting via a patent foramen ovale: efficacy of contrast transesophageal echocardiography. *Am J Med*. 1991;91:653–655.

29. Arat N, Sokmen Y, Ilkay E. Isolated right ventricular rupture: a rare complication of myocardial infarction. *Acta Cardiol*. 2007;62:413–416.

# Chapter 6
# Role of TEE in Acute Coronary Syndrome

Andrew P. Miller and Navin C. Nanda

## Introduction

Transesophageal echocardiography (TEE) can be useful in the diagnosis of and in assessing the complications of acute coronary syndromes (ACS) and myocardial infarction (MI).[1] Careful transesophageal imaging can provide insight into the anatomy of the coronary tree and yield conclusive evidence of coronary stenosis. TEE is often the diagnostic tool of choice to evaluate aortic dissection, which rarely but flagrantly can alter the treatment plan of patients with ACS. Similar to transthoracic imaging, TEE is capable of diagnosing any resulting wall motion abnormalities, aneurysm or pseduoaneurysm formation, and right ventricular infarction in ACS. When transthoracic imaging of a hemodynamically unstable or critically ill patient reveals apparent normal systolic function, a mechanical complication of MI should be considered. These complications of MI that can present later in the course of care, such as left ventricular free wall rupture, ventricular septal rupture, dynamic left ventricular outflow tract obstruction, mitral regurgitation from papillary muscle dysfunction or rupture, right ventricular papillary muscle rupture, and pericardial effusion, may be best appreciated with the TEE exam. Additionally, TEE may be particularly useful in the critical care unit in intubated or postoperative patients and others in whom transthoracic imaging may not be possible. If performed carefully, the TEE exam can be of importance in the cardiologist's armamentarium in patients with ACS.

## Coronary Stenosis

Evaluation of the proximal coronary tree, including the left main coronary (LMCA), left anterior descending (LAD), left circumflex (LCX), and right coronary (RCA) arteries, is possible with careful inspection during the TEE exam.[1-4] Stenosis may be

A.P. Miller (✉)
Cardiovascular Disease/Medicine, University of Alabama at Birmingham, Birmingham, AL, USA
e-mail: amiller@cvapc.com

E. Herzog, F.A. Chaudhry (eds.), *Echocardiography in Acute Coronary Syndrome*,
DOI 10.1007/978-1-84882-027-2_6, © Springer-Verlag London Limited 2009

**Fig. 6.1** Left main coronary artery stenosis. (**A**) An eccentric, highly reflectile atherosclerotic plaque (*upper arrow*) that produced >80% stenosis of the left main coronary artery (LMCA). The presence of normal-sized lumen beyond the stenosed area increases the diagnostic confidence, because it excludes the possibility of artificial narrowing produced by an oblique section through the coronary vessel. (**B**) Patients with severe mid left main stenosis with turbulent flow seen beyond the lesion. Pulsed Doppler interrogation reveals a high diastolic velocity. LA = left atrium; LAA = left atrial appendage; RA = right atrium; RVOT = right ventricular outflow tract. Reproduced with permission from Nanda and Domanski[1(p277)]

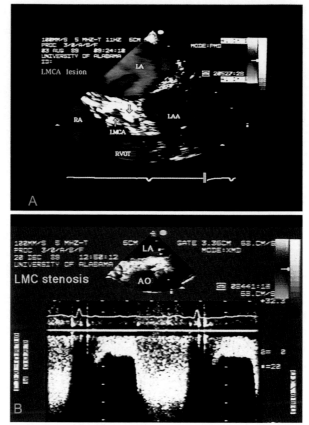

imaged directly and represented by compromise of the lumen, as seen in Fig. 6.1A. In this example of >80% stenosis of the LMCA, an eccentric, highly reflectile lesion is appreciated. To differentiate from an artifact produced by oblique imaging of the artery, normal lumen should be seen on both sides of the obstruction, as in this example. Poststenotic dilatation may be appreciated as well, and this often marks severe stenosis.

Doppler can be useful in confirming the diagnosis of proximal coronary stenosis and assessing its severity (Fig. 6.1B).[1–4] Turbulence by color Doppler can prompt further investigation. Pulsed Doppler interrogation will yield high diastolic velocities (>1 m/s) in stenotic lesions at rest. Provocative studies using stress agents can yield additional important clinical data. Using adenosine to induce maximum hyperemia may be valuable in assessing coronary flow reserve and has been validated against invasive flow wire techniques.[5]

In summary, by careful evaluation it is possible to image the entire LMCA, the proximal 2 cm of the LAD, the proximal 3 cm of the LCX, and the proximal 4 cm of the RCA in many patients.[2] Of these, the RCA is the most difficult to assess, owing to its anterior and immediate downward course. When performed in patients with ACS, TEE assessment of the coronary arteries is a skill that can yield important clinical results.

## Aortic Dissection

Unrecognized aortic dissection in the patient with ACS can yield tragic clinical consequences. Overall, the incidence of acute aortic dissection in the United States is 800 times lower than that of acute MI.[6] Thus, delaying time to reperfusion therapy in all patients with acute ST elevation MI would be a mistake.[7] However, symptoms that suggest aortic dissection should prompt further evaluation.

In the TEE exam of aortic dissection (reviewed elsewhere in this text), it is important to assess the ostium of the LMCA and RCA. Nearly 5% of patients presenting with type A aortic dissection will have an associated acute MI.[6] Whether the dissection extends to the coronary tree is the information imperative to proper surgical repair.

## Wall Motion Abnormalities

Evaluation of wall motion abnormalities, usually from the transgastric approach, is useful in assessing regions of ischemia or infarction.[1] In the intraoperative setting for both cardiac and noncardiac procedures, TEE offers monitoring that may

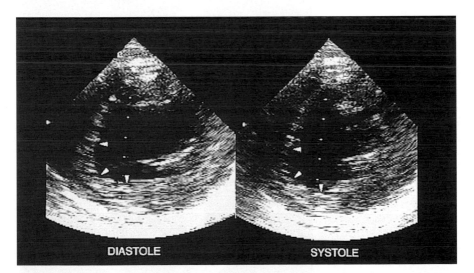

**Fig. 6.2** Left ventricular dysfunction. Marked hypokinesis of the anterior septum (*arrowheads*) is seen in this patient with ischemic heart disease. The inferior wall is also hypokinetic. Reproduced with permission from Nanda and Domanski[1(p284)]

provide the only clue for the presence of ACS.[8] In coronary revascularization procedures, TEE offers insight into the response to therapy, which can be magnificently appreciated during an intraoperative exam.

Wall motion abnormalities are usually best seen in short-axis views of the left ventricle from the transgastric approach, at the mid-papillary muscle level where segments corresponding to all three coronary arteries can be seen (Fig. 6.2). TEE assessment also involves an evaluation of overall left ventricular systolic function, and care should be taken to ensure that all segments are visualized, with the apical segment being the most difficult to image.

## Left Ventricular Aneurysm and Pseudoaneurysm Formation

Left ventricular aneurysm formation after MI (Fig. 6.3) results from regional contractile dysfunction and LV remodeling of the infarction and peri-infarction regions. To differentiate from pseudoaneurysm, left ventricular aneurysm is characterized

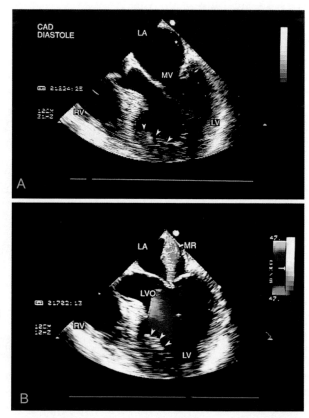

**Fig. 6.3** Left ventricular apical aneurysm. (**A**) A large apical aneurysm containing a thrombus (*arrowheads*) is shown. (**B**) Color Doppler examination shows the presence of associated mitral regurgitation (MR). LA = left atrium; LV = left ventricle; LVO = left ventricular outflow tract; MV = mitral valve; RV = right ventricle. Reproduced with permission from Nanda and Domanski[1(p286)]

by a broad neck, with the maximal internal width of the neck nearly equaling the maximal internal diameter of the aneurysm.[9]

In the setting of ACS, it is important to inspect for the presence of thrombus (Fig. 6.3A). Occurring in up to one-third of transmural anterior infarctions, more than half of LV thrombi form within 48 h and nearly all form within 1 week.[10] Though the length of anticoagulation is controversial, identification of LV thrombus warrants heparin therapy followed by warfarin for at least 3–6 months.[10]

Left ventricular aneurysm, due to both the magnitude of the associated infarction and the remodeling that follows, results in additional impairment in global ventricular function and geometry. Careful inspection during the TEE exam for associated functional impairment, such as significant mitral regurgitation (Fig. 6.3B), is warranted. In addition, the TEE exam may guide surgical interventions to restore or improve left ventricular geometry.

Left ventricular pseudoaneurysm (Fig. 6.4) is a false aneurysm that results from a left ventricular rupture contained by adherent pericardium or scar tissue. These lesions have narrow necks that communicate with the left ventricular cavity. In pseudoaneurysm, the maximal internal width of the neck is less than half that of the aneurysmal sac.[9] Owing to their traumatic origin, pseudoaneurysms may take serpentine paths and three-dimensional echocardiography may provide insight into their anatomy and wall structure.[11] Inherently unstable pseudoaneurysms have a propensity to rupture and should be resected even if discovered late in the clinical course after MI.

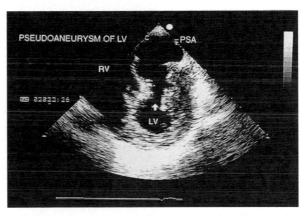

**Fig. 6.4** Left ventricular pseudoaneurysm. The *arrow* shows the communication of the left ventricle (LV) with the pseudoaneurysm which appears to be larger than the LV cavity. RV = right ventricle. Reproduced with permission from Nanda and Domanski[1(p288)]

# Right Ventricular Infarction

A well-recognized complication of inferior MI, right ventricular infarction is marked by right ventricular dilatation and hypokinesis/akinesis during the TEE exam.[12] This important clinical entity requires a different clinical approach, and when unrecognized can produce undesirable responses in the ACS patient. Only in rare instances would TEE be the diagnostic modality, since right ventricular infarction can be readily diagnosed by clinical signs, the electrocardiogram, and transthoracic echocardiography.

One complication of right ventricular infarction in which TEE may play a significant role is in patients with refractory hypoxemia due to shunting through an atrial septal defect or a patent foramen ovale.[13,14] When right atrial pressure increases to equal or exceed left atrial pressure, a right-to-left shunt can occur if an atrial septal defect or a patent foramen ovale exists. Contrast transesophageal echocardiography can be helpful in making the diagnosis and percutaneous closure can result in marked improvement in oxygenation.[13,14]

## Left Ventricular Free Wall Rupture

The most common mechanical complication of MI, left ventricular free wall rupture has been reported in up to 6% of patients prior to acute revascularization therapy.[15] In the modern era, rates of this complication have improved.[16] While

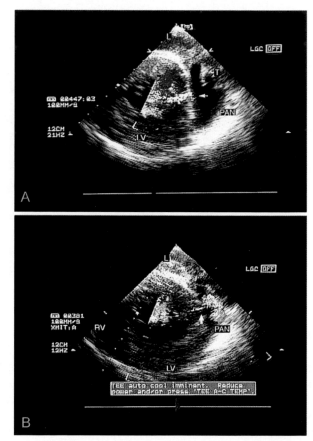

**Fig. 6.5** Contained slit-like cardiac rupture following acute myocardial infarction. Transgastric views. (**A,B**) Show a large and narrow color jet (*arrow*) within the left ventricle (LV) posterior wall. B also shows color flow signals partially filling the pseydoaneurysm cavity (PAN). RV = right ventricle; T = thrombus. Reproduced with permission from Rao[30]

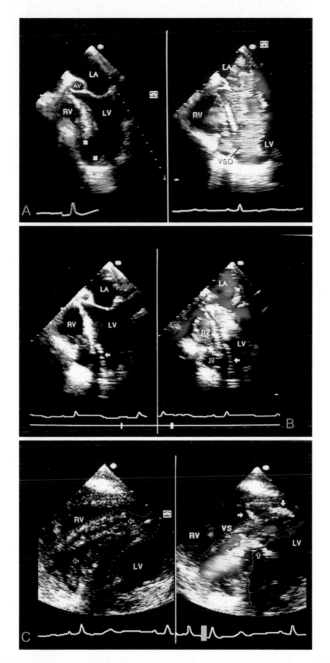

**Fig. 6.6**   Ventricular septal rupture after acute anterior myocardial infarction. (**A**) Apical five-chamber view. Flow signals are seen moving from the left ventricle (LV) into the right ventricle (RV) through the large apical defect (*arrows*). (**B**) The patch (*solid arrow*) used to close the defect. (**C**) Transgastric views (transverse plane imaging) from the same patient show marked enlargement and widening of the ventricular septum (VS), with large areas of echolucency consistent with

the most common presentation is out-of-hospital sudden death and the diagnosis is often made by postmortem exam, the diagnosis of free wall rupture should be considered in patients with acute clinical decline during the first 10 days after MI. Risk factors that should raise awareness include older age, female gender, first MI, single-vessel disease, transmural MI, anterior location, and absence of left ventricular hypertrophy. Complete rupture often results in hemopericardium and electromechanical dissociation, but smaller slit-like ruptures may result in slower bleeding and be accompanied by progressive signs of cardiogenic shock.

The most common echocardiographic finding in left ventricular free wall rupture is a pericardial effusion. Pericardial effusions containing echodense material (thrombus) neighboring a wall motion abnormality should raise suspicion for rupture (Fig. 6.5). Careful inspection with color flow Doppler can reveal the site of rupture. In addition, the use of contrast agents can improve sensitivity by demonstrating extravasation into the pericardial space.

## Ventricular Septal Rupture

Ventricular septal rupture is a less common mechanical complication of MI and occurs in about 0.2% of patients in the era of reperfusion therapy.[17] Ventricular septal rupture is usually associated with single-vessel disease (left anterior descending artery is most common) and occurs at the MI margin between thinned, necrotic and hyperdynamic, non-necrotic myocardium. Other risk factors include older age, female gender, hypertension, absence of smoking history, tachycardia, and Killip class 3 or 4.[17] Presenting with hemodynamic compromise and a new systolic murmur in most, ventricular septal rupture requires a prompt diagnosis.[18]

Anterior ventricular septal ruptures are more apically located, while inferior ruptures tend to occur toward the base and have a more complex course. Right ventricular infarction is commonly associated with inferoseptal rupture, and both portend a poor prognosis. While TTE can establish the diagnosis in most patients, TEE may be useful in those with poor transthoracic windows and during surgical intervention.

---

**Fig. 6.6** (continued) dissection (*horizontal open arrows* in **C**). Color Doppler imaging shows prominent color flow signals (maximal width 10 mm) moving from the LV into the ventricular septum (VS) (*vertical open arrow* in **C**) and occupying the large echolucent areas seen on the noncolor Doppler image. The prominent area of localized relatively high-velocity signals (flow acceleration) noted in the LV measured 9 mm at the site of the defect. No corresponding defect at the same level is seen on the right ventricular aspect, but two smaller sites of rupture, both 5 mm in size, are noted on the right side further posteriorly (*solid arrows* in **C**). These are associated with smaller areas of flow acceleration (1.5–2 mm). These defects are not delineated on the two-dimensional image but are visualized only during color Doppler examination. Therefore the patient has four defects in the VS, one very large and located in the apical region, and the other three much smaller and located more posteriorly. None of the findings noted in C was demonstrated by transthoracic echocardiography. LA = left atrium; VSD = ventricular septal defect. Reproduced with permission from Ballal et al.[20]

Imaging reveals a disrupted ventricular septum with left-to-right shunting by color flow Doppler (Fig. 6.6).[19, 20] Intravenous injection of agitated saline can demonstrate bubbles crossing into the left ventricle but is often marked by negative contrast of the right ventricle at the site of the defect. It is important to consider that defects may be underappreciated when they are very large and flow is of low velocity or when the rupture results in serpiginous tracts that produce multiple sites of entry into the right ventricle. In addition, posterior ventricular septal rupture may be sometimes only appreciated from the transgastric approach.

## Left Ventricular Outflow Tract Obstruction

In the setting of anteroapical MI with hyperdynamic basal segments, a rare complication of MI is left ventricular outflow tract obstruction.[21] The hemodynamic consequence of hyperdynamic basal septal contraction and systolic anterior motion of the mitral valve, this complication is more often seen in older women with hypertension and has also been described in Takostubo cardiomyopathy. Marked by a new systolic murmur and hemodynamic compromise that does not improve or worsens with inotropic therapy, this is another complication of MI that is best diagnosed with urgent bedside cardiac ultrasound.

Echocardiography reveals systolic anterior motion of the mitral valve, turbulent and high-velocity flow in the left ventricular outflow tract, and a dagger-shaped contour on continuous wave Doppler evaluation. Transthoracic imaging is usually adequate to make this diagnosis, but TEE is necessary in those with poor acoustic windows.

## Mitrial Regurgitation and Papillary Muscle Rupture

Papillary muscle rupture is the least common mechanical complication of acute MI. Usually (>90%) involving the posteromedial papillary muscle due to its single blood supply, rupture may be complete or just involve the muscular heads or tips and can occur in even small infarctions.[22] Patients with this disorder often present with acute volume overload and cardiogenic shock in the time period of 2–7 days after MI. Identification of papillary muscle rupture is a surgical emergency, with a 50% unoperated mortality rate over the first 24 h.[22] Due to tachycardia and a noncompliant left atrium in the acute phase of mitral regurgitation, the murmur of mitral regurgitation may be soft and transthoracic imaging may be inconclusive. The TEE exam offers significant incremental value in this clinical entity.

Echocardiographic features of papillary muscle rupture include hyperdynamic left ventricular function, a flail mitral leaflet with systolic prolapse into the left atrium, and severe mitral regurgitation. Though diagnostic, visualization of the ruptured papillary muscle head prolapsing into the left atrium (Fig. 6.7) may not be seen in about 35% of cases even with TEE.[23] Helpful clues include erratic motion

**Fig. 6.7** Left ventricular papillary muscle rupture. A classic finding of prolapse (*arrows*) of the ruptured papillary muscle head into the left atrium (LA) is noted. The ruptured head involved the anterior papillary muscle. Reproduced with permission from Moursi et al.[23]

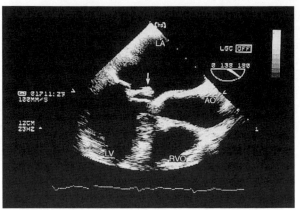

of a large echo density in the left ventricle (Fig. 6.8) and Doppler evidence of mitral regurgitation in all four pulmonary veins.

Rupture of the papillary muscle is not necessary to induce acute severe mitral regurgitation, which can be a result of ischemic dysfunction and respond to revascularization.[24] When associated with dilatation of the mitral annulus, the left atrium, and the left ventricle, functional mitral regurgitation may be long-standing and a subject of another chapter. When discovered in patients with ACS though, significant mitral regurgitation should be carefully considered, since insufficiency marks that a worse prognosis can progress with continued left ventricular remodeling after ischemic injury.[25,26]

**Fig. 6.8** Left ventricular papillary muscle rupture. Representation of transgastric view demonstrating erratic motion of the ruptured papillary muscle head (*arrow*) in the left ventricle (LV). The ruptured head, which involved the posterior papillary muscle, did not prolapse into the left atrium. RV = right ventricle. Reproduced with permission from Moursi et al.[23]

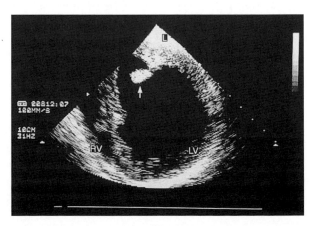

# Right Ventricular Papillary Muscle Rupture

Tricuspid insufficiency due to papillary muscle rupture is a rare clinical entity in ACS (Fig. 6.9).[27] More often seen spontaneously in neonates or from traumatic injury, right ventricular papillary muscle rupture has been reported in only a few cases.

**Fig. 6.9** Right ventricular papillary muscle rupture. Apical view. The ruptured papillary muscle (M) is visible in the right atrium (RA). The *arrow* points to an associated ventricular septal rupture. A = anterior tricuspid valve leaflet; LV = left atrium; LV = left ventricle; RV = right ventricle. Reproduced with permission from Maxted et al.[27]

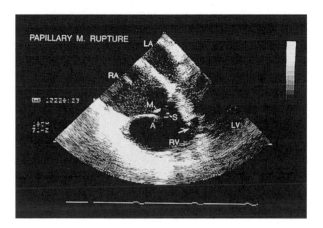

# Pericardial Effusion

As discussed above, the surgical emergencies of aortic dissection and left ventricular rupture may be represented by a pericardial effusion during the TEE exam. However, up to 28% of patients with acute MI may have a pericardial effusion, and hemopericardium comprises a minority of these.[28] Early postinfarction pericarditis often develops on day 2 or 3 after a transmural MI and the course is usually benign. Dressler's syndrome is a different clinical entity and usually develops during the second or third week after an acute MI, but may begin as early as 24 h after the MI. This syndrome can result in large effusions and rarely can produce cardiac tamponade.

During a TEE exam in the patient with ACS, a pericardial effusion should be viewed suspiciously, and aortic dissection or free wall rupture should be ruled out. The usual signs of cardiac tamponade should be evaluated, including pronounced respiratory variation of diastolic flow across the mitral and tricuspid valves, right atrial systolic collapse, right ventricular early diastolic collapse, and a dilated inferior vena cava with poor respiratory excursion. In patients after cardiac surgery, it is important to inspect for left ventricular collapse and a loculated posterior effusion. When these signs are absent, pericardial effusion may be a benign complication of acute MI.

# Conclusion

When performed in the operating room and in the cardiac care unit, TEE can add valuable information to the care of the ACS patient. Intraoperative TEE may provide only the diagnostic clue for ACS in the sedated patient with alterations in hemodynamics. In patients with aortic dissection, or the rare case of paradoxical embolus,[29] TEE may identify the etiology of ACS. In critically ill patients with sudden hemodynamic compromise in the hours to days after a transmural MI, TEE may be the diagnostic modality of choice to identify pseudoaneurysm, left ventricular free wall rupture, ventricular septal rupture, and papillary muscle rupture. These entities require prompt intervention and, thus, must not be missed.

# References

1. Nanda NC, Domanski MJ. *Atlas of Transesophageal Echocardiography*. Philadelphia: Lippincott Williams & Wilkins; 2007.
2. Samdarshi TE, Nanda NC, Gatewood RP, Jr., et al. Usefulness and limitations of transesophageal echocardiography in the assessment of proximal coronary artery stenosis. *J Am Coll Cardiol*. 1992;19:572–580.
3. Nanda NC, Gomez C, Liu M, et al. Transesophageal echocardiographic diagnosis of coronary stenosis in a stroke patient. *Echocardiography*. 1999;16:589–592.
4. Voros S, Nanda NC, Samal AK, et al. Transesophageal echocardiography in patients with ischemic stroke accurately detects significant coronary artery stenosis and often changes management. *Am Heart J*. 2001;142:916–922.
5. Redberg RF, Sobol Y, Chou TM, et al. Adenosine-induced coronary vasodilatation during transesophageal Doppler echocardiography: rapid and safe measurement of coronary flow reserve ratio can predict significant left anterior descending coronary stenosis. *Circulation*. 1995;92:190–196.
6. Hagan PG, Nienaber CA, Isselbacher EM, et al. The International Registry of acute Aortic Dissection (IRAD): new insights into an old disease. *JAMA*. 2000;283:897–903.
7. Kamp TJ, Goldschmidt-Clemont PJ, Brinker JA, Resar JR. Myocardial infarction, aortic dissection, and thrombolytic therapy. *Am Heart J*. 1994;128:1234–1237.
8. Hong Y, Orihashi K, Oka Y. Intraoperative monitoring of regional wall motion abnormalities for detecting myocardial ischemia by transesophageal echocardiography. *Echocardiography*. 1990;7:323–332.
9. Gatewood RP, Jr., Nanda NC. Differentiation of left ventricular pseudoaneurysm from true aneurysm with two dimensional echocardiography. *Am J Cardiol*. 1980;46:869–878.
10. Cregler LL. Antithrombotic therapy in left ventricular thrombosis and systemic embolism. *Am Heart J*. 1992;123:1110–1114.
11. Nekkanti R, Nanda NC, Ansingkar KG, McGiffin DC. Transesophageal three-dimensional echocardiographic assessment of left ventricular pseudoaneurysm. *Echocardiography*. 2002;19:169–172.
12. D'Arcy BJ, Nanda NC. Two-dimensional echo features of right ventricular infarction. *Circulation*. 1982;65:167–173.
13. Cox D, Taylor J, Nanda NC. Refractory hypoxemia in right ventricular infarction from right-to-left shunting via a patent foramen ovale: efficacy of contrast transesophageal echocardiography. *Am J Med*. 1991;91:653–655.
14. Bassi S, Amersey R, Andrews R. Right ventricular infarction complicated by right to left shunting through an atrial septal defect: Successful treatment with an Amplatzer septal occluder. *Heart*. 2005;91:e28.

15. Lopez-Sendon JGA, Lopez de Sa E, Coma-Canella I, et al. Diagnosis of subacute ventricular wall rupture after acute myocardial infarction: sensitivity and specificity of clinical, hemodynamic and echocardiographic criteria. *J Am Coll Cardiol*. 1992;19:1145–1153.
16. Becker R, Gore JM, Lambrew C, et al. A composite view of cardiac rupture in the United States National Registry of Myocardial Infarction. *J Am Coll Cardiol*. 1996;27:1321–1326.
17. Crenshaw B, Granger C, Birnbaoum Y, et al. Risk factors, angiographic patterns, and outcomes in patients with ventricular septal defect complicating acute myocardial infarction: GUSTO I (Global Utilization of Streptokinase and TPA for Occluded coronary arteries) trial investigators. *Circulation*. 2000;100:27–32.
18. Kishon Y, Iqbal A, Oh J, et al. Evolution of echocardiographic modalities in detection of postmyocardial infarction ventricular septal defect and papillary muscle rupture. *Am Heart J*. 1993;126:667–675.
19. Helmcke F, Mahan EF, Nanda NC, et al. Two-dimensional echocardiography and Doppler color flow mapping in the diagnosis and prognosis of ventricular septal rupture. *Circulation*. 1990;81:1775–1783.
20. Ballal RS, Sanyal RS, Mahan III EF, Nanda NC. Usefulness of transesophageal echocardiography in the diagnosis of ventricular septal rupture secondary to acute myocardial infarction. *Am J Cardiol*. 1993;71:367–370.
21. Armstrong W, Marcovitz P. Dyanmic left ventricular outflow tract obstruction as a complication of acute myocardial infarction. *Am Heart J*. 1996;131:827–830.
22. Nishimura R, Gersh B, Schaff HV. The case for an aggressive surgical approach to papillary muscle rupture following myocardial infarction: "From paradise lost to paradise regained." *Heart*. 2000;83:611–613.
23. Moursi MH, Bhatnagar SK, Vilacosta I, et al. Transesophageal echocardiographic assessment of papillary muscle rupture. *Circulation*. 1996;94:1003–1009.
24. Macander PJ, Roubin GS, Hsiung MC, Nanda NC. Transient severe mitral insufficiency during percutaneous transluminal coronary angioplasty: a case report. *Am Heart J*. 1991;122:1153–1156.
25. Birnbaum Y, Chamoun AJ, Conti V, Uretsky BF. Mitral regurgitation following acute myocardial infarction. *Coron Artery Dis*. 2002;16:337–344.
26. Hillis D, Moeller J, Pellika P. Prognostic significance of echocardiographically defined mitral regurgitation early after acute myocardial infarction. *Am Heart J*. 2005;150:1268–1275.
27. Maxted W, Nanda NC, Kim KS, Roychoudhury D, Pinhciro L . Transesophageal echocardiographic identification and validation of individual tricuspid valve leaflets. *Echocardiography*. 1994;11:585–591.
28. Gregoratos G. Pericardial involvement in acute myocardial infarction. *Cardiol Clin*. 1990;8:601–608.
29. Rovner A, Valika AA, Kovacs A, Kates AM. Possible paradoxical embolism as a rare cause for an acute myocardial infarction. *Echcoardiography*. 2006;23:407–409.
30. Rao A, Garimella S, Nanda NC, Chung SM. Transesophageal color Doppler echocardiographic diagnosis of cardiac rupture following acute myocardial infarction. *Echocardiography*. 1996;13:309–312.

# Chapter 7
# Newer Quantification Technique for the Left Ventricular Wall Motion Analyses

**Ajay S. Shah, Melana Yuzefpolsky, and Farooq A. Chaudhry**

## Introduction

One hundred and sixty years ago, the Austrian professor of mathematics Christian Doppler first described the Doppler principle for light. Applied to ultrasound this technique has been developed to an essential part of echocardiography. In contrast to two-dimensional echocardiography, Doppler signals are less affected by tissue between the region of interest and the transducer. Tissue Doppler imaging (TDI) and strain rate imaging (SRI) are new techniques providing velocities of normal and pathologic myocardial structures during the cardiac cycle.[1]

Usual indices of global LV function such as EF and volumes are load dependent and influenced by image quality, technical considerations, and measurement error. Ejection fraction reflects the sum contribution of several regions and does not provide information on regional function. Myocardial tagging with cardiac magnetic resonance (CMR) introduced the opportunity to noninvasively track regional myocardial mechanics.[2-4] TDI allows similar assessment by ultrasound.[5,6]

TDI depicts myocardial motion, measured as tissue velocities, at specific location in the heart. Tissue velocity indicates the rate at which a particular point moves toward or away from the transducer. Despite its validity in multiple cardiac pathologies,[7, 8] TDI is an imperfect measure of regional myocardial activity. It interrogates motion at a single point in the myocardium with transducer being the reference point and is influenced by translational motion and tethering. The term "tethering" is used to describe the dragging of akinetic basal segments toward the apex by normally functioning mid or apical segments. Strain and strain rate, however, allow us to measure myocardial deformation relative to the adjacent myocardium.

When considering the different modalities of echocardiography, the distinction between motion and deformation imaging is important. Displacement and velocity are *motion*, while strain and strain rate are *deformation*. A moving object does not undergo deformation so long as every part of the object moves with the same

A.S. Shah (✉)
Cardiology, St Luke's-Roosevelt Hospital Center, New York, NY, USA
e-mail: ashah@chpnet.org

E. Herzog, F.A. Chaudhry (eds.), *Echocardiography in Acute Coronary Syndrome*,
DOI 10.1007/978-1-84882-027-2_7, © Springer-Verlag London Limited 2009

velocity. The object may then be said to have pure translational velocity, but the shape remains unchanged. Over time, the object will change position – displacement. On the other hand, if different parts of the object have different velocities, the object has to change shape. Then, the motion of the different parts can be described by their velocity and displacement, while the whole object can be described as undergoing deformation.[9] This is illustrated below (Fig. 7.1).

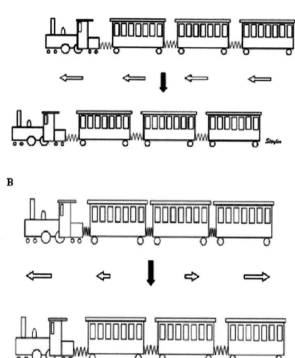

**Fig. 7.1** **(A)** The engine and coaches all run with the same velocity. Over a defined period of time, the train will change position (displacement), but not shape. Thus, the train shows both the velocity and the displacement, i.e., motion, but not deformation.[9] **(B)** The engine and the last coach pull away from each other. This lead to the whole train having different velocities, both in magnitude and direction, as indicated by *arrows*. There are different velocities within the train, and the coaches change position in relation to each other. Thus each part of the train has different motion, and the whole train is stretched, i.e., deformed[9]

Strain is a measure of tissue deformation and is defined as change in length normalized to the original length, also known as myocardial fiber shortening (Fig. 7.2). By this definition, strain is a dimensionless ratio and is often expressed in percent. Positive strain is lengthening or stretching and negative strain is shortening or compression, in relation to the original length.

Strain rate (SR) is the rate by which the deformation occurs, strain per time unit.

$$\dot{\varepsilon} = \Delta\dot{\varepsilon}/\Delta t$$

The unit of strain rate is $s^{-1}$. The strain rate is negative during shortening, positive during elongation. Myocardial thickening during systole is thus an example of a

**Fig. 7.2**  Strain measures tissue deformation and is defined as the change in dimension or length (L1–L0), normalized to the initial length L0 of the region of interest. For example, if the initial length of a myocardial segment is 10 cm, then shortening it by 2–8 cm indicates a strain of –20%. Likewise a lengthening of the segment to 12 cm indicates a strain of +20%. No change in length would suggest 0% strain. The rate at which any of these length (dimension) changes occur is strain rate

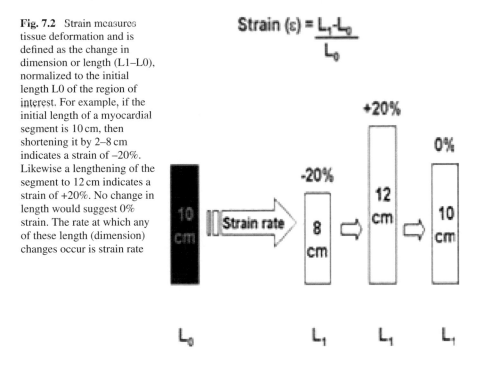

positive strain. Peak systolic strain rate represents the maximal rate of deformation in systole. Tissue Doppler velocities can be used to obtain an estimate of SR.

$$\dot{\varepsilon} = Va - Vb/d$$

Expression Va–Vb represents the difference of instantaneous myocardial velocities Va and Vb at measurement points a and b. Distance (d) specifies how far apart the two velocity points are at a time measurement (Fig. 7.3).[10]

If we assume that the time interval between consecutive frames is infinitesimally short, we can obtain strain by summing (integrating) SR values from a starting point t0 to an ending time point t. Indeed, SR seems to be a correlate of rate of change in pressure over time (dP/dt), a parameter that is used to reflect contractility, whereas strain is an analog of regional ejection fraction. As would be expected with ejection fraction, increasing preload is associated with increasing strain at all levels of wall stress, and increasing afterload is associated with a reduction of strain. Peak systolic strain rate is the parameter that comes closest to measuring local contractile function in clinical cardiology.[11]

The use of strain (deformation) to examine the properties of the heart is not a new concept. Mirsky and Parmley used strain to study the elastic properties of the myocardium.[12] Although myocardial strain is a three-dimensional tensor, it is usually simplified focusing on the three primary directions of strain in the heart. The

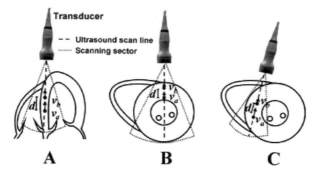

**Fig. 7.3** Schematic drawing demonstrating how strain rate is estimated from the difference in local tissue velocities Va and Vb over a distance (d). (**A**) Analysis of longitudinal shortening and lengthening in the ventricular septum using an apical four-chamber projection. (**B**) Analysis of radial thickening and thinning in the ventricular anterior wall using a short-axis view. (**C**) Analysis of circumferential shortening and lengthening in the ventricular septal wall using a short-axis view[10]

heart shortens and lengthens in the longitudinal direction, it thickens and thins in the radial direction, and it shortens and lengthens in the circumferential direction. A torsion or wringing motion is also present between the base and the apex of the heart (Fig. 7.4).[13] When viewed from the apex, the apex rotates counterclockwise, and the base rotates clockwise in systole (twisting), with the opposite motion (untwisting) in diastole. An example of typical SR and strain curves is provided below (Fig. 7.5).

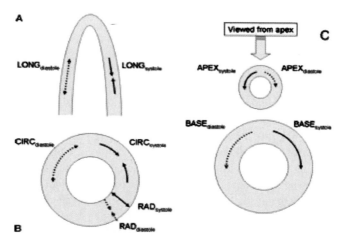

**Fig. 7.4** Graphic representation of the myocardial deformations: longitudinal (**A**), radial and circumferential (**B**), and torsional (**C**). *Solid lines*: direction of deformation in systole. *Dashed lines*: direction of deformation in diastole[13]

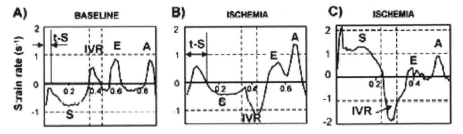

**Fig. 7.5**  Examples of longitudinal strain profiles in normal (**A**) and ischemic (**B** and **C**) myocardium. Reduced (**B**) or inverted (**C**) systolic (**S**) strain rate, delayed onset of systolic shortening (t-S), postsystolic shortening (negative strain rate) during isovolumic relaxation period (IVR), and reversed diastolic E/A strain rate ratio occur in acute ischemia

## Cardiomyopathies

Tissue velocities, strain rates, and strain are reduced in cardiomyopathies and potentially could be used for preclinical detection of several inherited cardiomyopathies. Early diastolic strain rates were significantly lower in asymptomatic, gene-positive patients with Friedrich's ataxia.[14] Abnormal systolic and diastolic tissue velocities are reported in Fabry's disease patients without ventricular hypertrophy.[15] Systolic strain and strain rates improved after enzyme-replacement therapy in Fabry's disease.[16]

Systolic SR during ventricular ejection and rapid ventricular filling was lower in restrictive cardiomyopathy compared with constrictive cardiomyopathy.[17] SR during isovolumic relaxation was positive in restrictive patients and negative in constrictive patients. Early diastolic SR (during rapid ventricular filling) was low in restrictive patients compared with constrictive patients and normal controls.[17]

Similarly, systolic SRs were lower in hypertrophic cardiomyopathy patients compared to athletes, hypertensive patients, or healthy subjects. Early diastolic strain is able to differentiate between hypertrophic cardiomyopathy and physiologic hypertrophy in athletes.[18] It also has been shown that advancing age is associated with a gradual decrease in systolic and early diastolic SR and a corresponding increase in late diastolic SR.[19, 20]

## Coronary Artery Disease

Detection of myocardial ischemia by visual assessment of wall motion is fraught with variability and low reproducibility.[21] Wall motion can be quantified by TDI or strain echocardiography, respectively. Low systolic tissue velocities correlate with angiographic or echocardiographic wall motion abnormalities.[22] Tissue velocities decrease with reduced regional perfusion, recover on reperfusion, and differentiate between trasmural and nontrasmural infarction.[23, 24] The advantage of strain/strain rate, as compared to regular echocardiography, is its ability to detect inducible ischemia at earlier stages than visual estimation of wall motion or wall thickening parameters.

The homogenous distribution of systolic SRs from apical to basal segments is lost during myocardial ischemia and infarction. The typical changes that are seen in strain rate profiles with acute ischemia are reduced or inverted systolic SR, predominant postsystolic SRs ( i.e., postsystolic shortening), delayed onset of systolic shortening, regional asynchrony in the onset of systolic contraction, reflecting early systolic bulging,[25, 26] and reversed diastolic E/A strain rate ratio[27–30] (Fig. 7.5).

Postsystolic shortening or thickening is a sensitive but not a very specific marker of ischemia and can be easily recognized by high, abnormal SR during the isovolumic relaxation period, often extending into the early filling period. Accurate timing of the aortic valve closure is critically important for correct recognition of postsystolic shortening. It has been shown that the extent of the myocardium that exhibits postsystolic shortening approximates the extent of the myocardium at ischemic risk[27–30] (Fig. 7.6).

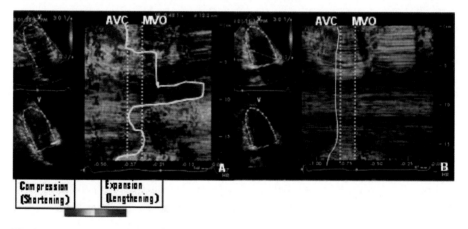

**Fig. 7.6** Example of longitudinal strain rate (SR) maps in apical long-axis view during infarction in the LAD territory (**A**) and postpercutaneous intervention to LAD (**B**). Negative SR (longitudinal shortening) is color-coded in *yellow-orange* and positive SR (longitudinal lengthening) in *cyan-blue*. During infarction, delayed onset, postsystolic shortening, and delayed onset of local lengthening are readily visible. Postpercutaneous intervention the strain rate is homogenously distributed from the apex to the base. The vertical lines indicate time of the aortic valve closure (AVC) and the mitral valve opening (MVO)

## Stress Echocardiography

Although clinically useful in its present form, the main limitation of stress echocardiography interpretation is the subjective visual analysis of endocardial motion and wall thickening and necessity of adequate training. Myocardial velocity may provide a more objective correlate of ischemia, reducing the expertise needed for interpreting stress echocardiography with improved reproducibility.

Changes in strain precede those in wall motion or tissue velocity during dobutamine stress and can differentiate stunned from ischemic myocardium.[31] Strain rate correlates with regional myocardial perfusion during dobutamine stress. Strain rate may be better than strain and both are likely superior to tissue velocity in detecting ischemia via stress echocardiography.[32] Systolic tissue velocities, strain rates, and to some extent strain increase with dobutamine stimulation in the normal subjects.[33, 34] This response is blunted in areas with stress-induced ischemia. Low systolic tissue velocity at maximal stress (<5.5 cm/s) predicts stress-induced ischemic wall motion abnormalities.[35] At rest, stunned, acutely ischemic myocardium and nontransmural infarction are associated with reduction of strain and SR, together with the presence of postsystolic shortening. Transmural infarction is associated with lower strain and SR and less postsystolic shortening than the other entities. Low-dose dobutamine increases the strain and SR and reduces the postsystolic shortening in stunned myocardium, but nontransmural infarcts show only a transient increase in SR, no change of strain, and increasing postsystolic thickening. Acutely ischemic tissue deteriorates and transmural infarction remains unchanged.

Viability assessment of DSE in combination with TDI improved accuracy and showed comparable results to thallium-201 tomography.[36, 37] In PET nonviable segment systolic peak velocities were significantly lower and demonstrated a reduced response during dobutamine stress compared to PET-viable segments.[38]

## Dyssynchrony Assessment

Patients with low ejection fraction, conduction abnormalities (prolonged QRS), and symptomatic heart failure refractory to optimal medical therapy experience significant benefits from cardiac resynchronization therapy (CRT).[39] However, about 30% of patients do not respond to CRT. This has to be attributed to the ill-defined selection criteria, which rely on QRS width as the only marker for dyssynchrony.[40] Mechanical dyssynchrony as determined by TDI may be superior to electrocardiography in predicting response to therapy.

In normal synchronous hearts, segmental systolic tissue velocities peak almost simultaneously (Fig. 7.7A). In dyssynchronous hearts, the lateral and/or posterior segments peak considerably later than the septum (Fig. 7.7B), which results in inefficient ejection. Pacing the delayed region allows synchronized mechanical activity and improves ejection (Fig. 7.7C).

The mechanical delay between the normal (early) and the late segments predicts response to resynchronization.[41] Among several proposed indices of mechanical dyssynchrony, the criteria commonly used in clinical practice are (1) septal to lateral wall delay >65 ms[40] and (2) the standard deviation systolic delay of time to peak systolic velocity of 12 segments >33 ms – Yu index.[42]

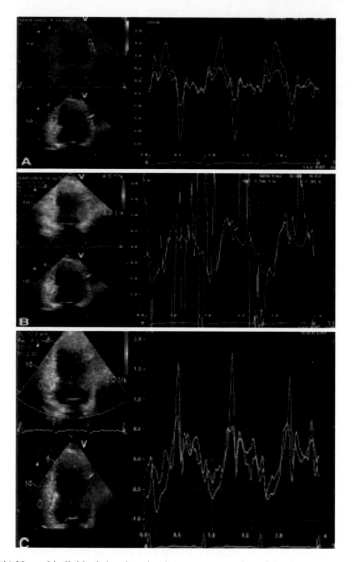

**Fig. 7.7** (**A**) Normal individual showing simultaneous contraction of the anteroseptum (*green* and *turquoise*) and the posterior (*yellow* and *red*) wall. (**B**) Tracing of a patient with heart failure and low ejection fraction prior to biventricular pacing demonstrates an early anteroseptal peak and a delayed lateral wall peak. The septal and lateral wall delay was 106 ms, which suggests significant mechanical dyssynchrony. (**C**) That is reduced to 14 ms after biventricular pacing

## Atrial Function

Atrial function has been examined by strain echo initially in amyloidosis[43] and subsequently in patients with atrial fibrillation, as an adjunct to appropriate selection of people for cardioversion. Atrial compliance is altered by atrial fibrillation before structural remodeling occurs. The degree of the impairment in atrial compliance assessed by strain and strain rate has been shown to be strongly predictive of maintenance of sinus rhythm.[44] The best predictive value for maintenance of sinus rhythm was obtained by peak systolic strain rate.

## Techniques and Limitations of the Strain Rate Imaging (SRI)

The velocity-regression technique has a number of potential pitfalls. First, the comparison of adjacent velocities is very sensitive to signal noise, and the quality of SR curves may vary depending on the curve used in obtaining the underlying velocity data. Optimizing the velocity signal should include avoidance of reverberation artifact (Fig. 7.8A) and ensuring adequate frame rate ($\geq 100$ frames/s). Improvements to the velocity signal by the use of harmonic imaging as well as both temporal and spatial averaging are important in optimizing the SR signal, although this comes at the cost of reducing spatial resolution.

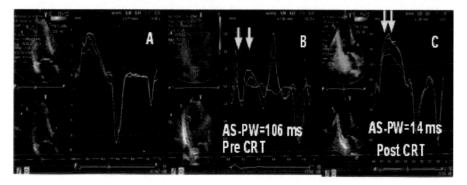

**Fig. 7.8** Pitfalls of tissue Doppler-derived strain rate. (**A**) Reverberation artifact shown in *yellow curve* compromises the strain rate signal, contrasted with an adjacent normal strain rate signal (*blue curve*). (**B**) Blood pool activity, noise strain rate curve (*yellow*) is compared with a smaller sample size, tracked to myocardial movement (*blue*). (**C**) The limited spatial resolution of tissue Doppler, *blue curve* (sample volume outside the cardiac contour), although noisy, is comparable with the *yellow curve* that is appropriately tracked to the wall

The second limitation relates to the limits on spatial resolution that are imposed by imaging at high temporal resolution. If the number of Doppler interrogating beams is limited in an effort to maximize temporal resolution, spatial resolution may be compromised. This may contaminate myocardial velocity signals with adjacent LV blood pool velocities, which are an important source of noise (Fig. 7.8B). In turn, this will compromise the strain rate signal (Fig. 7.8C). Tracking the sample throughout the cardiac cycle is also important to ensure that the sample remains with the myocardium.

Third, like all Doppler techniques, tissue velocity-based strain is sensitive to alignment. The application of this technique to areas where the axis of contraction changes along the scan line means that different vectors may be involved at each site, with consequent error in strain measurements.[45]

Fourth is the through plane motion. It should be remembered that myocardium undergoes wringing torsional motion so that the sample will inevitably move out of the scanning plane in the course of the cardiac cycle. This motion has little effect on systolic measurements, because peak SR occurs early in systole, but it may become important in the measurements of diastolic phenomena. Finally, angle changes during the cardiac cycle and with respiratory movement may contribute to drifting of the strain curve. This can be avoided by careful acquisition.

## Speckle Tracking

The basic principle of speckle tracking is based on the interference of the reflected ultrasound giving rise to an irregular random-speckled pattern. The random distribution of the speckles ensures that each region of the myocardium has a unique pattern. The speckles follow the motion of the myocardium, so when the myocardium moves from one frame to the next, the position of this unique pattern will shift slightly, remaining fairly constant. The speckles can be traced over time and speckle displacement is used to calculate tissue velocity and strain.[46] This method is relatively angle independent, because it is not based on Doppler principle. It is also performed at a much lower frame rates ( 40–90 frames/s) and may not be as accurate in timing mechanical events as Doppler-based imaging ( 100–250 frames/s).

## Velocity Vector Imaging

Velocity vector imaging is a novel quantitative echocardiographic technique that is applied to routine grayscale echocardiographic images. Velocity vector imaging can quantify left ventricular mechanical dyssynchrony and predict response to

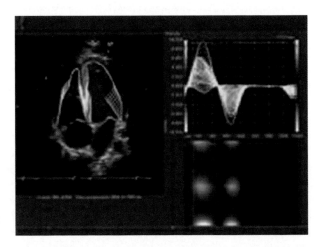

**Fig. 7.9** Depicting a normal velocity vector imaging

resynchronization therapy. Tissue velocities are determined by the automated track-ing of periodic B-mode image patterns on digital cine loops from standard apical four-chamber, two-chamber, and long-axis views, with the user tracing the mid left ventricular wall from a single frame. Dyssynchrony is determined as the greatest opposing wall peak longitudinal systolic velocity delay from the three views. Veloc-ity vector imaging has potential for clinical utility (Fig. 7.9).

## Conclusion

Over its 5-year history, SRI has provided a valuable physiological tool for under-standing myocardial mechanics. Unlike its parent methodology, tissue Doppler imaging, which has found a niche in the assessment of diastolic dysfunction and measurement of LV synchrony, the place of SRI in standard clinical practice remains incompletely defined. The most immediate clinical applications relate to myocar-dial viability and the identification of subclinical LV dysfunction, with the applica-tion of standard stress echocardiography and the quantification of resting function being more remote goals. Barriers to the clinical uptake of this technique include the requirements for significant understanding of complex methodology, techni-cal challenges of the acquisition and analysis, and lack of consensus regarding the superiority of any one among a number of potential measurements for different applications.[47]

## References

1. Yoshida T, Mori Y. Analysis of heart motion with ultrasonic Doppler method and its clinical application. *Am Heart J*. 1961;561:61–75.
2. Axel L, Doughert L. MR imaging of motion with spatial modulation of magnetization. *Radiology*. 1989;171:841–845.
3. Axel L, Gonclaves RC, Bloomgarden D. Regional heart wall motion: two dimensional analy-sis and functional imaging with MR imaging. *Radiology*. 1992;183:745–750.
4. Zerhouni EA, Parish DM, Rogers WJ, Yang A, Shapiro EP. Human heart: tagging with MR imaging – a method for noninvasive assessment of myocardial motion. *Radiology*. 1988;169:59–63.
5. Sutherland GR, Stewart MJ, Groundstroem KW, et al. Color Doppler myocardial imag-ing: a new technique for the assessment of myocardial function. *J Am Soc Echocardiogr*. 1994;7:441–458.
6. Heimdal A, Stoylen A, Torp H, Skjaerpe T. Real time strain rate imaging of the left ventricle by ultrasound. *J Am Soc Echocardiogr*. 1998;11:1013–1019.
7. Fleming AD, McDicken WN, Sutrherland GR, Hoskins PR, Assessment of color Doppler tissue imaging using test phantoms. *Ultrasound Med Biol*. 1994;20:937–951.
8. Miyatake K, Yamagishi M, Tanaka N, Uematsu M, Yamazaki N, Mine Y, Sano A, et al. New method for evaluating left ventricular wall motion by color coded tissue Doppler imaging: in vitro and in vivo studies. *J Am Coll Cardiol*. 1995;25:717–724.
9. Stoylen A. Introduction to strain and strain rate imaging of the heart for the novice researchers and curious clinicians. NTNU Norwegian University of Science and Technology. http://folk.ntnu.no/StoyLEN/StRAiNRATE

10. Pislaru C, Abraham TP, Belohlavek M. Strain and strain rate echocardiography. *Cur Opinion Cardiol*. 2002;17:443–454.

11. Greenberg NL, Firstenberg MS, Castro PL, et al. Doppler-derived myocardial systolic strain rate is a strong index of left ventricular contractility. *Circulation*. 2002;105:99–105.

12. Mirsky I, Parmley WW. Assessment of passive elastic stiffness for isolated heart muscle and the intact heart. *Circ Res*. 1973;33:233–243.

13. Abraham TP, Dimaano VL, Liang HY. Role of tissue Doppler and strain echocardiography in current clinical practice. *Circulation*. 2007;116:2597–2609.

14. Dutka DP, Donnelly JE, Palka P, Lange A, Nunez DJ, Nihoyannopoulos P. Echocardiographic characterization of cardiomyopathy in Friedreich's ataxia with tissue Doppler echocardiographically derived myocardial velocity gradients. *Circulation*. 2000;102:1276–1282.

15. Pieroni M, Chimenti C, Ricci R, Sale P, Russo MA, Frustaci A. Early detection of Fabry cardiomyopathy by tissue Doppler imaging. *Circulation*. 2003;107:1978–1984.

16. Weidemann F, Breunig F, Beer M, et al. Improvement of cardiac function during enzyme replacement therapy in patients with Fabry disease: a prospective strain rate imaging study. *Circulation*. 2003;108:1299–1301.

17. Palka P, Lange A, Donnelly JE. Differentiation between restrictive cardiomyopathy and constrictive pericarditis by early diastolic Doppler myocardial velocity gradient at the posterior wall. *Circulation*. 2000;102:655–662.

18. Lange A, Fleming AD. Differences in myocardial velocity gradient measured throughout the cardiac cycle in patients with hypertrophic cardiomyopathy, athletes and patients with left ventricular hypertrophy due to hypertension. *J Am Coll Cardiol*. 1997;30:760–768.

19. Palka P, Lange A, Fleming AD. Age related transmural peak mean velocities and peak velocity gradients by Doppler myocardial imaging in normal subjects. *Eur Heart J*. 1996;17:940–950.

20. Palka P, Lange A, Nihoyannopoulos P. The effect of long-term training on age related left ventricular changes by Doppler myocardial velocity gradient. *Am J Cardiol*. 1999;84: 1061–1067.

21. Hoffman R, Lethen H, Marwick T, et al. Analysis of interinstitutional observer agreement in interpretation of dobutamine stress echocardiograms. *J Am Coll Cardiol*. 1996;27:330–336.

22. Gorscan J III, Gulati VK, Mandarino WA, Katz WE. Color-coded measures of myocardial velocity throughout the cardiac cycle by tissue Doppler imaging to quantify regional left ventricular function. *Am Heart J*. 1996;131:1203–1213.

23. Derumeaux G, Loufoua J, Pontier G, Cribier A, Ovize M. Tissue Doppler imagiong differentiates transmural form nontransmural acute myocardial infarction after reperfusion therapy. *Circulation*. 2001;103:589–596.

24. Derumeaux G, Ovize M, Lpifoua J, Pontier G, Andre-Fouet X. Cribier A. Assessment of nonuniformity of transmural myocardial velocities by color coded tissue Doppler imaging: characterization of normal, ischemic, and stunned myocardium. *Circulation*. 2000;101: 1390–1395.

25. Jamal F, Kukulski T, Strotman J, et al. Quantification of the spectrum of changes in regional myocardial function during acute ischemia in closed chest pigs: an ultrasonic strain rate and strain study. *J Am Soc Echocardiogr*. 2001;4:874–884.

26. Pislaru C, Belohlavek M, Bae RY, et al. Regional asynchrony during acute myocardial ischemia quantified by ultrasound strain rate imaging. *J Am Coll Cardiol*. 2001;37: 1141–1148.

27. Tennant R, Wiggers CJ. The effect of coronary occlusion on myocardial contraction. *Am J Physiol*. 1935;112:351–361.

28. Doyle RL, Foex P, Ryder WA. Difference in ischemic dysfunction after gradual and abrupt coronary occlusion: effect of isovolumic relaxation. *Cardiovasc Res*. 1987;21:507–514.

29. Jones CJ, Raposo L, Gobson DG. Functional importance of the long axis dynamics of the human left ventricle. *Br Heart J*. 1990;63:215–220.

30. Leone BJ, Norris RM, Safwat A. Effects of progressive myocardial ischemia on systolic function, diastolic function, and load dependent relaxation. *Cardiovasc Res*. 1992;26:422–429.

31. Jamal F, Strotmann J, Weidemann F, et al. Noninvasive quantification of the contractile reserve of stunned myocardium by ultrasonic strain rate and strain. *Circulation*. 2001;104:1059–1065.

32. Weideman F, Jamal F, Kowalski M, et al. Can strain rate and quantify changes in regional systolic function during dobutamine infusion, B-blockade, and atrial pacing? Implications for quantitative stress echocardiography. *J Am Soc Echocardiogr*. 2002;15:416–424.

33. Gorsacn J III, Deswal A, Mankand S, et al. Quantification of the myocardial response to low dose dobutamine using tissue Doppler echocardiographic measures of velocity and velocity gradient. *Am J Cardiol*. 1998;81:615–623.

34. Voigt JU, Exner B, Schmiedehausen K, et al. Strain arte imaging during dobutamine stress echocardiography provides objective evidence of inducible ischemia. *Circulation*. 2003;107:2120–2126.

35. Madler CF, Payne N, Willkenshoff U, et al. Non-invasive diagnosis of coronary artery disease by quantitative stress echocardiography: optimal diagnostic models using off-line tissue Doppler in the MYDISE study. *Eur Heart J*. 2003;24:1584–1594.

36. Hanekom L, Jenkins C, Jeffries L, et al. Incremental value of strain rate analysis as an adjunct to wall motion scoring for assessment of myocardial viability using dobutamine echocardiography. A follow up study after revascularization. *Circulation*. 2005;112:3892–3900.

37. Le Feuvre C, Baubion N, Aubry N, Metzger JP, Vacheron A. Assessment of reversible dyssynergic segments after acute myocardial infarction: dobutamine echocardiography versus thallium-201 single photon emission computed tomography. *Am Heart J*. 1996;131(4): 668–675.

38. Hoffmann R, Altiok E, Nowak B, et al. Strain rate measurements by Doppler echocardiography allows improved assessment in myocardial viability in patients with depressed LV function. *J Am Coll Cardiol*. 2002;39:443–449.

39. Abraham WT, Fisher WG, Smith AL, et al. MIRACLE Study Group, Multicenter InSync Randomized Clinical Evaluation. Cardiac resynchronization in chronic heart failure. *N Engl J Med*. 2002;346:1845–1853.

40. Bax JJ, Bleecker GB, Marwick TH, et al. Left ventricular dyssynchrony predicts response and prognosis after cardiac resynchronization therapy. *J Am Coll Cardiol*. 2004;44:1834–1840.

41. Bax JJ, Abraham T, Barold SS, et al. Cardiac resynchronization therapy: part 2: issues during and after device implantation and unresolved questions. *J Am Coll Cardiol*. 2005;46: 2168–2182.

42. Yu CM, Fung WH, Lin H, Zhang Q, Sanderson JE, Lau CP. Predictors of left ventricular reverse remodeling after cardiac resynchronization therapy for heart failure secondary to idiopathic dilated or ischemic cardiomyopathy. *Am J Cardiol*. 2003;91:684–688.

43. Modesto KM, Disoenzieri A, Cauduro SA, et al. Left atrial myopathy in cardiac amyloidosis: implications of novel echocardiographic technique. *Eur Heart J*. 2005;26:173–179.

44. Di Salvo G, Caso P, Lo Piccolo R, et al. Atrial myocardial deformation properties predict maintenance of sinus rhythm after external cardioversion of recent-onset lonc atrial fibrillation: a color Doppler myocardial imaging and thransthoracic and transesophageal echocardiographic study. *Circulation*. 2005;112:387–395.

45. Urheim S, Edvardson T, Torp H, Angelsen B, Smiseth OA. Myocardial strain by Doppler echocardiography. Validation of a new method to quantify regional myocardial function. *Circulation*. 2000;102:1158–1164.

46. Leitman M, Lysyansky P, Sidenko S, et al. Two dimensional strains: a novel software for real time quantitative echocardiographic assessment of myocardial function. *J Am Soc Echocardiogr*. 2004;17:1021–1029.

47. Marwick TH. Measurement of strain and strain rate by echocardiography. *J Am Coll Cardiol*. 2006;47(7):1313–1327.

# Chapter 8
# 3D Echo in Acute Coronary Syndrome

**Kohei Fujimoto and Shunichi Homma**

The echocardiogram (echo) is a very important tool in assessing patients with coronary artery disease. Recently developed 3D echo has advantages over conventional 2D echo.

The evaluation of patients with chest pain is an important step in making diagnoses and clinical decisions. Although coronary angiography is the gold standard for the diagnosis of coronary artery disease, this is an invasive method. There are various noninvasive modalities to assess coronary artery disease. However, exercise electrocardiography has low reliability,[1] and myocardial scintigraphy is costly and has low reliability in certain cases such as those involving left main or multivessel coronary artery disease.[2] Thus, a simpler and more useful noninvasive modality seems to be ideal for these patients.

Exercise or pharmacological stress echo is used for the assessment of ischemic heart disease.[3] However, conventional 2D stress echo suffers from limited sensitivity and specificity and high interobserver variability, in part because of the limitations of 2D echo.[4] 3D echo would be especially useful in assessing ischemic heart disease since an accurate assessment of wall motion abnormality and asymmetric shape of the left ventricle (LV) is needed. The latest 3D echo systems are being to provide suitable images for clinical use.

Before the invention of real-time 3D echo, 3D echo took 10 min to acquire data and required significant offline data processing. The first real-time 3D echo (Volumetrics, Durham, North Carolina) used a sparse-array matrix transducer (2.5 or 3.5 MHz). Transducer consisted of 256 elements to generate a $60° \times 60°$ pyramidal volume within a single heartbeat. It shortened data acquisition time. As a result, 3D echo can be used for stress echo,[5,6] measuring accurate LV volume, mass or ejection fraction[7,8,9] in several clinical studies. However, the limitations of this device were suboptimal image quality and low frame rate. Recently, 3D echo has been developed in order to improve the image quality. Current 3D echo has been increasingly used for many clinical and research practice.

---

K. Fujimoto (✉)

Cardiology, Columbia University Medical Center, New York, NY, USA

e-mail: koheifujimoto@aol.com

E. Herzog, F.A. Chaudhry (eds.), *Echocardiography in Acute Coronary Syndrome*,     103
DOI 10.1007/978-1-84882-027-2_8, © Springer-Verlag London Limited 2009

## How to Record and Show 3D Images for Detecting Wall Motion Abnormality

There are several ways to record and show 3D images for the assessment of ischemia, as described below.

### *Real-Time Mode*

3D transducers and computer technology have improved so that real-time 3D (Philips Medical Systems, Andover, Massachusetts) images can now be generated. Both 3D transducer and computer technology have advanced to create matrix transducers with 3000 elements that can acquire a pyramidal image containing most cardiac structures.

Using real-time mode, it is possible to see an online 3D display of rendered images (Fig. 8.1). In this mode, not only can we change the 3D images by moving the probe, but we can also see the cross-sectional images of interest by moving the trackball on the machine using software. Though the image is too narrow to show the entire LV at once in this mode, we can use this mode for screening by moving the trackball.

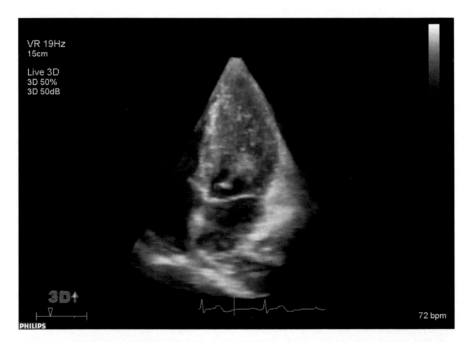

**Fig. 8.1** **Real-time mode**. The 3D echo image is displayed in real time by simply pushing the 3D switch using the matrix transducer

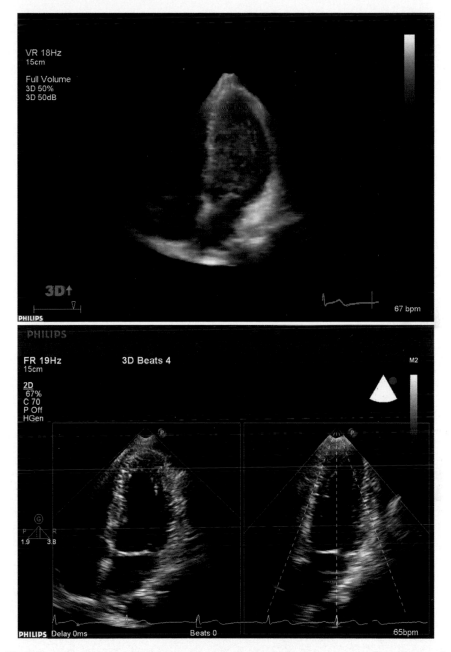

**Fig. 8.2   Full volume mode**. (**A**) The entire left ventricle is displayed by using full volume mode and collecting four pulse images. (**B**) The full volume image is collected using 2D images of the apical four-chamber and two-chamber view as references

## Full Volume Mode

Though it is difficult to show the entire LV in real-time mode, it is possible to show the entire LV by using full volume mode (Philips Medical Systems, Andover, Massachusetts) and collecting four pulse images (Fig. 8.2).

This mode provides an easy process for acquiring 3D data of the entire heart nearly in real-time. In addition, 2D images of the two-chamber view, four-chamber view, long-axis view, and short-axis view can be displayed by cutting the acquired full volume image. Thus far, this mode appears to be for assessing of wall motion abnormality. This mode allows us to measure LV ejection fraction, LV volume, and LV mass using all LV volume data. Moreover, we can record the wall motion of the entire LV at each stage of the dobutamine stress test.

## islice Mode

The islice mode (Philips Medical Systems, Andover, Massachusetts) is used to show multilevels of the short-axis image from the apex to the base of the heart (Fig. 8.3). After recording LV full volume data, it is possible to show multiple images of the

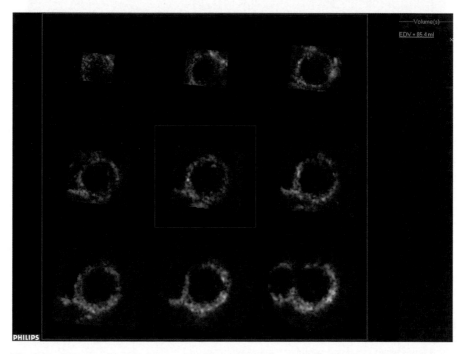

**Fig. 8.3    islice mode**. Full volume data recorded in full volume mode using an apical approach can be displayed as many short-axis slices. From the apex to the base, nine slices of the short-axis image are displayed

LV at the same time. It helps us quickly find the best views for diagnoses. This is useful in assessing the wall motion of the entire LV.

## Tri Plane Mode

GE (GE Vingmed Ultrasound, Horten, Norway) has also made it possible to show the images in a multiplanar mode with relatively high temporal resolution. Because of the recent improvements in matrix array transducer technology, imaging time is shortened without significantly compromising the quality of the images. This is due to the acquisition of multiple planes from one acoustic window instead of the entire LV volume. In addition, the transducer allows one to view the three planes simultaneously without any other adjustments once the image angles are set.

Tri plane imaging is a 3D technique that integrates data from three conventional 2D apical views. We can see 2D images of the apical four-chamber, two-chamber, and long-axis views simultaneously and in real time (Fig. 8.4). Unlike full volume mode, it is not necessary to hold one's breath during several pulses in tri plane mode.

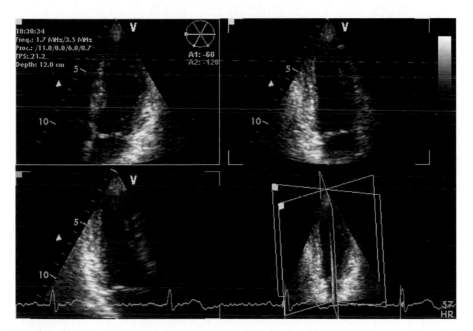

**Fig. 8.4   Tri plane mode**. The tri plane mode with apical approach shows 2D images of the apical four-chamber view (*upper left*), the two-chamber view (*upper right*), and the long-axis view (*lower left*) at the same time

## Assessing Left Ventricular Volume and Left Ventricular Ejection Fraction

Needless to say, measuring LV volume and LV ejection fraction is important. It is difficult to accurately assess the exact LV volume using the 2D modified Simpson's method in patients with ischemic heart disease. This is because such patients have wall motion abnormalities or aneurysms that make it difficult to show the true apex and negate the assumption used for LV volume in the 2D method.[10] However, all the LV data obtained using 3D can allow us to accurately calculate LV volume by searching for the real apex and showing the longest axis (Fig. 8.5). In the literature, it has been shown several times that 3D echo makes it possible to assess the exact LV volume both clinically and experimentally.[11,12,13] When calculating LV volume, it is necessary to trace the surface of the LV intima in several images. Recently developed software may prove useful to trace LV intima semiautomatically[14] (Fig. 8.5).

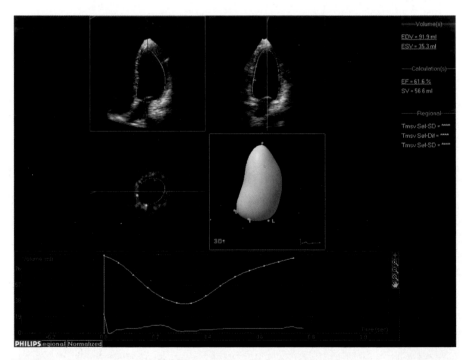

**Fig. 8.5    The recent software which calculates left ventricle volume**. By pointing out the apex and the mitral annulus in two views of one cycle, the endocardial border of the left ventricle can be traced automatically. End-diastolic volume, end-systolic volume, and ejection fraction are displayed in the *upper right corner*. The change in volume during a cycle is displayed in a graph at the *bottom*

## Observation of Wall Motion Abnormalities Using 3D Echocardiography

It is very important to assess the area of wall motion abnormality and LV function in order to evaluate the severity of the disease and prognosis.

Using 2D echo, the area and severity of wall motion abnormality and LV systolic function are assessed subjectively by an experienced physician. Experience is needed to reconstruct several images. However, using 3D echo, it may be easy to understand and assess the structure of the heart, as well as the area and severity of wall motion abnormality. 3D echo is especially appropriate for assessing wall motion in cases involving LV aneurysms.[7,15] Using the software, the image recorded in full volume mode can be colorized by wall motion for each LV segment[16] (Fig. 8.6). Showing the colorized graph may make it easy to assess wall motion more objectively.

## 3D Echocardiography for Ischemic Mitral Regurgitation

There are many reports about the utility of 3D echo for ischemic mitral regurgitation (MR). Previously, transesophageal 3D echo was used for evaluation of the mitral valve.[17,18] A sequence of 2D echos could be recorded, aligned, and reconstructed into a 3D data set. This methodology was limited by the need for off-line data processing to create and display the 3D images. However, transthoracic 3D echo is able to assess the mitral valve in real time.[19] The "surgeon's view" is one of the most currently used views in which to observe the mitral valve using 3D echo. This view can show us an image of the location and range of disease.

3D echo has played an important role in analyzing the mechanism of ischemic MR.[20–26] Using 3D echo, it has been shown that mitral valve leaflet tethering is an important factor for ischemic MR.[27,28] 3D echo can evaluate tethering and quantify tethering volume.[29–31] It is useful for the determination or evaluation of therapy for ischemic MR.[32,33]

We can evaluate the MR jet itself using 3D echo. Using 2D echo, we may underestimate the severity of MR with eccentric jet, but 3D echo can provide the exact origin and flow of MR. Though the PISA method of 2D echo used for the quantification of MR requires hemisphere acceleration flow, it has been reported that 3D echo assesses the real orifice area or volume of MR.[34,35]

There are two limitations of 3D echo with color Doppler. One limitation is that a patient is required to hold his or her breath for at least seven beats in order to get good images. Because this method requires ECG gating, the color data set is compiled by merging narrower pyramidal scans obtained over consecutive heartbeats. The other limitation is that we can only obtain a narrow-angle image. These technical issues need to be resolved.

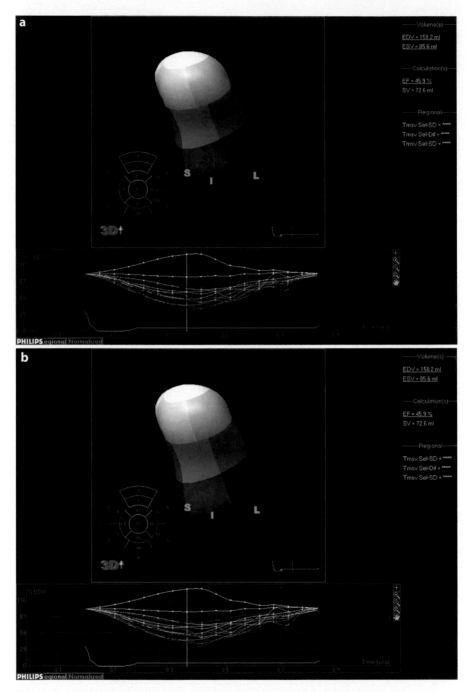

**Fig. 8.6** **The evaluation of focal wall motion abnormality using software**. This view was obtained from a patient with an old myocardial infarction. On the graph, the ratio of volume change is decreased in the white area, meaning that the wall motion is decreased in this area. In addition, end-systolic volume is bigger than end-diastolic volume in the *pale yellow* area, meaning that the wall motion is this area shows dyskinesis. (**A**) End systole; (**B**) End diastole

We have just begun to use the new real-time 3D transesophageal echo probe (Philips Medical Systems, Andover, Massachusetts), which is able to provide detailed real-time images.[36] It will offer useful information about ischemic MR.

## 3D Echocardiography for Complications of Myocardial Infarction

In the course of caring for patients with myocardial infarction (MI), we need to pay attention to complications. Several reports show that 3D echo is useful for evaluating complications of MI. It is very important to assess MR after MI because ischemic MR is an independent prognostic factor in patients with MI, and as previously mentioned, 3D echo is useful for assessing MR. LV aneurysm is another important complication of MI. We can evaluate wall motion abnormalities and volume of aneurysms precisely with 3D echo. Cardiac rupture resulting from aneurysm is one of the most dramatic complications after acute MI and is responsible for some in-hospital deaths.

3D echo might be used to help diagnose free wall rupture or pericardial effusion after MI. One study showed that preoperative real-time 3D color Doppler studies assisted surgical planning by clearly demonstrating the site and circular geometry of the myocardial rupture.[37] Ventricular septal perforation after MI can also be evaluated using 3D echo. Some studies illustrate the clinical usefulness of real-time 3D echo in defining the exact location of a post-MI ventricular septal defect.[38,39,40] Thrombus is also a well-known complication after MI. One report illustrates that 3D echo is beneficial for demonstrating the exact point of attachment of the thrombus to the LV wall and for providing more accurate assessment of thrombus mobility, which has prognostic indications.[41]

## Stress Test for Ischemic Heart Disease using 3D Echocardiography

In exercise or pharmacological stress echo, the advantage of 3D echo is rapid and simultaneous acquisition of images of all wall segments. Quick recording of the images at baseline and at peak stress is needed to precisely assess wall motion abnormalities. In order to assess LV wall motion, at least four different 2D images (parasternal long axis, parasternal short axis, apical two-chamber, and apical four-chamber views) are needed. It is technically difficult to record several images precisely and quickly using 2D echo. 3D echo can easily show 2D images of the apical four-chamber, two-chamber, and long-axis views at the same time using tri plane mode. It has been reported that the recording time is reduced when performing stress echo in multiplane mode.[4–6,42,43]

Using full volume mode, 3D echo can record the wall motion of the entire LV. Therefore, we can easily and accurately detect segmental wall motion abnormalities caused by stress and it might be possible to detect ischemia of a small area. This mode makes the recording time shorter than 2D echo recording time in pharmacological stress tests but maintains the accuracy of diagnosis found using 2D echo.[44,45]

However, this method still has some limitations. One limitation of this mode is that it is difficult to use the four images to reconstruct the 3D image if there are different time durations between four cycles of images because of arrhythmia. In addition, it is preferable for a patient to hold his or her breath while the images during four cycles are being taken. However, during exercise stress echo it is difficult to hold one's breath just after exercise. In such a case, the tri plane mode would be more useful because it is not necessary to hold one's breath.[43]

## Contrast Agent for 3D Echocardiography

### Contrast Echo for LV Opacification of 3D Images

Contrast agent is used with 3D echo in order to improve image quality.[46] Moreover, the usefulness of contrast agent during 3D stress echo was previously reported.[47,48] The use of contrast agent improves endocardial border visualization, leading to a more accurate interpretation of wall motion abnormalities.

### 3D Myocardial Contrast Echocardiography

One study showed that 3D echo with contrast agent can detect and quantify myocardial perfusion.[49] In the future, it may be used as a tool to detect myocardial ischemia.

## References

1. Gianrossi R, Detrano R, Mulvihill D, et al. Exercise-induced ST depression in the diagnosis of coronary artery disease. A meta-analysis. *Circulation*. 1989;80(1):87–98.
2. Christian TF, Miller TD, Bailey KR, Gibbons RJ. Noninvasive identification of severe coronary artery disease using exercise tomographic thallium-201 imaging. *Am J Cardiol*. 1992;70(1):14–20.
3. Marwick TH, Nemec JJ, Pashkow FJ, Stewart WJ, Salcedo EE. Accuracy and limitations of exercise echocardiography in a routine clinical setting. *J Am Coll Cardiol*. 1992;19(1):74–81.
4. Ahmad M, Xie T, McCulloch M, Abreo G, Runge M. Real-time three-dimensional dobutamine stress echocardiography in assessment stress echocardiography in assessment of ischemia: comparison with two-dimensional dobutamine stress echocardiography. *J Am Coll Cardiol*. 2001;37(5):1303–1309.
5. Takuma S, Cardinale C, Homma S. Real-time three-dimensional stress echocardiography: a review of current applications. *Echocardiography*. 2000;17(8):791–794.
6. Zwas DR, Takuma S, Mullis-Jansson S, et al. Feasibility of real-time 3-dimensional treadmill stress echocardiography. *J Am Soc Echocardiogr*. 1999;12(5):285–289.
7. Takuma S, Ota T, Muro T, et al. Assessment of left ventricular function by real-time 3-dimensional echocardiography compared with conventional noninvasive methods. *J Am Soc Echocardiogr*. 2001; 14(4):275–284.

8. Ota T, Kisslo J, von Ramm OT, Yoshikawa J. Real-time, volumetric echocardiography: use fulness of volumetric scanning for the assessment of cardiac volume and function. *J Cardiol.* 2001;37 Suppl 1:93–101.

9. Takuma S, Cabreriza SE, Sciacca R, Di Tullio MR, Spotnitz HM, Homma S. Determination of left ventricular mass by real-time three-dimensional echocardiography: in vitro validation. *Echocardiography.* 2000;17(7):665–674.

10. Lang RM, Bierig M, Devereux RB, et al. Recommendations for chamber quantification: a report from the American Society of Echocardiography's Guidelines and Standards Committee and the Chamber Quantification Writing Group, developed in conjunction with the European Association of Echocardiography, a branch of the European Society of Cardiology. *J Am Soc Echocardiogr.* 2005;18(12):1440–1463.

11. Kuhl HP, Schreckenberg M, Rulands D, et al. High-resolution transthoracic real-time three-dimensional echocardiography: quantitation of cardiac volumes and function using semiautomatic border detection and comparison with cardiac magnetic resonance imaging. *J Am Coll Cardiol.* 2004;43(11):2083–2090.

12. Arai K, Hozumi T, Matsumura Y, et al. Accuracy of measurement of left ventricular volume and ejection fraction by new real-time three-dimensional echocardiography in patients with wall motion abnormalities secondary to myocardial infarction. *Am J Cardiol.* 2004;94(5): 552–558.

13. Jenkins C, Bricknell K, Hanekom L, Marwick TH. Reproducibility and accuracy of echocardiographic measurements of left ventricular parameters using real-time three-dimensional echocardiography. *J Am Coll Cardiol.* 2004;44(4):878–886.

14. Jacobs LD, Salgo IS, Goonewardena S, et al. Rapid online quantification of left ventricular volume from real-time three-dimensional echocardiographic data. *Eur Heart J.* 2006;27(4):460–468.

15. Collins M, Hsieh A, Ohazama CJ, et al. Assessment of regional wall motion abnormalities with real-time 3-dimensional echocardiography. *J Am Soc Echocardiogr.* 1999;12(1): 7–14.

16. Corsi C, Lang RM, Veronesi F, et al. Volumetric quantification of global and regional left ventricular function from real-time three-dimensional echocardiographic images. *Circulation.* 2005;112(8):1161–1170.

17. Hozumi T, Yoshikawa J, Yoshida K, Akasaka T, Takagi T, Yamamuro A. Assessment of flail mitral leaflets by dynamic three-dimensional echocardiographic imaging. *Am J Cardiol.* 1997;79(2):223–225.

18. Ahmed S, Nanda NC, Miller AP, et al. Usefulness of transesophageal three-dimensional echocardiography in the identification of individual segment/scallop prolapse of the mitral valve. *Echocardiography.* 2003;20(2):203–209.

19. Sugeng L, Coon P, Weinert L, et al. Use of real-time 3-dimensional transthoracic echocardiography in the evaluation of mitral valve disease. *J Am Soc Echocardiogr.* 2006;19(4): 413–421.

20. De SR, Wolf I, Hoda R, et al. Three-dimensional assessment of left ventricular geometry and annular dilatation provides new mechanistic insights into the surgical correction of ischemic mitral regurgitation. *Thorac Cardiovasc Surg.* 2006;54(7):452–458.

21. Watanabe N, Ogasawara Y, Yamaura Y, et al. Geometric differences of the mitral valve tenting between anterior and inferior myocardial infarction with significant ischemic mitral regurgitation: quantitation by novel software system with transthoracic real-time three-dimensional echocardiography. *J Am Soc Echocardiogr.* 2006;19(1):71–75.

22. Watanabe N, Ogasawara Y, Yamaura Y, et al. Mitral annulus flattens in ischemic mitral regurgitation: geometric differences between inferior and anterior myocardial infarction: a real-time 3-dimensional echocardiographic study. *Circulation.* 2005;112(9 Suppl):I458–I462.

23. Watanabe N, Ogasawara Y, Yamaura Y, Kawamoto T, Akasaka T, Yoshida K. Geometric deformity of the mitral annulus in patients with ischemic mitral regurgitation: a real-time three-dimensional echocardiographic study. *J Heart Valve Dis.* 2005;14(4):447–452.

24. Otsuji Y, Handschumacher MD, Liel-Cohen N, et al. Mechanism of ischemic mitral regurgitation with segmental left ventricular dysfunction: three-dimensional echocardiographic studies in models of acute and chronic progressive regurgitation. *J Am Coll Cardiol*. 2001;37(2): 641–648.
25. Song JM, Kim MJ, Kim YJ, et al. Three-dimensional characteristics of functional mitral regurgitation in patients with severe left ventricular dysfunction: a real-time 3-dimensional color Doppler echocardiography study. *Heart*. 2008;94:590–596.
26. Levine RA, Hung J, Otsuji Y et al. Mechanistic insights into functional mitral regurgitation. *Curr Cardiol Rep*. 2002;4(2):125–129.
27. Otsuji Y, Handschumacher MD, Schwammenthal E, et al. Insights from three-dimensional echocardiography into the mechanism of functional mitral regurgitation: direct in vivo demonstration of altered leaflet tethering geometry. *Circulation*. 1997;96(6):1999–2008.
28. Song JM, Qin JX, Kongsaerepong V, et al. Determinants of ischemic mitral regurgitation in patients with chronic anterior wall myocardial infarction: a real time three-dimensional echocardiography study. *Echocardiography*. 2006;23(8):650–657.
29. Ryan L, Jackson B, Parish L, et al. Quantification and localization of mitral valve tenting in ischemic mitral regurgitation using real-time three-dimensional echocardiography. *Eur J Cardiothorac Surg*. 2007;31(5):839–844.
30. Song JM, Fukuda S, Kihara T, et al. Value of mitral valve tenting volume determined by real-time three-dimensional echocardiography in patients with functional mitral regurgitation. *Am J Cardiol*. 2006;98(8):1088–1093.
31. Watanabe N, Ogasawara Y, Yamaura Y, et al. Quantitation of mitral valve tenting in ischemic mitral regurgitation by transthoracic real-time three-dimensional echocardiography. *J Am Coll Cardiol*. 2005;45(5):763–769.
32. Sai-Sudhakar CB, Vandse R, Armen TA, Bickle KM, Nathan NS. Efficacy of chordal cutting in alleviating ischemic mitral regurgitation: insights from 3-dimensional echocardiography. *J Cardiothorac Surg*. 2007;2:39.
33. Yamaura Y, Watanabe N, Ogasawara Y, et al. Geometric change of mitral valve leaflets and annulus after reconstructive surgery for ischemic mitral regurgitation: real-time 3-dimensional echocardiographic study. *J Thorac Cardiovasc Surg*. 2005;130(5):1459–1461.
34. Iwakura K, Ito H, Kawano S, et al. Comparison of orifice area by transthoracic three-dimensional Doppler echocardiography versus proximal isovelocity surface area (PISA) method for assessment of mitral regurgitation. *Am J Cardiol*. 2006;97(11):1630–1637.
35. Sitges M, Jones M, Shiota T, et al. Real-time three-dimensional color Doppler evaluation of the flow convergence zone for quantification of mitral regurgitation: validation experimental animal study and initial clinical experience. *J Am Soc Echocardiogr*. 2003;16(1):38–45.
36. Pothineni KR, Inamdar V, Miller AP, et al. Initial experience with live/real time three-dimensional transesophageal echocardiography. *Echocardiography*. 2007;24(10):1099–1104.
37. Little SH, Ramasubbu K, Zoghbi WA. Real-time 3-dimensional echocardiography demonstrates size and extent of acute left ventricular free wall rupture. *J Am Soc Echocardiogr*. 2007;20(5):538–543.
38. Brandt RR, Elsaesser A, Hamm CW. Real-time three-dimensional echocardiographic diagnosis of postmyocardial infarction ventricular septal defect and guidance of transcatheter closure. *Heart*. 2007;93(5):551.
39. Gabriel H, Binder T, Globits S, Zangeneh M, Rothy W, Glogar D. Three-dimensional echocardiography in the diagnosis of postinfarction ventricular septal defect. *Am Heart J*. 1995;129(5):1038–1040.
40. Vengala S, Nanda NC, Mehmood F, et al. Live three-dimensional transthoracic echocardiographic delineation of ventricular septal rupture following myocardial infarction. *Echocardiography*. 2004;21(8):745–747.
41. Duncan K, Nanda NC, Foster WA, Mehmood F, Patel V, Singh A. Incremental value of live/real time three-dimensional transthoracic echocardiography in the assessment of left ventricular thrombi. *Echocardiography*. 2006;23(1):68–72.

42. Sugeng L, Kirkpatrick J, Lang RM, et al. Biplane stress echocardiography using a prototype matrix-array transducer. *J Am Soc Echocardiogr*. 2003;16(9):937–941.

43. Eroglu E, D'hooge J, Herbots L, et al. Comparison of real-time tri-plane and conventional 2D dobutamine stress echocardiography for the assessment of coronary artery disease. *Eur Heart J*. 2006;27(14):1719–1724.

44. Matsumura Y, Hozumi T, Arai K, et al. Non-invasive assessment of myocardial ischaemia using new real-time three-dimensional dobutamine stress echocardiography: comparison with conventional two-dimensional methods. *Eur Heart J*. 2005;26(16):1625–1632.

45. Aggeli C, Giannopoulos G, Misovoulos P, et al. Real-time three-dimensional dobutamine stress echocardiography for coronary artery disease diagnosis: validation with coronary angiography. *Heart*. 2007;93(6):672–675.

46. Malm S, Frigstad S, Sagberg E, Steen PA, Skjarpe T. Real-time simultaneous triplane contrast echocardiography gives rapid, accurate, and reproducible assessment of left ventricular volumes and ejection fraction: a comparison with magnetic resonance imaging. *J Am Soc Echocardiogr*. 2006;19(12):1494–1501.

47. Nemes A, Geleijnse ML, Krenning BJ, et al. Usefulness of ultrasound contrast agent to improve image quality during real-time three-dimensional stress echocardiography. *Am J Cardiol*. 2007; 99(2):275–278.

48. Pulerwitz T, Hirata K, Abe Y, et al. Feasibility of using a real-time 3-dimensional technique for contrast dobutamine stress echocardiography. *J Am Soc Echocardiogr*. 2006;19(5): 540–545.

49. Toledo E, Lang RM, Collins KA, et al. Imaging and quantification of myocardial perfusion using real-time three-dimensional echocardiography. *J Am Coll Cardiol*. 2006;47(1):146–154.

# Chapter 9
# Contrast Echocardiography in Acute Coronary Syndromes

Brian Nolan and Kevin Wei

## Introduction

The term "acute coronary syndrome (ACS)" encompasses a wide array of diagnoses from unstable angina to ST segment elevation myocardial infarction. Apart from its diversity, an ACS is a diagnosis that can be challenging to make because many other disease processes present with chest pain and confirmatory serology may take many hours to become positive.

Approximately 5–10 million chest pain (CP) patients present annually to an Emergency Department (ED) in the United States, of which only 10–30% will be eventually diagnosed with an ACS.[1-3] Looking for the "needle in the haystack" is both time-consuming and expensive. Current clinical methods which utilize the history, physical exam, and electrocardiogram (ECG) have poor sensitivity and specificity for identifying ischemia. The ECG is initially normal in 20% of patients who have acute myocardial infarction (AMI)[4] and remains normal in 5% of patients with this diagnosis.[4,5] Serum cardiac biomarkers are the gold standard for detecting AMI and have excellent utility in risk stratifying patients with CP.[6] Troponin I and T, however, have poor sensitivity for detecting AMI at initial presentation (23–66%) because they may take up to 6 h to become positive after the onset of ischemia. In unstable angina without myocellular necrosis, cardiac biomarkers may never become clinically detectable.[4] Awaiting the results of cardiac serum markers often delays the initiation of important medical therapies such as anticoagulation, platelet inhibition, or early invasive evaluation.

On the other hand, 2–8% of patients presenting with CP are discharged from the ED with an unrecognized ACS, with an estimated 30-day mortality of 10%.[7,8]

In patients presenting with unstable angina or a non-ST elevation myocardial infarction and a normal or nondiagnostic ECG for ischemia, an early diagnosis of ACS could significantly impact the institution of treatment. Furthermore, it may identify patients with noncardiac CP, leading to alternative diagnoses or earlier

K. Wei (✉)
Department of Internal Medicine/Cardiology, Oregon Health & Science University, Portland, OR, USA
e-mail: welk@ohsu.edu

E. Herzog, F.A. Chaudhry (eds.), *Echocardiography in Acute Coronary Syndrome*,
DOI 10.1007/978-1-84882-027-2_9, © Springer-Verlag London Limited 2009

discharge. Thus, much attention has been focused on the use of ancillary nonin-vasive imaging for the identification of myocardial ischemia.

Myocardial contrast echocardiography (MCE), which uses microbubble-based contrast agents as a tracer, has been an evolving tool since the 1960s. Apart from its ability to enhance the assessment of regional wall motion by opacifying the left ventricular (LV) cavity, it can provide a noninvasive evaluation of myocardial per-fusion. MCE is also the only portable imaging method available today. This chapter will illustrate many of the benefits that MCE can provide in a wide array of patients ranging from those with undifferentiated CP to those with a diagnosed AMI under-going reperfusion therapy.

## MCE Methodology

Microbubbles as perfusion agents have evolved over the last 10 years and have had significant impact on MCE. The use of air-filled microbubbles in MCE was initially limited by the rapid diffusion of air (mainly $N_2$ and $O_2$) down their concentration gradients into blood, resulting in a loss of microbubble size and backscatter signal. Because the scattering cross section of a microbubble is related to the sixth power of its radius, even small changes in radius would have a huge impact on the scattering cross section of a microbubble.[9] In recent years, these limitations have been over-come with the incorporation of high molecular weight gases with low diffusibility and solubility into the microbubble. The current second-generation agents available in the United States (Optison and Definity) contain perfluoropropane gas.

The microbubbles have a mean size of $<5 \mu m$ and possess unique properties for tracers currently used in imaging. They stay entirely in the intravascular space and do not alter hemodynamics. The microvascular behavior of microbubbles is also nearly identical to red blood cells,[10,11] making the microbubbles an ideal tool for the assessment of the spatial distribution of perfusion and for the quantification of myocardial blood flow (MBF).

Backscatter signals from microbubbles are processed into pixels of brightness, or acoustic intensity, in ultrasound. As shown in Fig. 9.1, the relationship between microbubble concentration and acoustic intensity is linear, which is important for the quantification of flow.[12] At high microbubble concentrations, the relation plateaus, and at even higher concentrations, there is a paradoxic decrease in acoustic intensity caused by attenuation of ultrasound by the microbubbles themselves.[12] Thus, assess-ments of MBF using MCE must be performed at concentrations of microbubbles that do not saturate the system, which can be achieved by maintaining myocardial enhancement visually lower than that of the LV.

The current method for the assessment of regional myocardial perfusion using MCE is the same as that for the quantification of MBF.[13] The actual imaging modalities, however, are beyond the scope of this chapter. During a constant infu-sion of microbubbles, their concentration reaches a steady state in the circulation, so microbubble washout and their subsequent replenishment in any myocardial

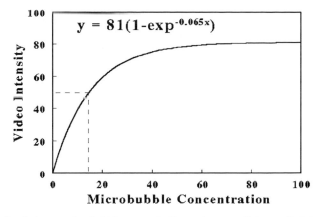

**Fig. 9.1** Relation between microbubble concentration and myocardial acoustic intensity. Redrawn from Skyba et al.[12]

microcirculatory unit are equal and dependent on MBF. The microbubbles can be destroyed by a high acoustic power pulse of ultrasound and the rate of replenishment of microbubbles represents MBF velocity.[13] When all the microvessels have been replenished with microbubbles, myocardial acoustic intensity represents capillary or myocardial blood volume (MBV).[13] These two terms can be used synonymously, as the vast majority of blood within the myocardium (~ 90% in systole) is contained in approximately 8 million capillaries.[14]

As discussed below, MBF velocity can be used to gain insight into the adequacy of antegrade perfusion in the setting of an ACS. For example, the presence of a critically stenosed or occluded epicardial coronary artery would be associated with reduced or absent MBF velocity in its perfusion bed.[15] Similarly, the assessment of MBV provides insight into capillary integrity – a sine qua non of the presence of residual myocardial viability.[16]

## Acute Chest Pain and MCE

Current tools used to evaluate patients presenting with acute CP are imperfect. As noted above, while up to 10 million patients visit the ED with chest pain, an ACS is confirmed in only 10–30%. Even though the majority of patients will be admitted to the hospital or observation units, an estimated 2–7% will be discharged and have subsequent acute coronary events. The appropriate diagnosis of ACS has implications not only to patient care but also to health-care resources and utilization of limited monetary funds. The sensitivity and specificity of our traditional tools have well-delineated limitations. The ECG has been demonstrated to be diagnostic in just 30–40% of patients with active myocardial ischemia.[17] In addition the biomarkers with greatest sensitivity are time delayed until hours after the onset of ACS.[18] Thus, a noninvasive method that can directly detect myocardial ischemia would be invaluable. Ischemia is defined as "a decrease in blood flow that results in tissue hypoxia." Thus, such a tool would need to detect either reduced perfusion to myocytes or the consequences of this abnormal perfusion. Ideally, such a tool would also have to be rapid, noninvasive, highly accurate, safe, and portable. MCE fits many of these criteria and has been shown to be of benefit in a wide array of scenarios.

## MCE in Patients with Suspected Cardiac Chest Pain

In patients with suggested ischemic CP, causes may include non-ST elevation myocardial infarction (NSTEMI), unstable angina, or transient ischemia. In patients with NSTEMI, subendocardial or patchy microvascular and myocellular necrosis results in both regional function abnormalities and abnormal myocardial perfusion which can be detected using MCE. In the event of only transient ischemia, myocardial perfusion defects may resolve, but abnormal regional function may still be present as a result of myocardial stunning. This abnormal regional function will be present despite the spontaneous restoration of antegrade flow.[19]

To understand the ability of MCE to detect acute myocardial ischemia, it is necessary to have a working knowledge of the relationship between resting MBF and regional wall thickening. Because of autoregulation, resting MBF remains normal even in the presence of up to 85% luminal diameter narrowing. When arteriolar vasodilatory reserve is exhausted, however, MBF will become dependent on perfusion pressure and will decrease below resting levels as stenosis severity progresses toward total occlusion. Because myocardial contractility is a major determinant of myocardial oxygen consumption, reduction in resting MBF is immediately followed by the development of a wall thickening abnormality[20] (Fig. 9.2). This relationship allows the evaluation of wall thickening as a measure of myocardial ischemia.

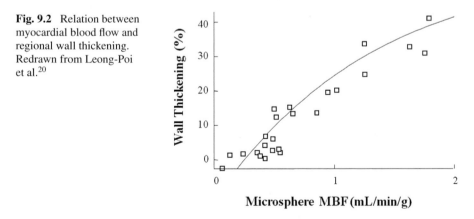

**Fig. 9.2** Relation between myocardial blood flow and regional wall thickening. Redrawn from Leong-Poi et al.[20]

The detection of ischemia using MCE can be identified within seconds of the initial event and may be present for hours thereafter. The presence of abnormal regional

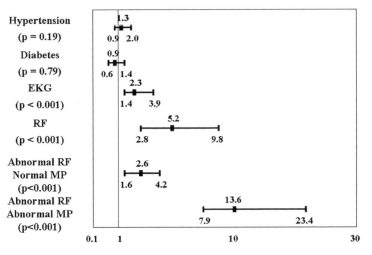

**Fig. 9.3** Multivariate logistic regression analysis of multiple variables for the prediction of early (48 h) cardiovascular events in patients presenting with suspected cardiac CP to the ED and no ST segment elevation on ECG. Different variables are shown with the corresponding odds ratio and confidence intervals

function with MCE has been shown in a large single center study to improve the detection of cardiac ischemia over traditional evaluation with ECG and biomarkers. As shown in Fig. 9.3, patients with abnormal myocardial function and myocardial perfusion were at a 14-fold higher risk of myocardial infarction, cardiac-related death, unstable angina, congestive heart failure, and revascularization within 48 h of presentation to the ED.[21] Normal regional function of MCE also has excellent negative predictive value. The incidence of nonfatal myocardial infarction or cardiovascular mortality within 24 h of evaluation was only 0.4% in these patients,[22] while patients discharged from EDs using routine evaluation have been shown to have an incidence of myocardial infarction of 2.3%.[23]

The early identification of ACS has a direct impact on patient care which may include earlier institution of definitive therapy, while alternative pathologic processes can be considered in patients who do not have cardiac chest pain, including more rapid patient disposition. By preventing unnecessary downstream resource utilization, there is also a significant impact on health-care dollars. The estimated cost of evaluating patients presenting with chest pain is in excess of 10 billion dollars annually.[24] Most of this cost is derived from the low threshold for admission of chest pain patients to "rule out" acute myocardial infarction. Because the incidence of infarction is exceedingly low in patients with a normal MCE, such patients could be discharged directly from the ED or could proceed immediately to stress testing prior to discharge. Despite the added cost of performing MCE on all patients with suspected cardiac chest pain, preventing unnecessary admissions has been shown to be a cost-efficient strategy.[25]

The following cases serve to demonstrate the positive and negative predictive value of MCE in patients presenting with chest pain to the ED.

## Case Study 1

A 60-year old man without prior cardiac history woke up at 5 AM with 5/10 dull retrosternal chest pain (CP), radiating to the left arm associated with diaphoresis. He denied associated symptoms such as dyspnea or nausea. The chest pain was not pleuritic, and the patient had no fever, cough, sputum production, or hemoptysis. He initially thought that the discomfort was reflux and took some antacids without relief. After 2 h, the patient presented to the ED with ongoing symptoms.

The patient had a history of hypercholesterolemia and was on atorvastatin 20 mg po daily. He was taking no other medications. He had no history of diabetes, tobacco abuse, or hypertension. There was no other significant past medical history.

On physical exam, the patient was in mild discomfort. He appeared his stated age. There was no cyanosis, pallor, clubbing, or jaundice. Heart rate was 70 bpm, blood pressure 110/60 when supine, respiratory rate was 16 per min. Oxygen saturation was 97% on room air. Respiratory exam was within normal limits. There was no reproducible discomfort to chest wall palpation. Jugular venous pulse was 1 cm above sternal angle with normal waveforms. The carotid upstroke and volume were normal without bruits. Apex beat was not palpable. On auscultation, S1 and S2 were normal, no S3 or S4 were heard in the ED. All pulses were 2+, with no subclavian, abdominal, or femoral bruits. There was no ankle edema. Neurologic exam was grossly normal. Stool guaiac exam was negative for occult blood.

The patient's electrocardiogram is shown in Fig. 9.4. A portable chest x-ray showed no mediastinal enlargement. Initial labs showed sodium of 138, potassium 3.7, chloride 105, CO2 23, BUN 16, creatinine 1.1. Glucose was 135, Ca 9, Mg 1.8, PO4 2.9, Hg 15, Hct 44, WBC 6.3, PLT 218. A lipid panel was drawn but was not available. PT 14, INR 1.1, PTT 32. The initial cardiac troponin I was <0.05 (negative).

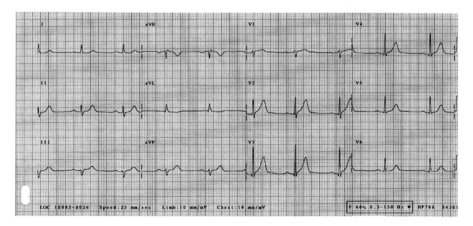

**Fig. 9.4** Presenting ECG for patient in Case 1. See text for details

The patient was given sublingual nitroglycerine three times with mild improvement in his pain, as well as intravenous morphine with some further improvement, but his symptoms did not completely resolve. A repeat 12-lead ECG showed no changes.

At this time, there is suspicion that the patient has ischemic cardiac CP, but no ECG or serologic evidence of AMI. Should he be treated empirically with antithrombotics or glycoprotein IIb–IIIa inhibitors at this time or should one wait for further serology? Should the patient be kept in the ED, or should he be admitted to the ward, step-down unit, or coronary care unit? Should he proceed directly to cardiac catheterization?

As shown in the discussion above, a MCE is indicated to help make a diagnosis of cardiac chest pain and to risk stratify the patient. The patient's echo showed that the mid to distal septum, anterior wall, and apex were akinetic (Fig. 9.5). In a patient with no prior history of MI, a new wall thickening abnormality confirms that his CP is related to cardiac ischemia. Perfusion imaging was also performed to evaluate the extent of residual viability in the anterior territory since the patient's presentation to the ED was delayed. This demonstrated a slow rate of replenishment

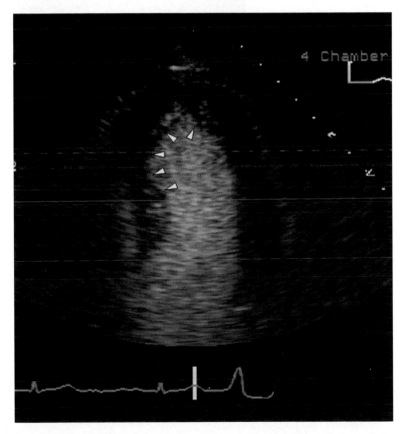

**Fig. 9.5**  Apical four-chamber view for patient in Case 1 using Definity for left ventricular opacification. The mid to distal septum and apex (*arrowheads*) was akinetic. See text for details

**Fig. 9.6** Myocardial
perfusion study for patient in
Case 1 demonstrating
extensive contrast
enhancement within the
akinetic area defined in
Fig. 9.5. See text for details

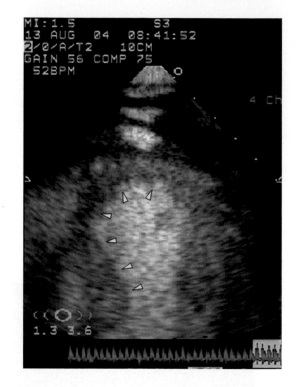

of microbubbles into the anterior territory (denoting either very slow antegrade flow
in the left anterior descending (LAD) artery due to a critical stenosis or a completely
occluded LAD with slow collateral flow). There was, however, nearly complete contrast enhancement of the entire akinetic territory, except for a small subendocardial
rim at a long pulsing interval of eight cardiac cycles – denoting extensive microvascular integrity and viability despite prolonged ischemia (Fig. 9.6). The patient was
therefore taken immediately to cardiac catheterization without need for further confirmatory serology, which revealed a critical mid-LAD stenosis that was successfully stented (Fig. 9.7). The patient was discharged in stable condition after 2 days.
This case illustrates the ability of MCE to rapidly diagnose and risk stratify patients
with cardiac CP.

## Case Study 2

A 41–year-old premenopausal female with a strong family history of CAD presents
to the ED with complaints of new-onset exertional CP over the last few days.
Episodes are located in the retrosternal area, with no radiation. Prior to the onset
of these symptoms, the patient was under a great deal of stress because her father
was very ill. The episodes appear to be increasing in frequency and severity and are
associated with dyspnea, but no nausea or diaphoresis. She works as a nurse in an

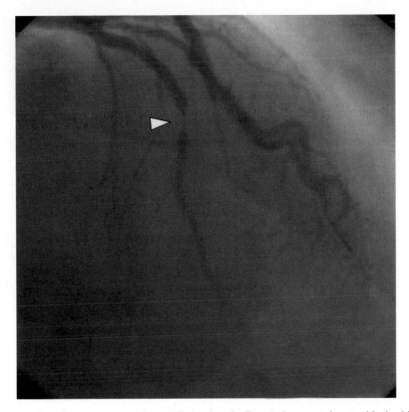

**Fig. 9.7** Selective coronary angiogram for patient in Case 1 demonstrating a critical mid left anterior descending artery stenosis. See text for details

ambulatory cardiology clinic and is very concerned about these symptoms. She is having ongoing CP in the ED. She has no other risk factors for coronary disease. She is on no medications. She reports no allergies. Her physical exam was normal. A 12-lead ECG was within normal limits. All labs (including a cardiac troponin I) have been drawn, and results are pending.

This patient has new-onset crescendo exertional chest pain and a strong family history for CAD. It is possible that she has unstable angina or is suffering an NSTEMI. However, the patient is clinically at low risk for cardiac ischemia because she is young, female, premenopausal, and has no cardiac risk factors. In this setting, a normal MCE would help to eliminate cardiac ischemia as a cause of her ongoing symptoms. An MCE was performed, which showed entirely normal LV systolic function and perfusion (Fig. 9.8).

Since an AMI was excluded by echo, the patient did not require a complete serological "rule out" in the ED. She was referred for an exercise stress sestamibi scan to assess for underlying occult CAD. The patient exercised to 12.9 mets, achieved peak HR of 188 beats per minute (105% maximal age-predicted heart rate), and SBP

**Fig. 9.8** Myocardial perfusion study for patient in Case 2 with the transmit focus placed at the level of the apex to prevent apical destruction artifact. There is some basal and mid lateral wall attenuation. Further imaging with the focus at the level of the mitral annulus demonstrated normal lateral wall contrast enhancement as well. See text for details

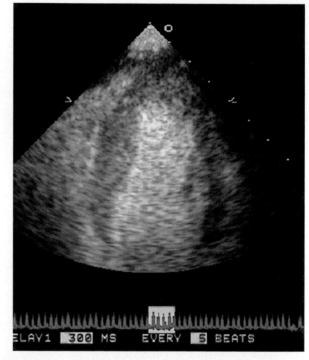

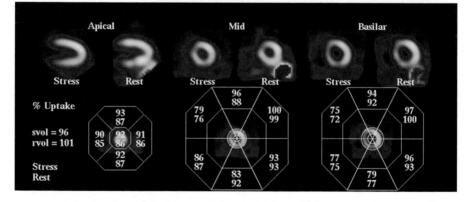

**Fig. 9.9** Rest and exercise stress [99m]Tc-sestamibi single photon emission computed tomograms from the patient in Case 2. See text for details

of 190. She had no CP during stress. Both the stress ECG and stress sestamibi scans were normal (Fig. 9.9).

Thus, this case illustrates the advantage of a normal MCE, which has a negative predictive value of ≥99% even in patients who present up to 12 h after their last episode of CP to the ED.[19]

## MCE in Patients with Established Cardiac Chest Pain

When a patient presents with ischemic chest pain and diagnostic changes on the ECG (ST segment elevation, new left bundle branch block, dynamic ST depression, or deep T-wave inversions), an MCE is not required for diagnosis and there are well-established guidelines for the management of patients with STEMI, NSTEMI, or unstable angina.

Nonetheless, MCE can be used to provide important adjunctive information that may be helpful for patient management or risk stratification. These include the ability of MCE to evaluate the effects of therapy – for example, to determine the success of thrombolysis; and MCE can be used to assess infarct size – or more importantly determine the extent of residual myocardial viability.

Patency in the infarct-related artery is not achieved in up to 30% of patients following thombolytic therapy. Establishing success or failure of reperfusion therapy is imprecise with clinical predictors such as relief of chest pain or resolution of ECG changes.[26] MCE has been used to evaluate the area at risk for myocardial necrosis before intervention and subsequently to evaluate success of reperfusion therapy early after coronary stenting. Patients with good myocardial contrast enhancement following intervention at 3–5 days led to eventual recovery of wall motion.[27] Of even greater importance is that MCE provides an assessment of reperfusion at a microvascular level. In up to 25% of patients with TIMI 3 flow in the epicardial coronary artery after primary angioplasty, there is significant "no-reflow" or "low-reflow" on MCE.[28] These patients had poor functional recovery of left ventricular function and greater infarct expansion, remodeling, and left ventricular dilation. They also have a greater incidence of heart failure, nonfatal myocardial infarction, and also higher mortality compared to patients with preserved microvascular perfusion during 1-year follow-up.[29]

Experimental studies in dogs have shown that the time course of cell death begins approximately 30–40 min after acute coronary occlusion and occurs initially in the subendocardium where ischemia is most severe.[30] Infarct size is determined by the size of the risk area (the territory "at risk" of necrosis in the absence of reperfusion), the duration of ischemia, and the amount of collateral blood flow.[31] As discussed above, MCE can establish infarct size after reperfusion by determining the spatial extent of the no-reflow zone. However, it may be clinically more useful to be able to predict eventual infarct size prior to reperfusion – e.g., if it can be established that a patient is going to have a very small infarct, management could potentially be more conservative. MCE can be used to predict infarct size, even prior to reperfusion, by assessing the adequacy of collateral blood flow within the risk area.[32] Myocytes can remain viable in the presence of MBF >20% of normal resting levels, which is also the amount of flow required to allow contrast enhancement on MCE. Territories with lesser degrees of flow are destined to necrose in the absence of reperfusion. The method is based on providing enough time for microbubble replenishment into the risk area after their destruction, so that slow collateral-derived flow can be imaged. Figure 9.10 shows short-axis images obtained in the presence of an occlusion of the left anterior descending coronary artery, during a continuous intravenous infusion of microbubbles. At the shortest pulsing interval, a clear demarcation is noted between the inferoposterior wall, which has normal myocardial perfusion, and the occluded anterior bed, which shows no contrast enhancement (9 o'clock to 1 o'clock, Panel A, Fig. 9.10). The hypoperfused zone at this PI represents the risk area. At a longer PI, border zones of the anterior myocardium supplied by collateral flow have started to replenish with microbubbles (panel B, Fig. 9.10). At a PI of 10 s, the entire risk area had become homogeneously opacified from collateral-derived MBF except for a small subendocardial rim. The spatial distribution of perfusion within the risk area identifies tissue that may be spared from necrosis despite persistent coronary occlusion. Thus, despite a prolonged 6-h occlusion in the animal shown in Fig. 9.10, only a small subendocardial infarct developed, as shown on the triphenyl-tetrazolium chloride-stained image (panel C, Fig. 9.10).[32]

**A.**                              **B.**                              **C.**

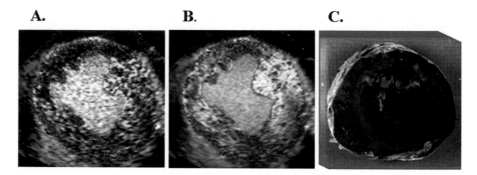

**Fig. 9.10**  MCE images at various pulsing intervals and ultimate infarct size by tissue staining in a dog undergoing 6 h of left anterior descending coronary artery occlusion. Although the risk area is large at a short pulsing interval of 2 s (**panel A**), infarct size on postmortem tissue staining occurred only in the subendocardium (**panel C**) because of collateral-derived MBF (**panel B**)

The extent of viability following intervention and stent placement can be predictive of the likelihood of recovery of resting systolic function and contractile reserve.[33,34] Residual myocardial viability has been shown to be an independent predictor of long-term cardiac events following myocardial infarction. During a 4-year follow-up period, following thrombolysis, the presence of myocardial viability on MCE predicted 99% survival versus 67% in patients without viability.[35] Thus, MCE is evolving as a powerful independent predictor of further cardiac events following ACS.

Early after reperfusion, there may be a sustained period of reactive hyperemia in the infarct bed. The use of MCE in this setting may result in underestimation of infarct size and overestimation of the degree of myocardial salvage.[36] Thus, the best timing for the evaluation of the extent of viability is approximately 3–5 days after reperfusion for prognostic information.

# Limitations of MCE

Limitations of MCE may include poor image quality in patients with suboptimal windows, which results in an inability to evaluate comprehensively for wall thickening abnormalities. In addition, the positive predictive value of MCE is lower than its negative predictive value because of the inability of MCE to differentiate acute from chronic wall motion abnormalities.[19] Logistical challenges also need to be addressed in order for MCE to be utilized effectively in acute CP patients. For example, many centers do not have staff available to perform and evaluate these studies at all hours. Finally, assessment of regional function and myocardial perfusion relies on subjective interpretation, which has known limitations.

Future investigation may overcome some of these described limitations. For example, utilization of specific targeted microbubbles may solve the dilemma between acute and chronic wall motion abnormality. Targeted microbubbles will enable the identification of inflammation and thus identify acute ischemia-perfusion injury.[37]

# Summary

MCE is a valuable and evolving noninvasive method for the evaluation of patients with chest pain and ACS. Appropriate utilization of this unique imaging tool allows expeditious evaluations of patients presenting with CP of unclear etiology. This will facilitate both an accurate diagnostic approach and a timely and cost-saving strategy in emergency centers. The high negative predictive value of MCE makes this an attractive imaging technique.

In addition to diagnostic information MCE can also add valuable prognostic information, including viability and functional recovery of LV function. The utilization of this modality requires an understanding of MBF and coronary physiology, as well as the infrastructure and personnel to acquire and interpret the appropriate imaging. MCE should be used in appropriate clinical scenarios and should not delay definitive treatment for patients presenting with STEMI or when traditional evaluation is consistent with NSTEMI.

# References

1. Strussman BJ. National Hospital Ambulatory Medicine Care Survey: 1995 emergency department summary. Advance data from vital and health statistics of the center for Disease Control Prevention National Center for Health Statistics. 1997;285:1–18.
2. Gibler WB, Lewis LM, Erb RE, et al. Early detection of acute myocardial infarction in patients presenting with chest pain and non-diagnostic ECGs: serial CK-MB sampling in the emergency department. *Ann of Emerg Med.* 1990;9:1359–1366.
3. Gibler WB, Young CP, Hedges JR, et al. Acute myocardial infarction in chest pain patients with non-diagnostic ECGs: serial CK-MB sampling in the emergency department. The emergency medicine cardiac research group. *Ann Emerg Med.* 1992;21:504–512.

4. Pope JH, Selker HP. Acute coronary syndromes in the emergency department: diagnostic characteristics, tests, and challenges. *Cardiol Clin*. 2005;23:423–426.
5. Haro LH, Decker WW, Boie ET, Wright RS. Initial approach to the patient who has chest pain. *Cardiol Clin*. 2006;24:1–17.
6. Hutter AM, Jr., Amsterdam EA, Jaffe AS. 31st Bethesda Conference. Emergency Cardiac Care. Task force 2: acute coronary syndromes: section 2B–chest discomfort evaluation in the hospital. *J Am Coll Cardiol*. 2000;35:853–862.
7. Pope JH, Selker HP. Diagnosis of acute cardiac ischemia. *Emer Med Clin Nor Amer*. 2003;21(1):27–59.
8. Lee TH, Rouan GW, Weisberg MC, et al. Clinical characteristics and natural history of patients with acute myocardial infarction sent home from the emergency room. *Am J Cardio.l* 1987;60:219–224.
9. DeJong N, Hoff L, Skotland T, Bom N. Absorption and scatter of encapsulated gas filled microspheres: theoretical considerations and some measurements. *Ultrasonics*. 1992;30: 95–103.
10. Keller MW, Glasheen W, Smucker ML, Burwell LR, Watson DD, Kaul S, Myocardial contrast echocardiography in humans. II. Assessment of coronary blood flow reserve. *J Am Coll Cardiol*. 1998;12(4):925–934.
11. Jayaweera AR, Edwards N, Glasheen WP, Villanueva FS, Abbott RD, Kaul S. In vivo myocardial kinetics of air-filled albumin microbubbles during myocardial contrast echocardiography. Comparison with radiolabeled red blood cells. *Circ Res*. 1994;74(6):1157–1165.
12. Skyba DM, Jayaweera AR, Goodman NC, Ismail S, Camarano G, Kaul S. Quantification of myocardial perfusion with myocardial contrast echocardiography during left atrial injection of contrast. Implications for venous injection. *Circulation*. 1994;90(3):1513–1521.
13. Wei K, Jayaweera AR, Firoozan S, Linka A, Skyba DM, Kaul S. Quantification of myocardial blood flow with ultrasound-induced destruction of microbubbles administered as a constant venous infusion. *Circulation*. 1998;97(5):473–483.
14. Wei K, Kaul S. The coronary microcirculation in health and disease. *Card Clin*. 2004;22(2):221–231.
15. Wei K, Ragosta M, Thorpe J, Coggins M, Moos S, Kaul S. Noninvasive quantification of coronary blood flow reserve in humans using myocardial contrast echocardiography. *Circulation*. 2001;103(21):2560–2565.
16. Wei K. Assessment of myocardial viability using myocardial contrast echocardiography. *Echocardiography*. 2005;22:85–94.
17. Short D. The earliest electrocardiographic evidence of myocardial infarction. *Br Heart J*. 1970;32:6–15.
18. Goldman BU, Hamm CW. Risk stratification in acute coronary syndrome. *Herz* 2001; 26(Suppl.1):24–29.
19. Kalvaitis S, Kaul S, Tong K, Rinkevich D, Belcik T, Wei K. Effect of time delay on the diagnostic use of contrast echocardiography in patients presenting to the emergency department with chest pain and no S-T segment elevation. *J Am Soc Echocardiogr*. 2006;19:1488–1493.
20. Leong-Poi H, Coggins MP, Sklenar J, Wei K, Lindner JR, Kaul S. Perfusion versus function: the ischemic cascade in demand ischemia: implications of single-vessel versus multivessel stenosis. *Circulation*. 2002;105(8):987–992.
21. Rinkevich D, Kaul S, Lepper W, et al. Regional left ventricular perfusion and function in patients presenting to the emergency department with chest pain and no ST segment elevation. *Eur Heart J*. 2005;26:1606–1611.
22. Tong LT, Kaul S, Wang X, et al. Myocardial contrast echocardiography versus thrombolysis in myocardial infarction score in patients presenting to the emergency department with chest pain and nondiagnostic electrocardiogram. *J Am Coll Cardiol*. 2005;46:920–927.
23. Pope JH, Aufderheide TP, Ruthazer R, et al. Missed diagnoses of acute cardiac ischemia in the emergency department. *N Engl J Med*. 2000;342:1163–1170.
24. Hutter AM Jr., Weaver WD. 31st Bethesda Conference. Emergency Cardiac Care. Task force 2: acute coronary syndromes: section 2A–prehospital issues. *J Am Coll Cardiol*. 2000;35(4):846–853.

25. Wyrick JW, Kalvaitis S, McConnell J, Belcik T, Horton K, Wei K. A Cost-Efficiency analysis for myocardial contrast echocardiography in chest pain patients in the emergency department. *J Am Soc Echocardiogr*. 2007;20:565 (abstract).

26. Califf RM, O'Neill W, Stacks RS, et al. Failure of simple clinical measurements to predict perfusion status after intravenous thrombolysis. *Ann Intern Med*. 1988;108:658–662.

27. Kaul S, Senior R, Firshke C, et al. Incremental value of cardiac imaging in patients presenting to the emergency department with chest pain and without ST-segment elevation: a multicenter study. *Am Heart J*. 2004;148:129–136.

28. Ito H, Okamura A, Iwakura K, et al. Myocardial perfusion patterns related to thrombolysis in myocardial infarction perfusion grades after coronary angioplasty in patients with acute anterior wall myocardial infarction. *Circulation*. 1996;93(11):1993–1999.

29. Ito H, Maruyama A, Iwakura K, et al. Clinical implications of the 'no reflow' phenomenon. A predictor of complications and left ventricular remodeling in reperfused anterior wall myocardial infarction. *Circulation*. 1996;93:223–228.

30. Reimer KA, Jennings RB. The "wavefront phenomenon" of myocardial ischemic cell death. Transmural progression of necrosis within the framework of ischemic bed size (myocardium at risk) and collateral flow. *Lab Invest*. 1979;40:633–644.

31. Schaper W, Frenzel H, Hort W. Experimental coronary artery occlusion, I: measurement of infarct size. *Basic Res Cardiol*. 1979;74:46–53.

32. Coggins MP, Sklenar J, Le DE, Wei K, Lindner JR, Kaul S. Noninvasive prediction of ultimate infarct size at the time of acute coronary occlusion based on the extent and magnitude of collateral-derived myocardial blood flow. *Circulation*. 2001;104(20):2471–2477.

33. Balcells E, Powers ER, Lepper W, et al. Detection of myocardial viability by contrast echocardiography in acute infarction predicts recovery of resting function and contractile reserve. *J Am Coll Cardiol*. 2003;41:827–833.

34. Janardhanan R, Swinburn JM, Greaves K, Senior R. Usefulness of myocardial contrast echocardiography using low-power continuous imaging early after acute myocardial infarction to predict late left ventricular recovery. *Am J Cardiol*. 2003;92:493–497.

35. Dwivedi G, Janardhanan R, Hayat S, Swinburn J, Senior R. Prognostic value of myocardial viability detected by myocardial contrast echocardiography early after myocardial infarction. *J Am Coll Cardiol*. 2007;50:327–334.

36. Villanueva FS, Glasheen WP, Sklenar J, Kaul S. Characterization of spatial patterns of flow within the reperfused myocardium by myocardial contrast echocardiography. Implications in determining extent of myocardial salvage. *Circulation*. 1993;88(6):2596–2606.

37. Christiansen JP, Leong Poi H, Xu F, Klibanov AL, Kaul S, Lindner JR. Non invasive imaging of myocardial reperfusion injury using leukocyte-targeted contrast echocardiography. *Circulation*. 2002;105:1764–1767.

# Chapter 10
# Cardiac Risk Prevention Strategies

Melana Yuzefpolsky, Olivier Frankenberger, and Eyal Herzog

Cardiovascular disease (CVD), which includes coronary heart disease (CHD), stroke, and peripheral vascular disease, is the leading cause of death and disability in most Western industrialized countries including the United States, dispersing across all ethnic, racial, and gender groups. Worldwide, it is estimated that death from CHD will increase 100% in men and 80% in women from 1990 to 2020, with majority of that increase coming from Asia, Africa, and Latin America.[1] Similarly, disability-adjusted life-years lost will increase 107% in men and 74% in women worldwide.[1]

Early recognition of the cardiovascular disease and aggressive treatment is of paramount importance. The ability of Doppler echocardiography to provide unique noninvasive information with minimal discomfort or risk coupled with its portability, immediate availability, and repeatability provides a unique diagnostic tool in prognostication of virtually all categories of cardiovascular disease. However, two-dimensional Doppler echocardiography is best used after a careful history, physical examination, electrocardiography, and risk assessment is performed.

The overall objectives of cardiovascular prevention are to reduce mortality and morbidity in those at high absolute risk and to assist those at low absolute risk to maintain this state, through a healthy lifestyle. Historical medical recordings as early as 2500 BC referred to the practice of Prevention. References to the importance of prevention are found in writings of Hippocrates and Osler, thus rendering the prevention concept important and certainly not new in practice of medicine.[2] However, it is not until 1961 when Kannel and colleagues in the Framingham Heart study gave modern medicine the term *risk factors* and their association with coronary heart disease. The major and independent risk factors for CHD are *cigarette smoking of any amount, elevated blood pressure, elevated serum total cholesterol and low-density lipoprotein cholesterol (LDL-C), low serum high-density lipoprotein cholesterol (HDL-C), diabetes mellitus, and advancing age.* Framingham heart study developed a quantitative relationship between these risk factors and CHD. The

O. Frankenberger (✉)
Cardiology, St. Luke's-Roosevelt Hospital, New York, NY, USA
e-mail: Ofranken@chpnet.org

E. Herzog, F.A. Chaudhry (eds.), *Echocardiography in Acute Coronary Syndrome*,
DOI 10.1007/978-1-84882-027-2_10, © Springer-Verlag London Limited 2009

total risk of a person can be estimated by a summing of the risks imparted by each of the major risk factors. Framingham score estimates the 10-year risk of cardiovascular events for persons without clinical manifestations of CHD. This risk score was modified by the National Cholesterol education program Expert Panel on Detection, Evaluation, and Treatment of High Blood Cholesterol in Adults (Adult Treatment Panel III or ATP III) for use in their recommendations for screening and treatment of dyslipidemia. The modifications include elimination of diabetes from the algorithm, broadening of the age range, inclusion of hypertension treatment, and age-specific points for smoking and total cholesterol.

The 10-year risk is defined as low <10% CHD risk, intermediate 10–20%, and high risk is >20%. Once CHD or its equivalents are established, Framingham scoring no longer applies. CHD equivalents include *symptomatic carotid artery disease, peripheral arterial disease, abdominal aortic aneurysm, and diabetes mellitus*. Other models have been developed in an attempt to provide better predictive accuracy for European patients. The largest of these is that developed by the SCORE project.[3]

The advantages of using the risk charts are the following:

- Intuitive and easy to use
- Takes account of multifactorial nature of CVD
- Estimates risk of all atherosclerotic CVD, not just CHD
- Allows flexibility in management – if an ideal risk factor level cannot be achieved, total risk can still be reduced by reducing other risk factors.
- Establishes a common language of risk for clinicians.

## Smoking

The overwhelming wealth of literature indicates that cigarette smoking increases the incidence of and mortality from CVD. Smoking accounts for more than 400,000 deaths annually in the United States and 1.6 million worldwide.[4] Despite the relative stability (25%) in prevalence of current smokers, rates of tobacco use are increasing among adolescents, young adults, and women.[5] Even among nonsmokers, we now recognize that inhaled smoke, whether from passive exposure or from cigar and pipe consumption, also increases coronary risk.

Smoking remains one of the most preventable risk factors in cardiology. In a recent review, smoking cessation reduced mortality from heart disease by 36% as compared with mortality in subjects who continued to smoke, an effect that did not vary by age, gender, or country of origin.[6] The importance of physician counseling for smoking cessation cannot be underestimated.

## *Methods of Cessation*

Both behavioral and pharmacologic approaches should be utilized to enhance smoking cessation. A simple behavioral approach (also referred to as 5As) for use in physician offices has been developed by National Cancer Institute and is also endorsed by British Thoracic Society.

A-ASK systematically. Identify all smokers at every opportunity.

A-ASSESS. Determine the person's degree of addiction and his/her readiness to stop smoking.

A-ADVISE. Urge all smokers to quit.

A-ASSIST. Create a smoking cessation plan including behavioral counseling, nicotine replacement therapy, and/or pharmacological intervention.

A-ARRANGE. A schedule of follow-up visits.

Patients can benefit from both clinician counseling and group setting. Hospitalized patients who smoke, especially those admitted with acute myocardial infarction, stand to benefit from this type of intervention. Smoking cessation counseling over the telephone or via a letter is also an effective means of communication.

Group counseling programs are offered widely. These typically include lectures, group interactions, exercises on self-recognition of one's habit, some form of tapering method leading to a "quit day," development of coping skills, and suggestions for relapse prevention.

Nicotine has been used as replacement therapy to help quitters go through the initial stages of smoking cessation. It is now available for administration in several ways: as a gum (nicotine polacrilex), via a transdermal patch, by nasal spray, or by inhaler. No nicotine delivery system is demonstrable superior to another, and all appear similarly effective.

Antidepressant medications have been used in aiding long-term smoking cessation, Bupropion being the most widely studied. A sustained-release formulation of the drug (Zyban) is licensed to be used in smoking cessation. The dose and duration of therapy is still not clear. Another new pharmacologic agent that may help in smoking cessation is *varenicline*, a nicotinic acetylcholine receptor agonist. It has been approved by the US FDA in May 2006. Patients start a 7-day dosing schedule and are instructed to quit smoking 1 week after starting varenicline. Treatment should be continued for 12 weeks before determining efficacy; patients who have successfully quit at 12 weeks can be continued for an additional 12 weeks. The most common side effects reported are nausea and abnormal dreams.

## Future Directions

*Rimonabant,* a selective CB1 cannabinoid receptor antagonist, has been developed as a treatment for both smoking cessation and obesity[7]; phase III human trials are ongoing. A separate experimental therapy uses a vaccine to generate antinicotine antibodies, which act within the central nervous system to inhibit the effects of nicotine.[8]

# Nutrition

Dietetics is an integral part of cardiovascular patient risk management. All patients having a CHD and those individuals at high risk should be given professional advice on the food and dietary options that reduce the cardiovascular risks.[9]

## Healthy Food Choices

- A wide variety of foods should be eaten.
- Caloric intake should be adjusted to avoid weight gain.
- Encourage: Fruits, vegetables, wholegrain cereals and bread, fish (especially oily), lean meat, and low-fat dairy products.
- Avoid saturated fats. Increase monosaturated and polyunsaturated fats from vegetable and marine sources to reduce total fat to <30% of caloric intake, of which less than 1/3 is saturated.
- Recommend reducing salt intake if blood pressure is raised.

Supplemental vitamin C, E, and beta carotene cannot be recommended in the primary prevention of CVD. Taking supplements without clinical benefits could, in theory, increase the risk if individuals mistakenly avoid therapeutic lifestyle changes or drug therapies with proven benefits.

Individuals who consume small to moderate amounts of alcohol have lower risks of CVD, including cardiovascular mortality.[10] The United States Dietary Guidelines recommend alcohol intake in moderation, if at all: one drink per day for women and up to two drinks per day for men. The type of alcoholic beverage does not appear to be important. Drinking should be strongly discouraged for individuals under the age of 40 who are at low risk of CVD, since the risks are likely to outweigh the benefits in this group.

Dietary recommendations should be defined individually, taking into account the local culture and the subject's risk factors – dyslipidemia, hypertension, diabetes, and obesity.

## Obesity

Obesity is associated with a number of risk factors for atherosclerosis and CVD, including hypertension, insulin resistance and glucose intolerance, high cholesterol, hypertriglyceridemia, low serum HDL cholesterol concentrations, and high plasma fibrinogen concentrations.[11,12] Data from the Framingham Heart Study and the Nurses' Health study have shown a positive association between body weight and coronary heart disease. The distribution of the body fat appears to be an important determinant as patients with excess central (visceral abdominal) fat are at greatest risk.[13]

Multiple indices of obesity are available for cardiovascular risk stratification: BMI, waist–hip circumference ratio (WHR), and simply waist circumference (WC). BMI has been extensively used to define the groups of body weight (kg/height (m$^2$)). According to the National Institutes of Health and the WHO, overweight is defined as BMI ranging from 25 to 29.9 kg/m$^2$ and obesity by BMI> 30 kg/m$^2$. Increasing BMI is highly associated with CVD. It has also been suggested by multiple expert panels to use WC as an additional indicator of metabolic risk within each category of BMI.[14,15]

Weight reduction is recommended for obese people (BMI>30 kg/m$^2$) and should be considered for those who are overweight (BMI>25 and <30 kg/m$^2$). Men with waist circumference of 94–102 cm and women with a waist circumference of 80–88 cm are advised not to increase their weight. Men above 102 cm and women above 88 cm should be advised to lose weight.[9]

Selection of treatment for overweight subjects is based upon an initial risk assessment. All should be evaluated for their readiness to change, as essential feature of those who are successful in losing weight. Those who are ready to lose weight should also receive basic information about behavior modification, diet, and exercise. It is likely that improvements in central fat metabolism occur with exercise even before weight reduction occurs.

Ten suggested steps for treating overweight and obesity in the primary care setting are as follows:

1. Measure height and weight.
2. Measure waist circumference.
3. Assess co-morbidities.
4. Should your patient be treated?
5. Which diet should you recommend?
6. Is the patient ready and motivated?
7. Discuss a physical activity goal.
8. Review the Weekly Food and Activity Diary.
9. Give the patient copes of the dietary information.
10. Enter the patient's information.

These strategies highlight the need to view the treatment of obesity in the context of a chronic disorder. Each individual needs ongoing follow-up, evaluation, and reinforcement.

## Drug Treatment for Overweight

Drug treatment has little additional value in weight reduction to diet and exercise. *Orlistat* inhibits intestinal lipases to prevent the hydrolysis and uptake of fat. Weight loss is usually modest, and gastrointestinal disturbances occur. *Sebutaramine* enhances a feeling of satiety after food by an effect of its metabolites which inhibit noradrenaline and serotonin uptake. *Rimonabant* is an endocannabinoid receptor antagonist that appears capable of inducing a modest but sustained weight loss in combination with calorie-controlled diet. It is still unclear if its promising effect on weight reduction and other factors will translate into hard points of cardiovascular mortality.

## Physical Activity

A number of observational studies have shown a strong inverse relationship between leisure time activity with energy expenditure, habitual exercise, and fitness with risk of coronary disease and death.[16,17] In primary prevention, appropriate physical activity would consist of 30 min or more of brisk walking four to six times a week. Endpoints indicating an adequate degree of activity include breathlessness, fatigue, and sweating. Achievement of goal heart rate is not necessary.

Exercise ECG testing has often been recommended for people who are sedentary but are considering a vigorous exercise program. However, the Lipid Research Clinic Coronary Prevention Trial found that, among 3617 asymptomatic men with elevated cholesterol, the cumulative incidence related to acute cardiac events was only 2% during a mean follow-up of 7.4 years.[18]

## *Management*

- Providers must stress that positive health benefits occur with almost any increase in activity; small amounts of exercise have an additive effect; exercise opportunities exist in the workplace, i.e., using stairs instead of the elevator.
- Try to find leisure activities that are positively enjoyable.
- 30 min of moderately vigorous exercise on most days of the week will reduce risk and increase fitness.
- Exercising with family or friends tend to improve motivation.
- Added benefits include a sense of well-being, weight reduction, and better self-esteem.
- Continued physician support and encouragement may help in the long term.

## Hypertension

Hypertension affects approximately 50 million individuals in the United States and approximately 1 billion individuals worldwide.[19] Data from the Framingham Heart Study suggest that individuals who are normotensive at 55 years of age have a 90% lifetime risk for developing hypertension.[20]

Elevated BP is a risk factor for CHD, heart failure, CVD, peripheral vascular disease, and renal failure in both men and women. In general, epidemiological studies of treated and untreated patients reveal that there is a gradually increasing incidence of coronary disease and stroke and cardiovascular mortality as the blood pressure rises above 110/75, with some notable differences in risk based upon age and underlying co-morbid conditions.[21] JNC VII, published in 2003, provides new classification of hypertension for adults aged 18 years or older. The classification is based on the mean of two or more properly measured seated BP readings on each of two or more office visits.

## Patient Evaluation

Evaluation of patients with documented hypertension has three objectives: (1) to assess lifestyle and identify other cardiovascular risk factors or concomitant disorders that may affect prognosis and guide treatment; (2) to reveal identifiable causes of high BP; and (3) to assess the presence or absence of target-organ damage and CVD.

The physical examination should include an appropriate measurements of BP, with verification in the contralateral arm; examination of the optic fundi; calculation of the body mass index, auscultation for carotid, abdominal and femoral bruits; palpation of the thyroid gland; thorough examination of the heart and lungs; examination of the abdomen for enlarged kidneys, masses, and abdominal aortic pulsation; palpation of the lower extremities for edema and pulses; and neurologic assessment.

Routine laboratory tests after initial evaluation include electrocardiogram; urinalysis; blood glucose and hematocrit, basic metabolic panel, estimate of glomerular filtration rate, and a fasting lipid profile. Additional testing for identifiable causes is not indicated unless BP control is not achieved.

## *Treatment: Who to Treat?*

Using the definitions from JNC VII in combination with ESC guidelines published in 2007, the following general approach can be used to determine which patients with hypertension require antihypertensive therapy.

All patients should undergo essential lifestyle modifications, including weight reduction for obese and overweight patients, physical activity, dietary sodium restriction, and moderation of alcohol consumption (Table 10.1). The decision to start antihypertensive drug treatment depends on the presence of CVD, diabetes, renal disease, and target-organ damage. When using the ESC guidelines, the SCORE estimate of total CVD risk is used to guide treatment choice (Table 10.2).

In the absence of end-organ damage, patients should not be labeled as having hypertension unless the blood pressure is persistently elevated over three to six visits

**Table 10.1** Recommendations for lifestyle modifications

| Modification | Recommendation | Approximate systolic BP reduction (mmHg) |
|---|---|---|
| Weight reduction | Maintain normal body weight (BMI, 18.5–24.9) | 5–20 mmHg/10 kg weight loss |
| Adopt DASH eating plan | Consume a diet rich in fruits, vegetables, and low-fat dairy products with a reduced content of saturated and total fat | 8–14 mmHg |
| Dietary sodium restriction | Reduce dietary sodium intake to not more than 100 mequiv./l (2.4 g of sodium or 6 g sodium chloride) | 2–8 mmHg |
| Physical activity | Engage in regular aerobic physical activity such as brisk walking ( at least 30 min per day, most days of the week) | 4–9 mmHg |
| Moderation of alcohol consumption | Limit consumption to not more than two drinks per day [1 oz or 30 ml ethanol (g, 24 oz beer, 10 oz wine, or 3 oz 80-roof whiskey)] in most men and not more than one drink per day in women and lighter-weight persons | 2–4 mmHg |

**Table 10.2** Blood pressure treatment guidelines based on the score index

| SCORE | Normal | Prehypertension | Stage 1 hypertension | Stage 2 hypertension |
|---|---|---|---|---|
| CVD risk | <120/80 mmHg | 130–139/80–89 mmHg | 140–159/90–99 mmHg | ≥160/100 mmHg |
| Low (<1%) | Lifestyle advice | Lifestyle advice | Lifestyle advice | Drug Rx if persists |
| Moderate (1–4%) | Lifestyle advice | Lifestyle advice | Consider drug Rx | Drug Rx if persists |
| Increased (5–9%) | Lifestyle advice | Consider drug Rx | Drug Rx | Drug Rx |
| Markedly increased (≥10%) | Lifestyle advice | Consider drug Rx | Drug Rx | Drug Rx |

within several months. During the initial evaluation period, patients should also be encouraged to measure their blood pressure at home or work.

Antihypertensive medications should generally be started if the systolic pressure is persistently ≥140 mmHg and the diastolic pressure is persistently ≥90 mmHg in the office and at home despite attempted nonpharmacologic therapy. Starting with two drugs may be considered in patients with a baseline blood pressure greater than 20/10 mmHg above goal. In patients with diabetes or chronic kidney disease, anti-hypertensive therapy is indicated when the systolic pressure is persistently above 130 mmHg and/or the diastolic pressure is above 80 mmHg. Extrapolating from prior trials, it is also suggested to keep the goal blood pressure ≤130/80 mmHg in patients with heart failure or coronary disease. Patients with office hypertension, normal values at home, and no evidence of end-organ damage should undergo ambulatory blood pressure monitoring to see if they are truly hypertensive.

## Flow Chart for Selecting Antihypertensive Medications

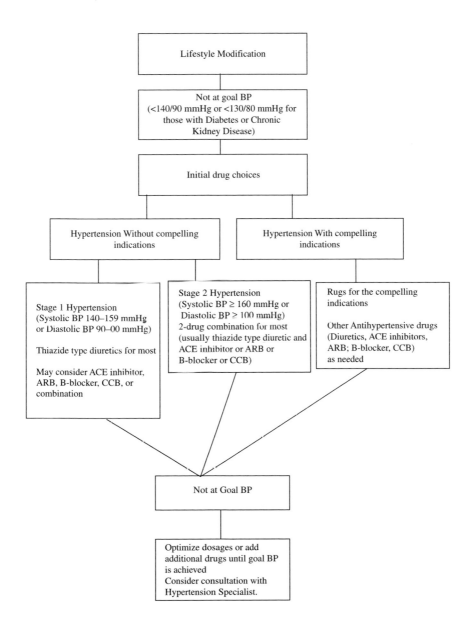

## *How to Treat?*

### Antihypertensive Medications

Two recent large-scale trials and meta-analyses have concluded that B-blockers may not protect against stroke, though they are equally effective in reducing coronary events and mortality.[22,23] It has also been proven that administration of B-blockers has been beneficial in patients with angina, heart failure, and recent MI. B-blockers should still be considered a valid option for initial and subsequent antihypertensive treatment strategies. However, they may induce weight gain, have adverse effect on lipid profile, and increase the incidence of new onset diabetes. Thiazide diuretics have also been shown to have diabetogenic and dyslipidemic effects.[24,25] Physicians should exercise caution when prescribing these medications to hypertensive patients with multiple metabolic risk factors, including the metabolic syndrome and its major components.

ACE inhibitors and angiotensin receptor antagonists have been particularly effective in reducing left ventricular hypertrophy and myocardial fibrosis. Additionally, they reduce microalbuminuria, proteinuria and help to preserve renal function, preventing progression to end-stage renal disease. Up to 35% increase in serum creatinine above baseline is expected with these medications and should not be used as a reason to withhold treatment.

### Follow-Up

Once the antihypertensive treatment has been initiated, patients should return for follow-up on a monthly basis until the optimal blood pressure has been achieved. More frequent follow-up may be required in patient with Stage 2 hypertension or with multiple co-morbidities. Serum potassium and creatinine should be checked at least once or twice a year. After blood pressure is in the target range, stable follow-up can be at 3- to 6-month intervals. Generally, antihypertensive treatment should be maintained indefinitely.

## Plasma Lipids

The relationship between elevated plasma cholesterol and atherosclerotic disease is well established. A 10% increase in serum cholesterol is associated with a 20–30% increase in risk for CHD. All patients with cardiovascular disease should be screened for serum cholesterol levels. Some controversy remains regarding screening in primary prevention. The National Cholesterol Education Program (NCEP) recommends routine screening of all adults older than 20 years, the American College of Physicians (ACP) recommends screening only men aged 35–65 and women 45–65 and the US Preventive Services Task Force recommends screening all men aged 35 and older and all women aged 45 and older. To establish treat-

**Table 10.3**   Cholesterol treatment guidelines based on the risk category

| Risk category | LDL-C goal | Initiate TLC | Consider drug therapy |
|---|---|---|---|
| High risk: CHD or CHD risk equivalents; 10-year risk>20% | <100 mg/dl (optional goal: <70 mg/dl) | ≥100 mg/dl | ≥100 mg/dl (<100 mg/dl; consider drug options) |
| Moderately high risk: 2+ risk factors (10–year risk, 10%–20%) | <130 mg/dl | ≥130 mg/dl | ≥130 mg/dl (<130 mg/dl; consider drug options) |
| Moderate risk: 2+ risk factors (10-year risk, 10–20%) | <130 mg/dl | ≥130 mg/dl | ≥160 mg/dl |
| Lower risk:0–1 risk factor | <160 mg/dl | ≥160 mg/dl | ≥190 mg/dl (160–189 mg/dl: LDL-lowering drug optional) |

ment goals for the patients with no known coronary disease, the 10-year risk for developing CHD should be carried out using modified Framingham risk scoring (Table 10.3).

The two major modalities of LDL-lowering therapy are *therapeutic lifestyle changes* (*TLC*) and *drug therapy*. Essential features of TLC are reduced intake of saturated fats (<7% of total calories) and cholesterol (<200 mg per day); therapeutic options for enhancing LDL lowering such as plant stanols/sterols (2 g/day) and increased viscous (soluble) fiber (10–25 d/day), weight reduction, and increased physical activity. If dietary therapy does not achieve the target LDL level, drug therapy should be started.

The current armamentarium of lipid-lowering drugs includes inhibitors of hydroxyl-3-methyl-glutaryl-CoA reductase (statins), fibrates, bile acid sequestrates (anion exchange resins), niacin (nicotinic acid), and selective cholesterol absorption inhibitors (ezetimibe). Statins have been shown not only to reduce hyperlipidemia but also to reduce cardiovascular events, mortality, the need for coronary artery bypass grafting, and various forms of coronary angioplasty. High-dose statins also seem to halt progression or induce regression of coronary atherosclerosis. Therefore, they are recommended as the first choice.

Selective cholesterol absorption inhibitors can be used in combination with statins in patients not reaching treatment goals. Bile acid sequestrates also decrease total and LDL cholesterol but tend to increase triglycerides. Fibrates and nicotinic acid are used primarily for triglyceride lowering and increasing HDL cholesterol, while fish oils (omega-3-fatty acids) are used for triglyceride lowering. In some patients, goals cannot be reached even on maximal lipid-lowering therapy, but they will still benefit from treatment to the extent to which cholesterol has been lowered. Increased attention to other risk factors can reduce total risk (Table 10.4).

**Table 10.4** Drugs affecting lipoprotein metabolism

| Drug class | Lipid effects | Side effects | Contraindications |
|---|---|---|---|
| Statins (HMG CoA reductase inhibitors) | LDL-↓ 18–55%; HDL-↑ 5–15%; TGL-↓ 7–30% | Myopathy; increased liver enzymes | Absolute: active or chronic liver disease; relative: concomitant use of certain drugs |
| Bile acid sequestrants | LDL-↓ 15–30%; HDL-↑ 3–5%; TGL-no change or increase | Gastrointestinal distress; constipation; decreased absorption of other drugs | Absolute: dysbetalipoproteinemia, TG > 400 mg/dl; relative: TG > 200 mg/dl |
| Nicotinic acid | LDL-↓ 5–25%; HDL-↑ 15–35%; TGL-↓ 20–50% | Flushing; hyperglycemia; hyperuricemia; upper GI distress; hepatotoxicity | Absolute: chronic liver disease (sever gout); relative: diabetes; hyperuricemia; peptic ulcer disease |
| Fibric acids | LDL-↓ 5–20% (may be increased in patients with high TGL); HDL-↑ 10–20%; TGL- ↓ 20–50% | Dyspepsia; gallstones; myopathy; unexplained non-CHD deaths in WHO study | Absolute: severe renal disease, severe hepatic disease |

## *Elevated Triglycerides*

A recent meta-analysis of prospective studies indicated that elevated triglycerides are an independent risk factor for CHD.[26] ATP III proposed the following classification of serum triglycerides:

- Normal triglycerides: <150 mg/dl
- Borderline-high triglycerides: 150–199 mg/dl
- High triglycerides: 200–499 mg/dl
- Very high triglycerides: ≥500 mg/dl

In patients with high triglycerides (≥200 mg/dl), *non-HDL cholesterol* [total cholesterol minus HDL cholesterol] becomes a secondary target of therapy with the goal non-HDL cholesterol 30 mg/dl higher than that for LDL cholesterol. The primary aim of therapy for all persons with elevated triglycerides is to achieve the target goal for LDL cholesterol. When triglycerides are *borderline high* (150–199 mg/dl), emphasis should also be placed on weight reduction and increased physical activities. For *high* triglycerides (200–499 mg/dl), non-HDL cholesterol becomes a secondary target therapy. There are two approaches to drug therapy. First, the non-HDL cholesterol goal can be achieved by intensifying therapy with an LDL-lowering drug and second, nicotinic acid or fibrate can be added. In rare cases in which triglycerides are *very high* (≥500 mg/dl), the initial aim of therapy is to prevent acute

pancreatitis through triglyceride lowering. This approach includes weight reduction, low-fat diet, physical activity, and drug therapy. Only after triglyceride levels
have been lowered to <500 mg/dl should attention turn to LDL lowering to reduce
risk for CHD.

## *Low HDL*

Low HDL is a strong independent predictor of CHD. Low HDL is defined as a level
<40 mg/dl. There are no specific goals for raising HDL. Although clinical trials
suggest that raising HDL will reduce risk, the evidence is insufficient to specify a
goal for therapy. Treatment for isolated low HDL with fibrates and nicotinic acid
should be reserved for persons with CHD and CHD risk equivalents.

## Diabetes

The National Cholesterol Education Program report from the United States and
guidelines from Europe consider type 2 diabetes to be a CHD equivalent, thereby
elevating the patient to the highest risk category.[27]

Maintaining tight control of blood sugar in either type 1 or type 2 diabetes has
a clear benefit on microvascular complications.[28] In relation to macrovascular disease the picture is less clear. In type 1 diabetes, the effects of long-term optimized
metabolic control on the risk of developing CVD have been demonstrated.[29] This
could be an effect mediated through the effect of microvascular complications. In
type 2 diabetes, the evidence from studies strongly indicates an effect of glucose
control on risks of CVD. Recommended treatment targets for patients with type 2
diabetes are HgbA1C ≤6.5 if feasible, fasting/preprandial <110 mg/dl, and post-
prandial <135 mg/dl.

## Conclusion

One of the major objectives of a CVD detection program should be to identify those
apparently healthy individuals who have asymptomatic arterial disease in order to
slow the progression of atherosclerotic disease, to induce regression, and in particular to reduce risk of clinical manifestations. For coronary artery disease, the consequences of coronary atherosclerosis can be objectively assessed noninvasively, using
a variety of techniques such as bicycle or treadmill exercise, ECG testing, stress
echocardiography, or radionuclide scintigraphy. These techniques are routinely used
in diagnostic work-up programs.

# References

1. Murray CJL, Lopez AD. The global burden of disease in 1990. In: Murray CJL, Lopez AD, Harvard School of Public Health, World Health organization, World Bank, eds. *The Global Burden of Disease: A Comprehensive Assessment of Mortality and Disability form Disease, Injuries, and Risk Factors in 1990 and Projected to 2020*, Cambridge, MA: Harvard School of Public Health, 1996:247–293.
2. Strauss MD. *Familiar Medical Quotations*. 1st ed. Boston, MA: Little, Brown, and Company, 1968:1
3. Conroy RM, Pyorala K, Fitzgerald AP, et al. Estimation of ten-year risk of fatal cardiovascular disease in Europe: the SCORE project. *Eur Heart J*. 2003:24:987–1003.
4. Fellows Y, Trosclair A. Annual smoking-attributable mortality, years of potential life list, and economic costs-United States, 1995–1999. *MMWR Morb Mortal Wkly Rep*. 2002;51:300.
5. Trosclair A, Husten C. Cigarette smoking among adults-United States, 2000. *MMWR Morb Mortal Wkly Rep*. 2002;51:642.
6. Critchley JA, Capewell S. Mortality risk reduction associated with smoking cessation in patients with coronary heart disease: a systemic review. *JAMA*. 2003;86:290
7. Gelfand E. Rimonabant: a cannabinoid receptor type 1 blocker for management of multiple cardiometabolic risk factors. *JACC*. 2006;47:1919–1926.
8. Hall W. The prospects for immunotherapy in smoking cessation. *The Lancet*. 2002; 260(9339):1089–1091.
9. Graham I, Atar D, Borch-Johnsen B. European guidelines on cardiovascular disease prevention in clinical practice: executive summary. Fourth Joint Task Force of the European Society of cardiology and other societies on cardiovascular disease prevention in clinical practice. *EHJ*. 2007;28:2375–2414.
10. Klatsky AL. Risk of cardiovascular mortality in alcohol drinkers, ex-drinkers and nondrinkers. *Am J Card*. 1990;66(17):1237–1242.
11. Wajchenberg B. Subcutaneous and visceral adipose tissue: their relation to the metabolic syndrome. *Endocr Rev*. 2000;21:697–738.
12. Carr M, Brunzell JD. Abdominal obesity and dyslipidemia in the metabolic syndrome: importance of type 2 diabetes and familial combined hyperlipidemia in coronary artery disease risk. *J Clin Endochrinol Metab*. 2004;89:2601–2607.
13. Despres J, Moorjani S, Lupien PJ, Tremblay A, Nadeau A, Bouchard C, Regional distribution of body fat, plasma lipoprotein, and cardiovascular disease. *Atherosclerosis*. 1990;10: 497–511.
14. World Health Organization Consultation of Obesity. *Obesity: Preventing and Managing the Global Epidemic*. Geneva, Switzerland: Division of Non-communicable diseases, Programmed of Nutrition, Family and Reproductive Health, WHO; 1998.
15. National Heart, Lung, and Blood Institute Obesity Education Initiative Expert Panel. Clinical guidelines on the identification, evaluation, and treatment of overweight and obesity in adults. *Obes Res*. 1998;6:51S–209S.
16. Caspersen C, Bloemberg B. The prevalence of selected physical activities and their relation with coronary heart disease risk factors in elderly men, The Zutphen Study 1985. *Am J Epidemiol*. 1991;133(11):1078–1092.
17. Paffenbarger JR, Wing AL. Physical activity as an index of heart attack risk in college alumni. *IS J Epidemiol*. 1995;142(9):889–903.
18. Rifkind BM. Lipid research clinics coronary primary prevention trial: results and implications. *Am J Cardiol*. 1984;54(5):30C–34C.
19. The JNC 7 report. *JAMA* 2003;289(19):2560–2572.
20. Vasan RS, Beiser A, Seshadri S, et al. Residual lifetime risk for developing hypertension in middle aged women and men: The Framingham Heart Study. *JAMA*. 2002;287:1003–1010.
21. Douglas JC, Bakris GL, Epstein M, et al. Management of high blood pressure in African Americans: consensus statement of the Hypertension in African Americans Working

Group of the International Society of Hypertension in Blacks. *Arch Intern Med*. 2003; 163:587.

22. Messerli FH, Grossman E, Goldbourt U. Are B-blockers efficacious as a first line therapy for treatment of hypertension in the elderly? A systematic review. *JAMA*. 1998;279:1903–1907.

23. Lindholm LH, Carlberg B. Should B-blockers remain first choice in the treatment of primary hypertensions? A meta-analysis. *Lancet*. 2005;366:1545–1553.

24. ALLHAT Officers and Coordinators for the ALLHAT collaborative research group: Major outcomes in high-risk hypertensive patients randomized to angiotensin-converting enzyme inhibitor or calcium channel blocker vs. diuretic: The Antihypertensive and Lipid Lowering treatment to prevent Heart Attack Trial (ALLHAT) *JAMA*. 2002;288:2981 2997.

25. Hanson L, Lindholm LH, Ekbom T, et al. Randomized trial of old and new antihypertensive drugs in elderly patients: cardiovascular mortality and morbidity in the Swedish trial in old patients with hypertension-2 study. *Lancet*. 1999;34:1129–1133.

26. Cullen P. Evidence that elevated triglycerides are an independent coronary heart disease risk factor. *Am J Cardiol*. 2000;86(9):943–949.

27. Third report of the National Cholesterol education program (NCEP) Expert Panel on detection, evaluation and treatment of high blood cholesterol in adults (Adult Treatment Panel III): Final report. US Department of Health and human services; Public Health Service; National institute of health; National Heart, Lung, and Blood institute. *Circulation*. 2002;106:3143.

28. Intensive blood-glucose control with sulfonylureas or insulin compared with conventional treatment and risk of complications in patients with type 2 diabetes (UKPDS 33). UK prospective diabetes study (UKPDS) Group. *Lancet*. 1998;352:837.

29. Effect of intensive diabetes management on macrovascular events and risk factors in the Diabetes Control and Complications Trial. *Am J Cardiol*. 1995;75:894.

# Chapter 11
# The "Ischemic Cascade"

Asimul Ansari and Jyothy Puthumana

## Introduction

The ischemic cascade refers to a predictable sequence of events that occurs in the myocardium after the onset of ischemia.[1] Myocardial perfusion is determined by coronary blood flow and myocardial oxygen consumption. Any imbalance in this supply and demand relationship may result in myocardial ischemia. The mechanical, electrographic, and clinical events that follow the development of ischemia were formally described in 1985 by Hauser et al.[2] and were later termed the "ischemic cascade."[3] Classically the observable changes occur sequentially (Fig. 11.1) starting with perfusion abnormalities leading to abnormalities in wall function, then

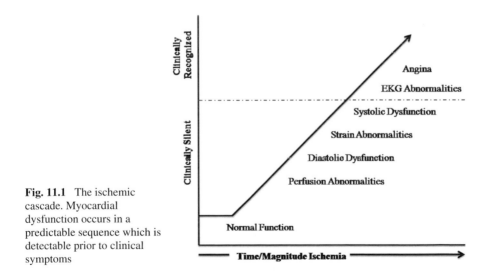

**Fig. 11.1** The ischemic cascade. Myocardial dysfunction occurs in a predictable sequence which is detectable prior to clinical symptoms

A. Ansari (✉)
Department of Cardiology, Northwestern Memorial Hospital, Chicago, Illinois, USA
e-mail: ansari01@gmail.com

E. Herzog, F.A. Chaudhry (eds.), *Echocardiography in Acute Coronary Syndrome*,
DOI 10.1007/978-1-84882-027-2_11, © Springer-Verlag London Limited 2009

ischemic electrocardiogram (ECG) changes, and finally angina.[4] Echocardiography has the ability to detect these pathophysiologic changes in the myocardium at the most initial stages and therefore is more sensitive than history, physical examination, and ECG for identification of myocardial ischemia.[5]

Echocardiography for the diagnosis of suspected acute ischemia is most helpful in subjects with a high clinical suspicion but non-diagnostic electrocardiograms, as it is the only technique available that allows real-time assessment of myocardial function. Additionally, through stress modalities, it offers assessment and risk stratification in patients who present to the ED with chest pain.

It has been well documented that ischemia from coronary stenosis (supply) can occur without clinically recognizable signs such as electrocardiograph (ECG) changes or symptoms such as angina.[6,7] It is also known that earlier recognition and treatment of ischemia improves outcomes.[8,9] Recent data suggest that the ischemic cascade is also observed with demand ischemia.[10] Interestingly, there is also evidence that the temporal sequence of events may overlap. Recognition of the concept of the ischemic cascade allows clinicians to focus on the preceding underlying pathophysiologic factors rather than the clinically recognizable end result.[3]

## Coronary Anatomy and Myocardial Perfusion

While the angiogram is still considered by most physicians to be the "gold standard" for defining coronary anatomy, careful investigations have revealed many inherent deficiencies.[11,12] According to Topol, investigators began questioning the accuracy and reproducibility of coronary angiography as early as the 1960s.[13] Initial studies established that visual interpretation exhibited clinically significant intra-observer and inter-observer variability, with differences in the estimation of stenosis severity approaching 50%.[13-15] Noninvasive stress tests, such as echocardiography, are often performed not only to detect coronary stenosis but also to determine whether intermediate coronary lesions previously identified by angiography are physiologically important.

The coronary circulation is functionally composed of the epicardial coronary arteries (>500 μm) and the microvasculature: prearterioles (500–100 μm) and the arterioles (<100 μm).[16] These smaller vessels effectively divide the coronary circulation into vascular micro-domains which have separate auto-regulatory ability to ensure oxygenation can meet the physiologic demand.[17] The coronary arteries, located epicardially, provide unrestricted blood flow unless limited by stenoses. Conversely, the prearterioles, located subepicardially, have the ability to dilate or constrict based on changes in central aortic pressure. The arterioles, located subendocardially, auto-regulate on the basis of metabolic factors released by the myocardium in response to increased oxygen consumption.[10,11,18]

Under normal conditions, myocardial blood flow is determined by both the epicardial coronary vessels and the subendocardial microvasculature and functions to maintain the cardiac cellular metabolism. The heart is entirely dependent on this blood flow and cannot tolerate an oxygen deficit.[19] The large epicardial coronary arteries provide almost no resistance to blood flow under normal conditions. However, as a stenotic lesion develops in these vessels, a drop in perfusion pressure occurs across the stenosis. This causes auto-regulatory signals to stimulate the microvasculature to dilate to compensate for the reduced distal arterial perfusion pressure, maintaining the normal amount of blood flow. Consequently, when most patients with coronary arterial obstructions are resting, they have no ischemia and therefore no angina.[20] In animal models, there is no impairment of baseline blood flow until about 90% of the cross-sectional area of the artery (or 80–90% of the true angiographic diameter) is obstructed.[21–23] Additionally, with the collateral circulation from the other epicardial vessels, at baseline there may not be any decrease in blood flow irrespective of the percent stenosis in a single artery.

In comparison, under stress conditions when there is increased myocardial metabolic demand, blood flow can increase approximately fourfold from the normal level in order to meet oxygen requirements, when a flow-limiting stenosis is not present.[24] This amount of hyperemia represents the vasodilator reserve of the coronary arterial system and is again mediated by dilation of the microvasculature and a corresponding decrease in resistance. In the stenotic blood vessel, however, the capacity of the microcirculation to dilate further is limited, and the oxygen requirement of the myocardium may exceed coronary blood supply, resulting in ischemia.[20] It has been assumed that during maximal hyperemia, the microvasculature is maximally dilated and the decrease in hyperemic flow is due to resistance offered by the epicardial coronary stenosis.[25] In human models, flow during hyperemia in the patients with stenoses of less than 40–50% of the luminal diameter (60% of the cross-sectional area) was not significantly different from flow in the controls. Among the patients with stenoses of 40% or more, flow during hyperemia and coronary vasodilator reserve progressively decreased as the degree of stenosis increased. For stenoses equal to 80% (90% of the cross-sectional area), flow during hyperemic conditions is not increased above baseline; there is absence of coronary vasodilator reserve.[23]

It has become increasingly evident that true blood flow limitation, and therefore the potential to develop ischemia, cannot truly be fully assessed without interpretation of the physiologic impact of the lesion. Multiple methods have been derived in an attempt to quantify physiologic blood flow limitation whether epicardial coronary, microvascular, or both. The initial conceptualization of this process, the coronary flow reserve (CFR), was submitted in 1974 by Gould et al. and is defined as the maximal hyperemic blood flow to resting blood flow ratio.[21] Different invasive methods have been introduced for the assessment of CFR, including Doppler wire, coronary pressure wire/fractional flow reserve (FFR), and estimated pressure gradient velocity ($dp_{v50}$).[26,27] However, these methods require interventional cardiologists to manage the measurements in a catheterization lab. Therefore, noninvasive modalities have been developed and include radionuclide cardiac imaging, magnetic resonance imaging (MRI) perfusion imaging, and most recently myocardial contrast echocardiography (MCE). Previous evaluation of suspected ischemia by echocardiography was limited to 2D echo. While 2D echo has been shown to have effectiveness in the risk stratification of patients with suspected ischemic syndromes, it has been described as having slightly lower sensitivity (88%) compared to nuclear imaging (92%).[28,29] At present, echocardiography may be able to diagnose perfusion impairment which is significantly abnormal.

It is critical to understand and assess the physiologic burden of coronary stenoses rather than rely on the degree of anatomic obstruction. As discussed above, patients with physiologically significant stenoses, and therefore ischemia, are at increased risk for clinical events, while those with even angiographically severe lesions, yet no physiologic consequence, are at much lower risk.[30]

## Ischemic Cascade Perfusion Abnormalities

One of the most significant advances in echocardiography has been the development of micro bubble contrast agents, which allow noninvasive perfusion assessment of the myocardium up to the level of the microvasculature.[31] MCE has the ability to demonstrate both myocardial blood volume and velocity on a regional basis.[32] The commercially available contrast agents are composed of a thin shell of lipids containing an inert gas and are of smaller diameter than red blood cells. Imaging can then be performed with bolus of contrast or continuous infusion, using either destructive or non-destructive protocols.[33]

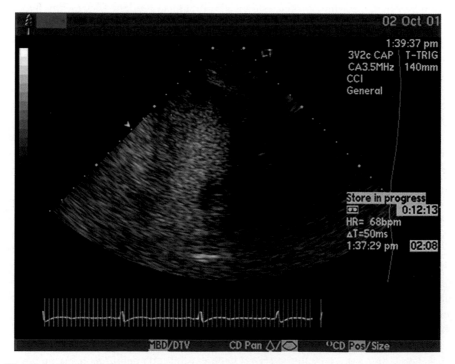

**Fig. 11.2** Myocardial contrast perfusion echo demonstrating apical subendocardial hypoperfusion/ischemia

In the evaluation of chest pain patients with non-diagnostic ECG changes seen in the emergency department, MCE was able to classify intermediate modified thrombolysis in myocardial infarction (TIMI) score patients into low and high risk for acute coronary syndrome (ACS) prior to availability of serum cardiac enzymes.[34] Currently contrast agents are not FDA approved specifically for perfusion imaging; however, improvement of visualization of the endocardial border and thus facilitating recognition of wall motion abnormalities increases the sensitivity of this testing methodology.[35]

The additive data on perfusion have shown increased accuracy in detection and regionalization of ischemia compared to dobutamine stress echocardiography (DSE) primarily at intermediate (84 vs. 20%) stages but also for both single vessel (81 vs. 53%) and multi-vessel CAD (95 vs. 76%).[40] MCE also had a higher negative predictive value compared to DSE[36] and offers better spatial resolution and therefore visualization of subendocardial ischemia compared to nuclear imaging (Fig. 11.2).[36]

Finally, direct visualization of the epicardial coronary arterial blood flow with Doppler echo has been proven to be technically feasible[37]; however, the practicality of this application in the acute setting has not been demonstrated.

## Diastolic Dysfunction

Abnormalities in diastolic function are classically one of the earliest observable signs of myocardial ischemia and are independent and persist longer than changes in systolic function. Doppler echocardiography has emerged as the principal clinical tool for the assessment of ventricular diastolic function, and its sensitivity to detect ischemia, whether from epicardial stenosis or microvascular disease, has been validated in many clinical studies.[38 40] Doppler flow indices have been used to evaluate different parameters of diastolic function, including left ventricular (LV) filling pressure, compliance, and relaxation.[41,42] In comparison to filling and compliance, ventricular relaxation is an active process. Diastolic function may rarely be visually observed, but can be measured quantitatively by M-mode, pulse Doppler of mitral inflow, and more recently by Doppler tissue imaging (DTI).

Impairment of relaxation is usually the first indication of diastolic dysfunction and can occur abruptly. Within seconds of the development of ischemia, reduction in E-wave velocity and an increase in A-wave velocity occur and can be noted on mitral inflow (Fig. 11.3).[46] Subendocardial fibers in the left ventricle are oriented along the long axis of the LV and are most susceptible to the early manifestations of ischemia. Hence detection of shortening (systole) and lengthening (diastole) abnormalities would be a sensitive indicator of early ischemia. Doppler tissue imaging (DTI) using pulsed Doppler technique selectively detects low-range Doppler shifts in tissue signals and detects regional myocardial velocities. Using this tool, longitudinal abnormalities of decreased systolic excursion (S') or reduced velocities during early (E') and late diastole (A') with or without a reversal of the E' to A' ratio can be used to detect ischemia (Fig. 11.4).

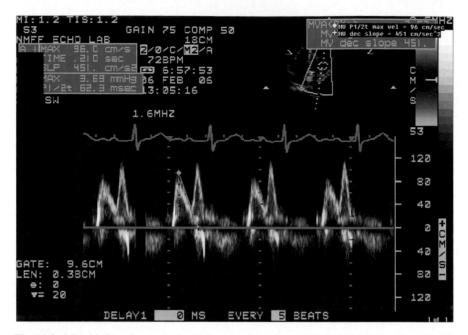

**Fig. 11.3** Mitral inflow demonstrating E/A reversal consistent with impaired relaxation–diastolic dysfunction

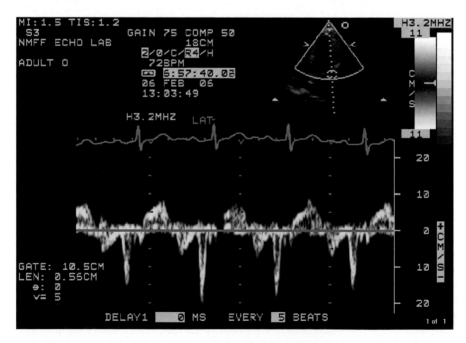

**Fig. 11.4** Tissue Doppler imaging of mitral annulus with E′/A′ reversal

Using this tool in dobutamine stress echo, investigators have been able to increase the sensitivity of detecting functionally significant coronary lesions as identified by a decrease in peak systolic excursion, decrease in early diastolic relaxation velocities, and reversal of E′ to A′ ratios.[46] DTI imaging appears to be less dependent on preload when compared to mitral inflow parameters and is useful for the evaluation of regional myocardial function; however, tethering from surrounding normal segments may limit its accuracy. Tissue velocity curves can be obtained off-line using color-coded 2D DTI images and can improve the reproducibility and accuracy of these measurements.

## Strain

The sequence of contraction and thickening abnormalities in response to ischemia that can be evaluated by echocardiography has been well documented.[43] Ischemia reduces early systolic thinning and delays the onset of systolic thickening, resulting in the phenomenon of post-systolic thickening (PST). Even the trained eye cannot visualize or time mechanical events shorter than 90 ms. Post-systolic thickening lasts for about 50–60 ms and therefore cannot be discerned by the naked eye.

In order to overcome the limitations of DTI related to angle of interrogation, cardiac motion, and rotation, strain (S) and strain rate (Sr) imaging have been developed to measure regional deformation in systole and diastole. Strain is defined as change in length normalized to the original length (Fig. 11.5), and the rate at which this occurs is called the strain rate. Ischemia-related changes in peak S and Sr have been shown to be detectable earlier than either DTI abnormalities or wall motion abnormalities, and these measures are thus important tools early in the evaluation of the ischemic cascade. Sr has been shown to be independent of preload and afterload and is therefore a highly accurate measure of regional function. Normal S and Sr values for longitudinal and radial strain have been defined by Kowalski et al. Peak radial strain in normal subjects is higher than longitudinal strain (50–70 vs. 20–30%) (Fig. 11.6).[44] S and Sr curves thus obtained can then be timed with cardiac cycle. Several studies have shown that a reduction in the peak systolic S and Sr with significant increase in PST is a sensitive marker of ischemia.[46]

**Fig. 11.5** Calculation of strain (ε). $L_0$ = original length. $\Delta L$ = change in length[53]

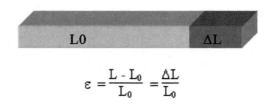

$$\varepsilon = \frac{L - L_0}{L_0} = \frac{\Delta L}{L_0}$$

In the setting of balloon occlusion during PCI, segments at risk (without adequate collaterals) have an acute >50% reduction in peak S and Sr with immediate occurrence of PST that is not noted in the non-ischemic segments (Fig. 11.7).[45]

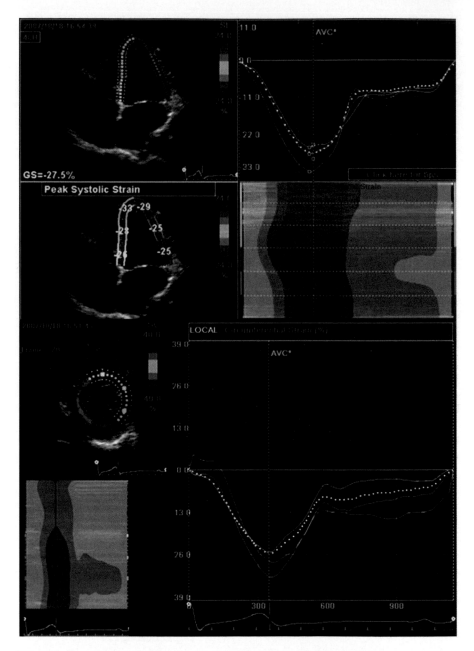

**Fig. 11.6** Normal longitudinal and circumferential strain by 2D strain method

Non-Doppler 2D strain is a newer and easier modality of obtaining S and Sr measurements by tracking speckles (natural acoustic markers) frame to frame in the ultrasonic images in two dimensions. Since it is not based on tissue Doppler, the

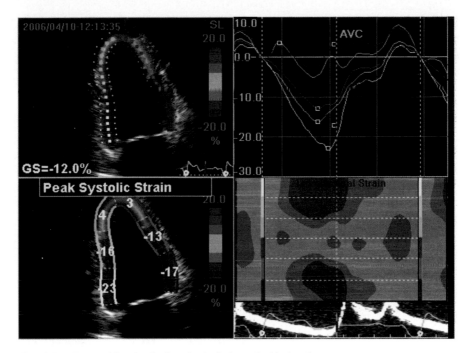

**Fig. 11.7** Abnormal longitudinal strain depicting apical ischemia

measurements are angle independent. Non-Doppler 2D strain is simple to perform and requires acquisition of only a single cardiac cycle (figure) and has been validated against tissue Doppler-derived S and Sr.

## Wall Motion Abnormalities

In 1929, Tenet and Wiggers published their observations that ligation of a coronary artery results in almost instantaneous loss of regional contractility.[46] Transient myocardial dysfunction is the most easily recognized and specific marker of ischemia. Echocardiography is the only technique available that allows real-time assessment of stress-induced reduction in systolic wall thickening. The location of regional wall motion abnormalities correlates well with the distribution of the artery involved.[47] When echocardiography is performed soon after presentation to the emergency department (ED) or during a chest pain episode, wall motion abnormalities are detected in 90–95% of transmural infarctions and in 80–90% of subendocardial infarctions. Additionally, the specificity of echocardiography is approximately 80–90%.[48] An absence of wall motion abnormalities has excellent negative predictive value.[49]

In patients with coronary artery disease (CAD), those with negative stress echo had very low need of further cardiac evaluation (visits in ED 3%, readmissions

2%)[50] and clinical events (negative predictive value of stress echocardiography was 99% after $13 \pm 12.2$ months follow-up).[51] In addition to wall motion abnormalities, failure to decrease cavity size or an increase in end-diastolic dimension has been used to detect physiologically significant single or multi-vessel stenoses in CAD patients.

## Conclusion

The ischemic cascade predicts the sequence of myocardial dysfunction after the onset of ischemia. Echo can accurately and quickly evaluate each component of the ischemic cascade resulting in earlier diagnosis of both acute coronary syndromes and CAD. The use of echocardiography for the suspected acute ischemia in the setting of chest pain has received a class I ACC/AHA recommendation.[52] In cases of CAD, ischemia may be identified with stress echocardiography while still clinically silent. Progressive advancements in echo technology such as MCE and strain imaging will continue to improve identification, risk stratification, and outcomes in these patients.

## References

1. Feigenbaum H, Armstrong WF, Ryan T. *Feigenbaum's Echocardiography*. Philadelphia: Lippincott Williams & Wilkins; 2005.
2. Hauser AM, Vellappillil G, Ramos RG, Gordon S, Timmis GC. Sequence of mechanical, electrocardiographic and clinical effects of repeated coronary artery occlusion in human beings: echocardiographic observations during coronary angioplasty. *J Am Coll Cardiol.* 1985;5: 193–197.
3. Nesto RW, Kowalchuk MD. The ischemic cascade: temporal sequence of hemodynamic, electrocardiographic and symptomatic expressions of ischemia. *Am J Cardiol.* 1987;57:23C–30C.
4. Harbinson M, Anagnostopoulos CD. *Nonivasive Imaging of Myocardial Ischemia. Principles of Pathophysiology Related to Noninvasive Cardiac Imaging.* London: Springer; 2006.
5. Lewis WR. Echocardiography in the evaluation of patients in chest pain units. *Cardiol Clin.* 2005;23:531–539.
6. Gottlien SO, Weisfildt ML, Ouyang P, Mellits ED, Gerstenblith G. Silent ischemia as a marker for earl unfavorable outcomes in patients with unstable angina. *N Engl J Med.* 1986;314: 1214–1219.
7. Geft IL, Gishbein MC, Ninomiya K, et al. Intermittent brief periods of ischemia have a cumulative effect and may cause myocardial necrosis. *Circulation.* 1982;66:1150–1153.
8. Beller GA. Myocardial perfusion imaging for detection of silent myocardial ischemia. *Am J Card.* 1988;61(12):22F–28F.
9. Kaul S, Senior R, Frischke C, et al. Incremental value of cardiac imaging in patients presenting to the emergency department with chest pain and without ST-segment elevation: a multicenter study. *Am Heart J.* 2004;148:129–136.
10. Leong-Poi H, Rim S, Le E, Fisher NG, Wei K, Kaul S. Perfusion versus function: the ischemic cascade in demand ischemia. *Circulation.* 2002;105:987–992.
11. Arnett EN, Isner JM, Redwood CR, et al. Coronary artery narrowing in coronary heart disease: comparison of cineangiographic and necropsy findings. *Ann Intern Med.* 1979;91:350–356.

12. Grodin CM, Dyrda I, Pasternac A, Campeau L, Bourassa MG, Lespérance J. Discrepancies between cineangiographic and post-mortem findings in patients with coronary artery disease and recent myocardial revascularization. *Circulation*. 1974;49:703–709.
13. Topol EJ, Nissen SE. Our preoccupation with coronary luminology: the dissociation between clinical and angiographic findings in ischemic heart disease. *Circulation*. 1995;92:2333–2342.
14. Zir LM, Miller SW, Dinsmore RE, et al. Interobserver variability in coronary angiography. *Circulation*. 1976;53.627–632.
15. Galbraith JE, Murphy ML, Desoyza N. Coronary angiogram interpretation: interobserver variability. *JAMA*. 1981;240:2053–2059.
16. Camici PG, Crea F. Coronary microvascular dysfunction. *N Engl J Med*. 2007;356:830–840.
17. Chilian WM. Coronary microcirculation in health and disease: summary of an NHLBI workshop. *Circulation*. 1997;95:522–528.
18. Kuo L, Davis MJ, Chilian WM. Myogenic activity in isolated subepicardial and subendocardial coronary arterioles. *Am J Physiol*. 1988;255:H1558–H1562.
19. Sigwart U, Grbic M, Parot M, Goy JJ, Essinger A, Fischer A. Ischemic events during coronary artery balloon obstruction. In: Rutishauser W, Roskamm H, eds. *Silent Myocardial Ischemia*. Berlin: Springer-Verlag; 1984:29–36.
20. Wilson, RF. Assessing the severity of coronary-artery stenoses. *N Engl J Med*. 1996;334:1735–1737.
21. Gould KL, Lipscomb K, Hamilton GW. Physiologic basis for assessing critical coronary stenosis: instantaneous flow response and regional distribution during coronary hyperemia as measures of coronary flow reserve. *Am J Cardiol*. 1974;33:87–94.
22. Pijls NHJ, de Bruyne B, Peels K, et al. Measurement of fractional flow reserve to assess the functional severity of coronary-artery stenoses. *N Engl J Med*. 1996;334:1703–1708.
23. Uren, NG, Melin, JA., De Bruyne, B, Wijns, W, Baudhuin T, Camici PG. Relation between myocardial blood flow and the severity of coronary-artery stenosis. *N Engl J Med* 1994;330:1782–1788.
24. Rigo F, Gherardi S, Galderisi M, Cortigiani L. Coronary flow reserve evaluation in stress-echocardiography laboratory. *J Cardiovasc Med*. 2006;7:472–479.
25. Sanjiv K, Hiroshi I. Microvasculature in acute myocardial ischemia: part I evolving concepts in pathophysiology, diagnosis, and treatment. *Circulation*. 2004;109:146–149.
26. Vicario ML, Cirillo L, Storto G. Influence of risk factors on coronary flow reserve in patients with 1-vessel coronary artery disease. *JNM*. 2005;46(9):1438–1443.
27. Marques KMJ, vanFenige MJ, Sprujit HJ, et al. The diastolic flow velocity-pressure gradient relation and $dp_{V50}$ to assess the hemodynamic significance of coronary stenosis. *Am J Physiol Heart Circ Physiol*. 2006;291:H2630–H2635.
28. Gani F, Diwaker J, Lahiri A. The role of cardiovascular imaging techniques in the assessment of patients with acute chest pain. *Nucl Med Commun*. 2007;28:441–449.
29. Kontos MC, Jesse RL, Anderson FP, Schmidt KL, Ornato JP, Tatum JL. Comparison of myocardial perfusion imaging and cardiac troponin I in patients admitted to the emergency department with chest pain. *Circulation*. 1999;99:2073–2078.
30. Lesser JL, Wilson RF, White CW. Physiologic assessment of coronary stenoses of intermediate severity can facilitate patient selection for coronary angioplasty. *J Coronary Artery Dis*. 1990;1:697–705.
31. Wei K, Lindner J. Contrast ultrasound in the assessment of patients presenting with suspected cardiac ischemia. *Crit Care Med*. 2007;35:S280–289.
32. Monaghan MJ. Stress myocardial contrast echocardiography. *Heart*. 2003;89:1391–1393.
33. Tsutsui JM, Xie F, McGrain AC, et al. Comparison of low-mechanical index pulse sequence schemes for detecting myocardial perfusion abnormalities during vasodilator stress echocardiography. *Am J Cardiol*. 2005;95(5):565–570.
34. Tong KL, Kaul S, Wang XQ, et al. Myocardial contrast echocardiography versus thrombolysis in myocardial infarction score in patients presenting to the emergency department with chest pain and a nondiagnostic electrocardiogram. *J Am Coll Cardiol*. 2005;46(5):920–927.

35. Gentile F, Trocino G, Todd S. New technologies applied to stress echocardiography: myocardial contrast echocardiography. J Cardiovasc Med. 2006;7:491–497.
36. Elhendy A, O'Leary EL, Xie F, McGrain AC, Anderson JR, Porter TR. Comparative accuracy of real-time myocardial contrast perfusion imaging and wall motion analysis during dobutamine stress echocardiography for the diagnosis of coronary artery disease. J Am Coll Cardiol. 2004;44(11):2185–2191.
37. Iliceto S, Marangelli V, Memmola C, Rizzon P. Transesophageal Doppler echocardiography evaluation of coronary blood flow velocity in baseline conditions and during dipyridamole-induced coronary vasodilation. Circulation. 1991;83:61–69.
38. El-Said M, Roeland J, Fioretti PM, et al. Abnormal left ventricular early diastolic filling during dobutamine stress Doppler echocardiography is a sensitive indicator of significant coronary artery disease. J Am Coll Cardiol. 1994;24:1618–1624.
39. Wijns W, Serruys PW, Slaager CJ, et al. Effect of coronary occlusion during percutaneous transluminal angioplasty in humans on left ventricular chamber stiffness and regional diastolic pressure-radius relations. J Am Coll Cardiol. 1986;7:455–463.
40. Lee KW, Blann AD, Lip GY. Impaired tissue Doppler diastolic function in patients with coronary artery disease: relationship to endothelial damage/dysfunction and platelet activation. Am Heart J. 2005;150(4):756–766.
41. Garcia MJ, Thomas JD, Klein AL. New Doppler echocardiographic applications for the study of diastolic function. J Am Coll Cardiol. 1998;32:865–875.
42. Pirracchio R, Cholley B, De Hert S, Solal AC, Mebazaa A. Diastolic heart failure in anaesthesia and critical care. Br J Anaesth. 2007;98(6):707–721.
43. Leone BJ, Norris RM, Safwar A, Foëx P, Ryder A. Effects of progressive myocardial ischemia on systolic function, diastoli dysfunction and load dependent relaxation. Cardiovasc Res. 1992;26:422–429.
44. Kowalski M, Kukulski T, Jamal F, et al. Can natural strain and strain rate quantify regional myocardial deformation? A study in healthy subjects. Ultrasound Med Biol. 2001;27:1087–1097.
45. Kukulski T, Jamal F, D'Hooge J, Bijnens B, De Scheerder I, Sutherland GR. Acute changes in systolic and diastolic events during clinical coronary angioplasty: a comparison of regional velocity, strain rate and strain measurement. J Am Soc Echocardiogr. 2002;15:1–12.
46. Jain D, Zaret BL. Nuclear imaging techniques for the assessment of myocardial viability. Cardiol Clin. 1995;13:43–57.
47. Banka VS, Bodenheimer MM, Helfant RH. Relation between progressive decreases in regional coronary perfusion and contractile abnormalities. Am J Cardiol 1977;40(2):200–205.
48. Zabalgoitia M, Ismaeil M. Diagnostic and prognostic use of stress echo in acute coronary syndromes including emergency department imaging. Echocardiography. 2000;17(5):479–493.
49. Sabia P, Afrookteh A, Touchstone DA, Keller MW, Esquivel L, Kaul S. Value of regional wall motion abnormality in the emergency room diagnosis of acute myocardial infarction. A prospective study using two-dimensional echocardiography. Circulation. 1991;84(3 Suppl):I85–92.
50. Ingkanisorn WP, Kwong RY, Bohme NS, et al. Prognosis of negative adenosine stress magnetic resonance in patients presenting to an emergency department with chest pain. J Am Coll Cardiol. 2006;47(7):1427–1432.
51. Bedetti G, Pasanisi EM, Tintori G, et al. Stress echo in chest pain unit: the SPEED trial. Int J Cardiol. 2005;102(3):461–467.
52. Cheitlin, MD, Armstrong, WF, Aurigemma, GP, et al. ACC/AHA/ASE 2003 guideline for the clinical application of echocardiography. Available at: www.acc.org/qualityandscience/clinical/statements.htm
53. Teske AJ, De Boeck BW, Melman PG, Sieswerda GT, Doevendans PA. Echocardiographic quantification of myocardial function using tissue deformation imaging, a guide to image acquisition and analysis using tissue Doppler and speckle tracking. Cramer MJCardiovasc Ultrasound. 2007;5:27.

# Chapter 12
# How to Perform Stress Echocardiography

Bette Kim and Farooq A. Chaudhry

There are different modalities of stress echocardiography which can be used in the evaluation of patients with coronary artery disease. For patients who are able to exercise, treadmill and supine bicycle stress echocardiograms are preferred techniques. For patients unable to exercise, pharmacologic stress testing using dobutamine, dipyridamole, or adenosine is an alternative method to provoke ischemia. These various stress modalities will be discussed in detail (Table 12.1).

**Table 12.1** Methods to induce Stress

| Exercise | Pharmacological |
|---|---|
| Treadmill | Dobutamine |
| Supine bicycle | Dipyridamole |
| Isometric | Adenosine |

The basic principle of stress echocardiography is the identification of new wall motion abnormalities that occur in the presence of ischemia. This involves the comparison of baseline echocardiographic images obtained under resting conditions with those obtained immediately post-exercise in the case of treadmill or peak exercise in the case of bicycle protocol. Parasternal long and short axis as well as apical two, three, and four chamber views are acquired at baseline and post-stress testing. The left ventricle is divided into 16 segments as per the recommendation of the American Society of Echocardiography. All images are digitized in a continuous loop format utilizing a quad-screen format to facilitate the detection of new segmental wall motion abnormalities. The digitizer allows for the capture of a complete cardiac cycle that is then continuously played on a cine loop format for ease of analysis. The best post-exercise image is selected and compared with the baseline image by side to side comparison in the quad-screen image format[1] (Fig. 12.1).

B. Kim (✉)
Division of Cardiology, St. Luke's-Roosevelt Hospital Center, New York, NY, USA
e-mail: bekim@chpnet.org

E. Herzog, F.A. Chaudhry (eds.), *Echocardiography in Acute Coronary Syndrome*, 161
DOI 10.1007/978-1-84882-027-2_12, © Springer-Verlag London Limited 2009

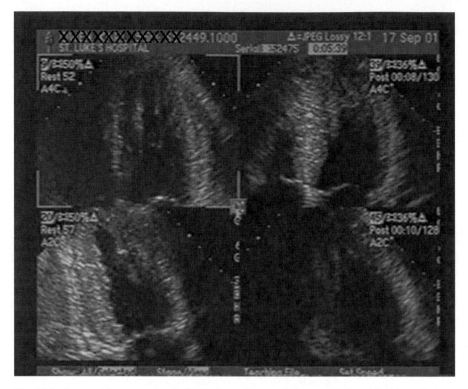

**Fig. 12.1** Rest and Post-exercise shuffled echocardiographic images displayed in the quad-screen format

## Treadmill Versus Bicycle Exercise Protocol

The most commonly used method for provoking ischemia in patients able to exercise is treadmill testing. The sensitivity of exercise testing is strongly dependent upon attaining adequate heart rate and cardiovascular workload. The use of treadmill or bicycle methods of exercise requires the patient to achieve a target heart rate of 85% of the age-predicted maximum heart rate or attain a workload of at least 6 METS in order to achieve satisfactory sensitivity. In patients who can achieve these workloads, exercise testing is the method of choice to provoke myocardial ischemia. Studies have shown that treadmill exercise testing results in higher heart rates compared with bicycle exercise. However, systolic blood pressure increases are more pronounced with bicycle exercise compared to treadmill exercise. Despite these differences, these two tests are probably comparable as the double products are similar.[1] The advantage of supine bicycle stress testing include imaging at peak stress as well as the easy identification of Doppler abnormalities which occur with peak exercise such as left ventricular outflow tract obstruction, mitral regurgitation, or tricuspid regurgitation.

The most common treadmill protocol used is the Bruce protocol, although other protocols such as the modified Bruce or Naughton can be used depending upon the level of fitness of the patient. According to standard stress testing protocol, the patient has continuously ECG monitoring with exercise, and blood pressure is checked every 3 min. With treadmill exercise, the post-exercise images are obtained ideally within less than 1 min.

The exercise test should be terminated if any of the following occur:

1. Severe symptoms such as chest pain or dyspnea
2. Severe ST depressions
3. Hemodynamically significant arrhythmia
4. Severe hypertensive response (BP > 220/120 mmHg)
5. Hypotension (a decrease of >20 mmHg)

## Pharmacologic Stress Echocardiogram: Dobutamine

For those patients who cannot exercise, dobutamine, dipyridamole or adenosine stress echocardiograms can alternatively be performed. By far, dobutamine is the most common pharmacologic agent used to provoke ischemia in stress echocardiograms. Dobutamine is a synthetic catecholamine that binds to beta 1 and beta 2 receptors. The affinity of dobutamine for beta 1 cardiac muscle receptors results in positive inotropic and chronotropic effects. Therefore, dobutamine induces myocardial ischemia in patients with flow-limiting coronary stenosis by increasing left ventricular contractility, heart rate, wall stress, and therefore myocardial oxygen demand. Dobutamine has a short half-life and is rapidly metabolized once the infusion is discontinued. Any adverse side effects or arrhythmias can usually be quickly terminated by discontinuation of the drip or by intravenous beta blockers.[2]

Dobutamine protocol:

1. The patient is asked not to eat for 4–6 h prior to the dobutamine stress echocardiogram.
2. Baseline heart rate, blood pressure, and electrocardiogram are obtained. Peripheral intravenous access is obtained. Baseline echocardiographic images are obtained in the standard views as described earlier.
3. Dobutamine infusion is started at 5 mcg/kg/min if the patient has underlying wall motion abnormalities to assess for viability; otherwise, the infusion is begun at 10 mcg/kg/min and increased in a stepwise manner by 10 mcg/kg/min every 3 min to a maximum infusion rate of 50 mcg/kg/min. If the patient's heart rate response to dobutamine is suboptimal, atropine can be given in 0.25 mg increments to a maximum dose of 2 mg beginning at the 30–40 mcg/kg/min dose of dobutamine. In those patients who do not take beta blockers, handgrip exercise

as well as leg exercises beginning at the 30–40 mcg/kg/min stage of dobutamine has been shown to decrease the time to achieve target heart rate and decrease the need for atropine.[3]

4. Blood pressure and EKG obtained with each stage of dobutamine.
5. Standard echocardiographic images are obtained at rest, low-dose dobutamine, peak dose dobutamine, and in recovery. These images along with baseline images are digitized and displayed in a quad-screen format (Fig. 12.2).

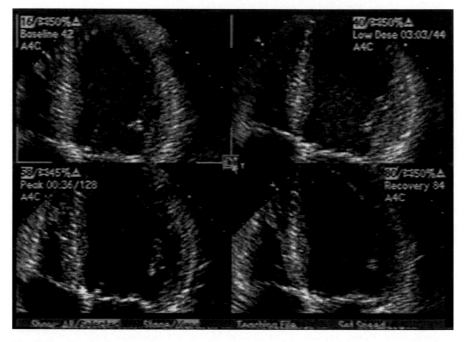

**Fig. 12.2** Shuffled Dobutamine echocardiographic images in the quad-screen format with the resting image in the *upper left*, low-dose image displayed in the *upper right*, peak stress image in the *lower left*, and the recovery image in the *lower right*

Indications for dobutamine infusion termination:

1. Reaching 85% of age-predicted maximum heart rate
2. Development of new wall motion abnormalities
3. Maximum dobutamine dose
4. Severe symptoms
5. Ventricular tachycardia or supraventricular tachycardia
6. Severe ST depressions
7. Severe hypertension (BP > 220/120 mmHg)
8. Hypotension (a decrease of 20 mmHg from the previous level of infusion should be used as a guide, but terminating the infusion should be at the discretion of the physician monitoring the test)

## Adenosine and Dipyridamole Stress Echocardiography

Both adenosine and dipyridamole are potent vasodilators. Adenosine increases intracellular cyclic adenosine monophosphate (cyclic AMP) and cyclic guanosine monophosphate (cyclic GMP) which results in smooth muscle relaxation. Dipyridamole works by blocking the uptake of adenosine by endothelial cells which thus leads to an increase in the concentration of adenosine within the myocardial and arterial walls. In myocardial regions perfused by normal coronary arteries, blood flow increases in both endocardial and epicardial layers reflecting normal coronary flow reserve. With a critical coronary stenosis, flow may increase in the epicardium but fall in the subendocardium distal to the flow-limiting stenosis.[4]

Adenosine and dipyridamole stress echocardiography are not preferred pharmacologic stress echo modalities. Dobutamine stress echocardiography has far greater sensitivity to detect coronary artery disease and is better tolerated compared with adenosine and dipyridamole protocols. The sensitivity of dobutamine stress echocardiography is 76% (95% CI, 59–93%) compared with adenosine (40%; CI, 21–59%; $p < 0.001$) and dipyridamole (56%; CI, 37–75%; $p = 0.019$).[5] However, using adenosine and dipyridamole in conjunction with myocardial contrast perfusion echocardiography is a promising technique to detect significant coronary artery disease.[6]

Adenosine and dipyridamole stress echocardiography protocol consists of the standard two-dimensional parasternal long and short axis as well as apical two, three, and four chamber views acquired at baseline and post-stress testing. The patient is monitored with continuous electrocardiographic monitoring during the infusion. Vital signs are monitored every 2 min throughout the protocol and into recovery. Adenosine is infused at 140 mcg/kg/min and some centers have used a level as high as 200 mcg/kg/min for 6 min. Dipyridamole is infused at 0.56 mg/kg to as high as 0.84 mg/kg at some centers over 4–6 min. Wall motion is recorded during the last 3 min of the adenosine infusion and between 2 and 5 min after completion of the dipyridamole infusion.

Contraindications for adenosine or dipyridamole stress echocardiography include the following:

1. Severe asthma with active wheezing
2. Systolic BP of less than 90 mmHg
3. Second or third degree heart block
4. Use of dipyridamole or aminophylline medications within the last 24 h
5. Ingestion of caffeinated foods within 12 h of the test
6. Unstable angina or acute coronary syndrome

Adenosine and dipyridamole infusions can cause a modest increase in heart rate and a modest decrease in blood pressure. Minor side effects of adenosine and dipyridamole infusions include flushing, chest pain, dyspnea, dizziness, and nausea. A small incidence of transient AV block has been described. The infusion of adenosine or dipyridamole should be terminated in the setting of severe hypotension, symptomatic, persistent second or third degree heart block, wheezing, or severe chest pain. Aminophylline can be used to reverse symptoms related to the dipyridamole infusion. Because of the very short half-life of adenosine, aminophylline is rarely required to treat symptoms.[4]

# Conclusion

There are several different stress echocardiographic protocols which can be used in the diagnosis of coronary artery disease. For those patients able to exercise, treadmill or bicycle stress echocardiograms are the preferred modalities. Symptoms obtained with exercise as well as ECG changes, blood pressure response, and workload achieved are all important clinical and prognostic parameters which should be incorporated with the cardiac imaging results. Pharmacologic stress should be reserved for those patients who cannot attain an adequate workload. Dobutamine stress echocardiography is the preferred pharmacologic stress echocardiographic modality compared with adenosine or dipyridamole. Dobutamine echocardiography is more sensitive than adenosine or dipyridamole to detect coronary artery disease and is better tolerated. However, adenosine and dipyridamole may play a greater role in stress echocardiography when myocardial contrast perfusion echocardiography becomes clinically available.

# References

1. Lambert KL, Sehgal R, Danao N, McNeal M, Tommaso C, Chaudhry FA. Principles and techniques of stress echocardiography. *Video J Echopcardiog*. 1993;3:5–11.
2. Valentini V, Greenfield S, McDermott E, McNeal M, Danao N, Chaudhry FA. Principles and techniques of pharmacologic stress echocardiography. *Video J Echocardiog*. 1993;3:82–89.
3. Yao S-S, Moldenhauer S, Sherrid MV. Isometric handgrip exercise during dobutamine-atropine stress echocardiography increases heart rate acceleration and decreases study duration and dobutamine and atropine dosage. *Clin Cardiol*. 2003;26:238–242.
4. Chaudhry FA. Adenosine stress echocardiography. *Am J Cardiol*. 1997;79:25–29.
5. Martin TW, Seawoth JF, Johns JP, Pupa LE, Condos WR. Comparison of adenosine, dipyridamole, and dobutamine in stress echocardiography. *Ann Int Med*. 1992;116:190–196.
6. Dijkmans PA, Senior R, Becher H, et al. Myocardial contrast echocardiography evolving as a clinically feasible technique for accurate, rapid and safe assessment of myocardial perfusion: the evidence so far. *J am Coll Cardiol*. 2006;48(11):2168–2177.

# Chapter 13
# Principles of Interpretation of Stress Echocardiography

**Kameswari Maganti and Vera H. Rigolin**

Stress echocardiography was introduced in the early 1980s and has matured into a robust, versatile, widely available, reliable, and cost-effective technique utilized for noninvasive imaging of the heart. In combination with a variety of stressors, stress echocardiography provides a means for the detection of ischemia by assessment of regional wall motion abnormalities. In addition to its utility in detection and accurate risk stratification of patients with suspected and established coronary artery disease, it has a role in assessment of severity of valvular heart disease by providing valuable physiological hemodynamic data and also has a proven role in the assessment of myocardial viability in patients with dyssynergic segments as well as with left ventricular dysfunction.

This chapter will provide an overview of the interpretation of stress echocardiography.

## Pathophysiology

With dynamic exercise or inotropic stress, the normal response is an increase in heart rate, endocardial excursion, systolic wall thickening, and ejection fraction with a decrease in systolic dimensions and volumes. An abnormal response typically is noted as new or worsening wall motion abnormalities, increase in the left ventricular cavity size, or a decrease in ejection fraction. Regional wall motion abnormalities usually precede ST segment changes and chest pain, but follow diastolic dysfunction and regional perfusion abnormalities. This ischemic cascade is delineated in Fig. 13.1.

K. Maganti (✉)
Cardiology, Northwestern University, Chicago, IL, USA
e-mail: k-maganti@northwestern.edu

E. Herzog, F.A. Chaudhry (eds.), *Echocardiography in Acute Coronary Syndrome*,     167
DOI 10.1007/978-1-84882-027-2_13, © Springer-Verlag London Limited 2009

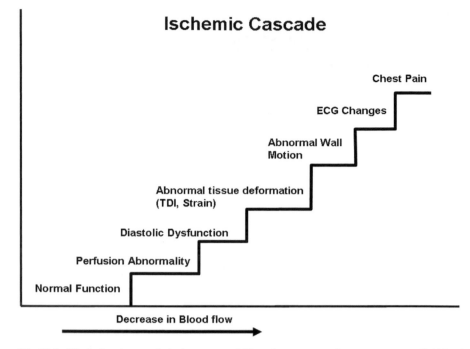

**Fig. 13.1** The ischemic cascade is demonstrated. Note the sequence of events as myocardial blood flow diminishes. The first abnormality noted is in myocardial perfusion. Diastolic dysfunction and myocardial deformation then follow. Abnormal wall motion then occurs, which is visually noted in an abnormal stress echo. The final abnormalities to occur are ECG changes followed by chest pain

## Methodology of Stress Echocardiography

The interpretation of stress echo begins with the knowledge of what type of stress test is being performed and the clinical response of the patient to the stressor.

Stress echocardiography may be performed using dynamic exercise (treadmill or bicycle) or pharmacologic stress in patients who are unable to exercise or when viability information is desired. Rarely, pacing stress using either a transvenous pacer or a transesophageal atrial pacer is used as an alternative to exercise.[1] In patients capable of exercising, dynamic exercise is preferred to pharmacologic stress as it provides information pertaining to exercise capacity which allows better prognostic discrimination. The selection of pharmacologic stress is mostly determined by local expertise.

With treadmill exercise stress echocardiography, the Bruce protocol is the most commonly used exercise protocol in the United States. With treadmill exercise, it is critical that post-exercise images are obtained within 1 min after cessation of the test. Unfortunately, resolution of wall motion abnormalities can occur quickly following the cessation of exercise, which reduces the sensitivity of the test. This may be obviated by the use of upright images which may be performed immediately at peak exercise in some patients.[2] Upright or supine bicycle stress echocardiography is attractive as it has the advantage of imaging the heart at peak exercise. The bicycle protocol is similar to the one for treadmill exercise in that exercise intensity can be increased every 3 min. The differences, however, are that image acquisition can be made at each stage of exercise and can be performed while the patient is still exercising. Performing the stress echo in this fashion permits adequate assessment at ischemic thresholds and a concurrent increase in the sensitivity for detection of coronary artery disease.[3]

Pharmacologic stress agents include dobutamine which is most widely used in the United States and vasodilator agents such as adenosine and dipyridamole which are less commonly used. Dobutamine, a sympathomimetic agent, has a unique method of action. At low doses, there is an increase in myocardial perfusion preferentially by recruitment of viable myocardium which thereby results in an increase in myocardial contractility. At high dose, however, there is an increase in myocardial oxygen demand and consumption due to increases in inotropic state, heart rate, and blood pressure.[4] If there is a flow-limiting stenosis, a demand/supply mismatch ensues, resulting in a new wall motion abnormality. Dobutamine is used as an infusion starting at 5 or 10 mcg/kg/min and is incrementally increased every 3–5 min till a maximal dose of 50 mcg/kg/min. Atropine is often used in conjunction with dobutamine for heart rate augmentation. Atropine may be given in incremental doses beginning at 0.25 mg and up to a total of 2.0 mg.

Vasodilator agents such as adenosine and dipyridamole are less commonly used for pharmacologic stress testing in the United States. These induce ischemia by induction of coronary steal which occurs in the setting of severe or extensive coronary artery disease.

## Image Acquisition/Stress Echo Protocols

A baseline exam with 2D, M mode, and, if indicated, Doppler assessment is performed using transthoracic harmonic imaging with two parasternal (long and short axis views) and two to three apical baseline views (four, two, and three chamber views). Transesophageal stress imaging is reserved for the rare patients with poor image quality[5] as the use of contrast for endocardial border delineation had in general obviated its need.

The peak exercise stress images are acquired immediately after the cessation of exercise. It is preferable that the images are acquired within 1 min after cessation of exercise and that they are acquired at or above 85% of the maximal predicted heart rate for age. In the dobutamine studies, the images are acquired at baseline, at each stage of the dobutamine infusion, and in recovery. Rest and stress images are arranged side by side for comparison and digital archiving. This allows for comparison of regional function as well as assessment of timing of contraction.

The rapid advances in image acquisition, image processing and digital display, and the development of harmonic and contrast imaging have certainly spurred the widespread use of stress echocardiography.[6-8] However, the interpretation stress echo is greatly dependent on image quality and rapid acquisition of post-exercise images. Continued problems with image quality in certain subsets of patients and technical expertise needed for image interpretation continue to be its biggest disadvantages. The use of an echo contrast agent should be considered in patients with poor image quality to assure the best diagnostic accuracy.

## Image Analysis

Interpretation of stress echocardiography is one of the most challenging aspects of echocardiography, and the standard approach is qualitative. The need for appropriate training and experience[9-11] as well as problems faced with reproducibility especially when many centers are involved[12] continues to be the biggest shortcomings of this modality. The reproducibility of the subjective interpretation of stress echocardiograms at a single, high-volume center with experienced readers is very good.[13,14] As the accuracy of stress echocardiography is based on evaluation of myocardial thickening and endocardial motion, it is essential that all the wall segments be adequately visualized.

The interpretation of stress echo is based on the subjective analysis of regional wall motion, left ventricular shape, and volume and ejection fraction at rest and after stress. The baseline images should be carefully inspected for any baseline wall motion abnormalities that may suggest prior myocardial infarction or hibernating myocardium. Baseline wall motion abnormalities may also be present for reasons other than coronary artery disease, such as a left bundle branch block, a paced rhythm, or a nonischemic cardiomyopathy. The other major advantage of stress echo compared to other imaging modalities is its ability to evaluate the other cardiac structures such as the valves and the pericardium. Close inspection of the entire heart often provides clues to the etiology of the patient's symptoms. In addition, previously unknown structural abnormalities can be detected that preclude safe exercise testing, such as severe aortic stenosis, hypertrophic cardiomyopathy, and large pericardial effusions. Fig. 13.2 shows an example of a patient who presented for a stress echo with previously unknown aortic stenosis.

The normal response to both pharmacological stress and exercise is an increase in myocardial excursion and a decrease in left ventricular end-systolic volume. The latter is noted visually as a decrease in left ventricular cavity size. Attention should also be paid to the right ventricular size and function. Fig. 13.3 shows an example of a normal stress echo. Regional wall motion analysis of the left ventricle should be performed in a systematic fashion with assessment of endocardial excursion in each segment.

The 2005 American Society of Echocardiography (ASE) Chamber Quantification Guidelines suggest that either a 16- or a 17-segment model of the left ventricle

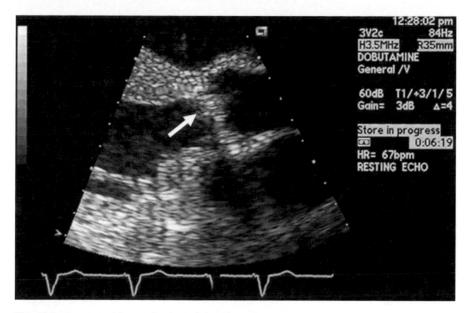

**Fig. 13.2** Parasternal long axis view of a patient who presented for a dobutamine stress echo for the evaluation of chest pain. He was found to have severe aortic stenosis, which was previously unknown (shown by *arrow*)

may be used for the assessment of regional wall motion (Fig. 13.4). The 17-segment model includes an "apical cap," a segment beyond the level that the LV cavity is seen. The 17-segment model is recommended if myocardial perfusion is evaluated or if echocardiography is compared with another imaging modality.[15] Regional wall motion is assessed by evaluating the basal, mid, and apical segments of each wall in a systematic fashion. The left ventricle can also be analyzed according to coronary artery distribution (Fig. 13.5). However, due to variability in coronary anatomy, accurate identification of the culprit coronary artery is not always possible, particularly when differentiating ischemia between the right coronary artery and the left circumflex.

Evaluation of left ventricular function is performed by calculation of wall motion score index, which is a unitless number that is directly proportional to the regional wall function. Each of the 16–17 myocardial segments is assigned a score in the following fashion: normal or hyperkinesis = 1, hypokinesis = 2, akinesis (negligible thickening) = 3, dyskinesis (paradoxical systolic motion) = 4, and aneurysmal (diastolic deformation) = 5. Wall motion score index can be derived as a sum of all scores divided by the number of segments visualized.[15] The rest and stress images are then compared.

Hypokinesis is defined as a decrease in endocardial thickening, but with some preservation. Hypokinesis has been arbitrarily defined as less than 5 mm of endocardial excursion. Akinesis is defined as complete absence of endocardial thickening and excursion. Dyskinesis is defined as systolic thinning and outward motion of the

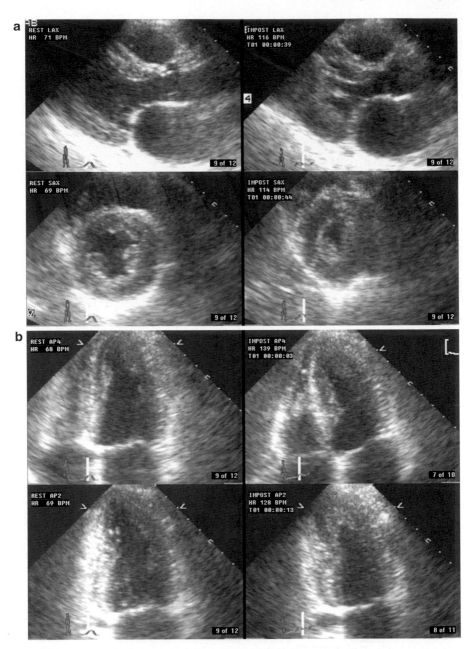

**Fig. 13.3** Rest and stress images of a patient with a normal stress echo. Frames are at end systole. **Panel A** shows the parasternal views. **Panel B** shows the apical views. Note the increase in endocardial thickening and the decrease in left ventricular cavity size post-exercise. Also note the preservation of the triangular shape of the left ventricle after exercise

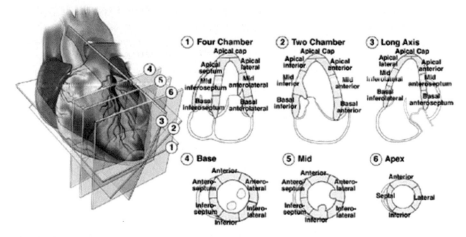

**Fig. 13.4** Segmental model of the left ventricle recommended for regional wall motion analysis by the American Society of Echocardiography. Reproduced with permission[15]

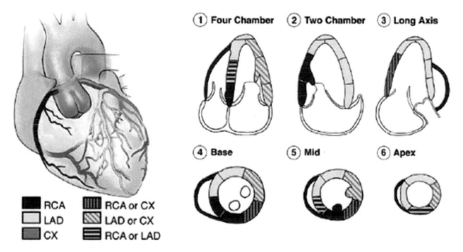

**Fig. 13.5** Segmental model of the left ventricle divided into the three major coronary artery territories. Reproduced with permission[15]

endocardium during systole.[16] An aneurysm is defined as a regional area of akinesis or dyskinesis and scar that has abnormal geometry in both systole and diastole.[17] The detection of regional wall motion abnormalities can often be challenging due to tethering of abnormal segments by adjacent normal regions. Close attention to endocardial thickening rather than motion alone can help obviate this problem and avoid false-negative readings. False-positive wall motion abnormalities can be a result of early relaxation, which is often a normal variant. Early relaxation occurs in a segment with normal early systolic excursion but early relaxation compared to other adjacent segments. Noting the normal early systolic contraction can help interpret this finding correctly. Translational motion of the heart from extra cardiac structures, such as the diaphragm or the liver, can also result in false-positive readings. The clue to the absence of ischemia in such cases is the presence of normal systolic thickening.

A normal response is augmentation of contractile function in all segments along with a decrease in left ventricular chamber size. The detection of ischemia is also aided by evaluating myocardial shape. When viewing the left ventricular chamber from the apical views, a triangular shape of the left ventricular cavity is appreciated. This is well appreciated in Fig. 13.3B. With exercise or pharmacologic stimulation, the size of the left ventricular cavity should decrease, but the triangular shape should be maintained. Fig. 13.6A and B provides an example of a patient with severe left circumflex stenosis. Note the increase in cavity size and loss of the triangular shape in the apical images post-exercise.

Lack of hyperkinesis of the myocardium and failure of left ventricular end-systolic volume to decline is always an abnormal finding. An increase in end-systolic volume post-exercise is often associated with multi-vessel coronary disease. Fig. 13.7 provides an example of a patient with two-vessel coronary artery disease with significant stenosis noted in the left anterior descending as well as the right coronary arteries. Although such findings often represent coronary ischemia, there are other factors that can result in similar findings. These include a severely hypertensive response to exercise, the presence of a nonischemic cardiomyopathy, beta blocker therapy, left bundle branch block, submaximal exercise, or a delay in acquiring the post-exercise images.[16] Therefore, the interpretation of the results needs to include a comprehensive knowledge of all aspects of the patient and the circumstances of the test itself. Fig. 13.8 demonstrates a false-positive stress echo of a patient with a hypertensive response to exercise and an increase in cavity size post-exercise.

An increase in left ventricular volumes can be seen as a normal response in patients undergoing supine exercise bike testing. Elevation of the legs during exercise increases venous return, so an increase in ventricular volumes at peak exercise may be a normal finding. However, cavity size should rapidly decrease once exercise is stopped.[16]

Determination of ischemia involves identification of a new or worsening wall motion abnormality. The different myocardial responses to stress are elucidated in Table 13.1. Ischemia is defined as a normal segment worsening wall motion post-stress. A resting wall motion abnormality that remains unchanged post-exercise suggests the presence of a myocardial infarction.

To better serve the referring physician, in addition to interpretation of test as normal or abnormal, the site, extent, and severity of abnormality should be described as well as the ischemic threshold. The report must also include the baseline and stress assessment of global and regional systolic function, segmental wall motion, protocol used, the exercise time or dose of pharmacologic agent used, the maximum heart rate achieved, whether the level of stress was adequate, the blood pressure response, the reason for test termination, any cardiac symptoms during the test, and electrocardiographic changes or significant arrhythmias.[11]

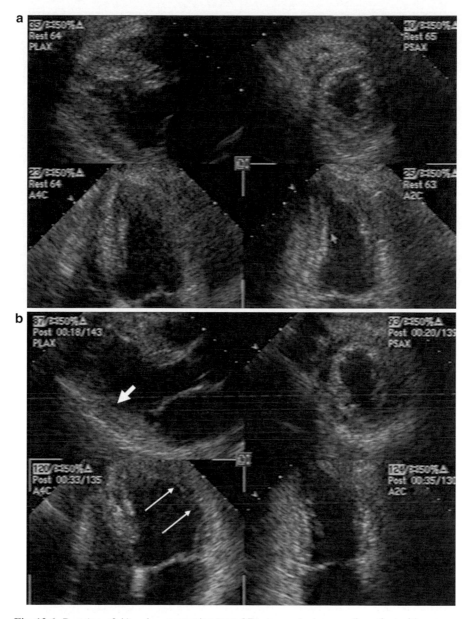

**Fig. 13.6** Rest (**panel A**) and post-exercise (**panel B**) stress echo images of a patient with a severe stenosis of the left circumflex artery. Note the decrease in wall thickening of the anterolateral and inferolateral walls (*arrows*). In addition, there is an increase in cavity size and loss of the triangular shape of the left ventricle in the apical views post-exercise

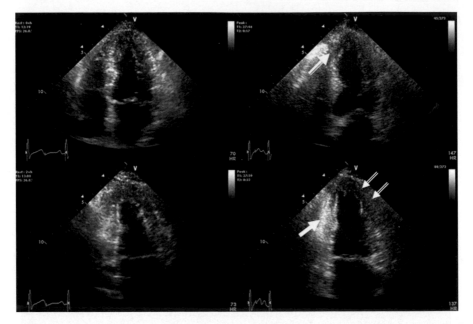

**Fig. 13.7** Pre and post-exercise end-systolic frames of the apical images of a patient who presented for a stress echo for evaluation of chest pain and shortness of breath. Note the cavity dilatation post-exercise. In addition, there is new hypokinesis of the apical anterior wall (*double arrow*), the apical septum (*large arrow*), and failure of the inferior wall to augment its contraction (*single, small arrow*). The findings are suggestive of severe disease in the mid left anterior descending artery and the proximal right coronary artery

**Table 13.1** Interpretation of response to stress echocardiography

| Response | Baseline/rest | Low dose | Peak stress |
|---|---|---|---|
| Normal | Normal | Normal, hyperkinetic | Hyperkinetic |
| Ischemic | Normal | Normal, hypokinetic/akinetic | Hypokinetic/Akinetic |
| Ischemic | Hypokinetic | Hypokinetic/Akinetic | Hypokinetic/akinetic compared to baseline |
| Ischemic: Viability+ | Resting WMA | Improvement | Hypokinetic/akinetic compared to baseline c |
| Nonischemic: Viability+ | Resting WMA | Improvement | Continued improvement |
| Infarction | Resting WMA | No change | No change |

Given the various limitations that are inherent to the current stress testing methodologies, techniques proposed to improve accuracy of stress echocardiography have included peak exercise imaging,[13,14] 3D imaging,[18] myocardial contrast perfusion imaging,[19,20] combined stress modalities,[21] and methods to quantify regional wall motion, including acoustic quantification and color kinesis, which

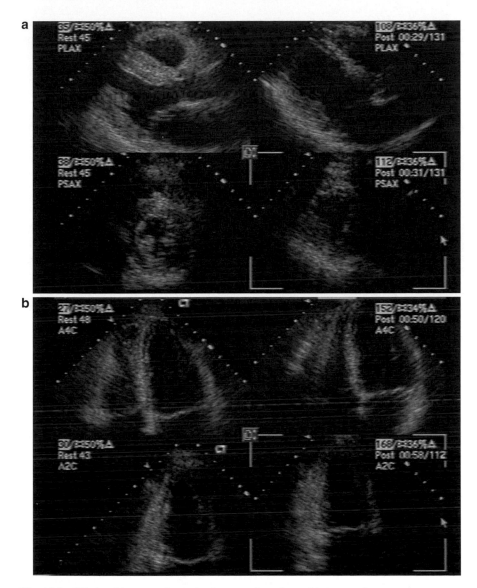

**Fig. 13.8** Side by side rest and exercise images of a patient with a severe hypertensive response to exercise. Note the cavity dilatation post-exercise. Coronary angiography later showed normal coronary arteries

involve tracking the blood and myocardial tissue interface.[22] Tissue Doppler and strain rate imaging have provided quantifiable and reproducible assessment of regional myocardial contractile function. The advantage of higher temporal resolution makes these procedures attractive for interpretation of subtle abnormalities that are undetected by the naked eye.[23] Whether the newer methods add anything additional to the current interpretation by an experienced interpreter needs to be further defined, and future studies are needed to document improvement over existing methods.

## Accuracy of Stress Echocardiography for the Detection of Coronary Artery Disease

### Diagnostic Utility in Coronary Artery Disease

Stenosis severity as well as plaque morphology seems to determine the results of dobutamine and dipyridamole stress testing, whereas the results of exercise stress echocardiography, although separately influenced by plaque morphology, are predominantly influenced by stenosis severity. With simple lesion morphologies, dobutamine and particularly dipyridamole with a lower ischemic potential may not reach ischemic threshold, while exercise may achieve it due to the higher inherent ischemic potential. On the other side in patients with a complex lesion of similar severity, the ischemic threshold may be reached by all three tests due to the lower ischemic threshold of the lesion. Integrated evaluation of angiographic variables has shown that the coronary arteriographic cutoff of luminal diameter stenosis at which wall thickening abnormalities occur is 54% for exercise, 58% for dobutamine, and 60% for dipyridamole.[24,25]

The primary factors that alter the sensitivity and specificity of stress echo are listed in Table 13.2. Other factors that reduce the sensitivity include distal atherosclerotic lesions, concurrent antianginal medications, the presence of collaterals, and, in the case of exercise, too much time taken to acquire post-exercise images (Fig. 13.9).

The diagnostic accuracy of stress echo is greatly affected by the presence of concentric remodeling of the left ventricle. In a study by Smart et al., patients with increased wall thickness and small chamber size showed a disproportionate increase

**Table 13.2** Factors that impact the accuracy of interpretation of stress echocardiograms

| False-positive studies | False-negative studies |
| --- | --- |
| Hypertensive response to stress | Submaximal stress |
| Microvascular disease, e.g., diabetes, syndrome X, left ventricular hypertrophy, etc. | Poor image quality |
| Cardiomyopathies | Concentric remodeling |
| Paradoxical septal motion, e.g., post-cardiac surgery, LBBB, etc. | Hyperdynamic state accompanying significant Ar or MR |
| Coronary spasm | L circumflex disease |
| Localized basal inferior wall motion abnormalities | Mild coronary stenoses |
| Overinterpretation | Single vessel disease |

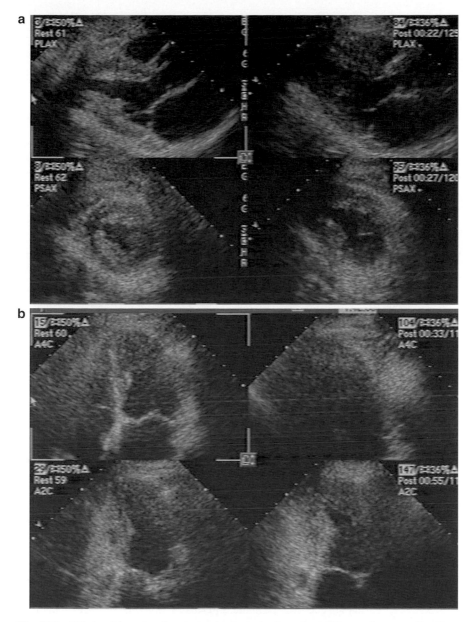

**Fig. 13.9** Side by side rest and post-exercise images of a patient with poor image quality. Post-exercise image acquisition was delayed due to difficulty in acquiring the images. The study was read as normal. Coronary angiography later showed severe left main stenosis

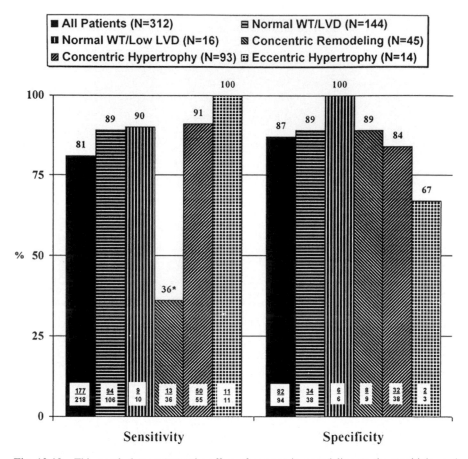

**Fig. 13.10** This graph demonstrates the effect of concentric remodeling on the sensitivity and specificity of dobutamine stress echocardiography. Note the marked decrease in sensitivity in the patients with concentric remodeling. WT = wall thickness, LVD = left ventricular minor axis dimension. Reproduced with permission[26]

in false-negative dobutamine stress echo studies (Fig. 13.10). The authors postulate that a blunted increase in systolic wall stress with dobutamine may account for this finding.[26]

Studies comparing the accuracy of nuclear perfusion imaging and stress echocardiography have shown that the tests have similar sensitivities for the detection of coronary artery disease (CAD) in the same patient population, but stress echocardiography has higher specificity.[25–29] Myocardial perfusion imaging detects a relative reduction in myocardial blood volume that occurs earlier than wall thickening abnormality in the ischemic cascade. Despite this, there was no significant difference between the two techniques in the sensitivity for location of CAD and in the prediction of multi-vessel CAD.[30]

In a pooled analysis of 18 studies in 1304 patients who underwent exercise or pharmacologic stress echocardiography in conjunction with thallium or technetium-labeled radioisotope imaging, sensitivity and specificity were 80 and 86% for echocardiography and 84 and 77% for myocardial perfusion imaging, respectively.[11,27] The lack of significant difference in sensitivity between myocardial perfusion imaging and stress echocardiography may be explained by two major factors: Myocardial perfusion imaging requires a difference of at least 35% decrease in myocardial blood volume before a relative perfusion defect is appreciated, with a poor spatial resolution about 12 mm. Conversely, echocardiographic wall thickening abnormalities are assessed independently in each vascular territory with a far greater spatial resolution of about 2 mm.[31] The factors that impact the accuracy of stress echocardiography are outlined in Table 13.2.[32–37]

## Diagnostic Utility in Symptomatic Women

ECG stress testing remains the oldest and most used modality to diagnose coronary artery disease in both men and women. However, ECG stress testing has been reported to have diminished accuracy in women due to more frequent resting ST-T abnormalities, diminished voltage, and the effect of estrogen on the ST segments.[38–53] The addition of echocardiographic imaging to ECG stress testing has been shown in numerous studies to improve the diagnostic accuracy over ECG stress testing alone.[54,55] When the data are combined from various studies on nearly 1000 women, stress echo was found to have a sensitivity of 81% (89% for multivessel disease), a specificity of 86%, and an overall accuracy of 84%.[54,56–67]

Dobutamine echo reliably detects significant obstructive disease in women who are unable to exercise. The studies evaluating the utility of DSE for the detection of CAD in women have demonstrated sensitivities ranging from 75 to 93% and specificities of 79–92%, with an overall accuracy of 82–88%.[58, 59, 62, 63, 67, 68] The diagnostic accuracy of both exercise and dobutamine stress echo is gender neutral, with similar accuracies for both men and women.

## Dobutamine Echocardiography for the Assessment of Myocardial Viability

Myocardial viability refers to dysfunctional myocardium that is potentially reversible. The differentiation between dysfunctional yet viable versus nonviable myocardium poses significant diagnostic challenges since both appear similar in the resting state. Several techniques have been proposed to detect myocardial viability in order to determine the best candidates for coronary revascularization. Such techniques include dobutamine stress echocardiography, thallium rest–redistribution, positron emission tomography (PET), and magnetic resonance imaging.

The interpretation of wall motion in dobutamine stress echo is challenging due to the frequent presence of markedly dysfunctional myocardium at rest. Viability is defined as a dysfunctional segment at rest that improves contractile function by at least one grade in response to dobutamine. Ischemia is defined as deterioration in contractile function. An improvement in contractility (viability) followed by ischemia is called the biphasic response. This is appreciated in Fig. 13.11. This response is the most specific for the improvement in wall motion following revascularization.[69] The various types of responses to dobutamine are listed in Table 13.1.

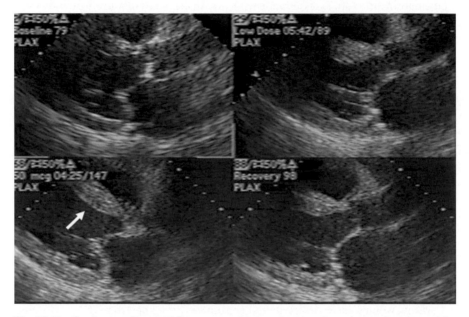

**Fig. 13.11** Quad-screen image of the parasternal long axis view of a patient undergoing a dobutamine viability study. The *left upper panel* is the resting image. The *right upper panel* is during low-dose dobutamine administration. Note the improvement in wall motion and the decrease in cavity size. The *left lower panel* is during peak dobutamine administration. Now there is an increase in cavity size due to hypokinesis of the anteroseptum. The improvement in contractile function followed by deterioration (viability + ischemia) is referred to as the biphasic response. The *right lower panel* was taken during recovery

A review of data from 402 patients in 15 studies revealed that the sensitivities and specificities for dobutamine predicting regional wall motion after revascularization range from 74 to 95%.[70–83]

Compared to the other techniques, dobutamine echo is less sensitive but more specific for the detection of viability.[84,85] The difference in accuracy may be explained by the mechanistic differences between dobutamine echo and the other techniques. For example, dobutamine echo measures viability using contractile reserve whereas thallium measures cell membrane activity. Blood flow and flow reserve may be reduced so that contractile function is lost while transmembrane

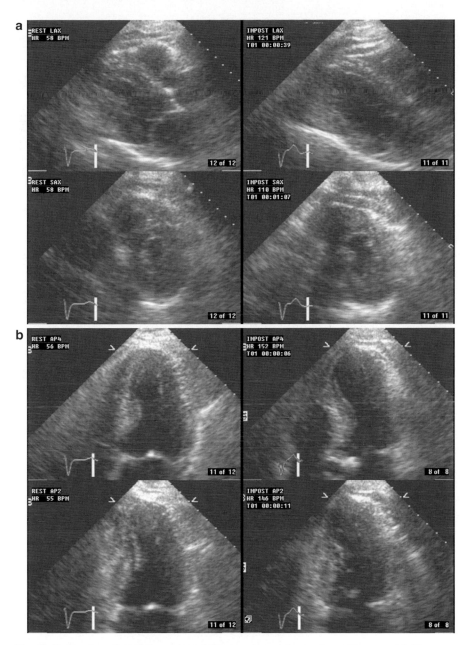

**Fig. 13.12** Pre (**panel A**) and post (**panel B**)-stress images in a patient with severe AS. The stress test was done since the patient claimed to be asymptomatic. Note the increase in cavity size. The patient also had a decrease in blood pressure during exercise that led to the termination of exercise at 5 min on a Bruce protocol. The patient was subsequently referred for valve replacement surgery

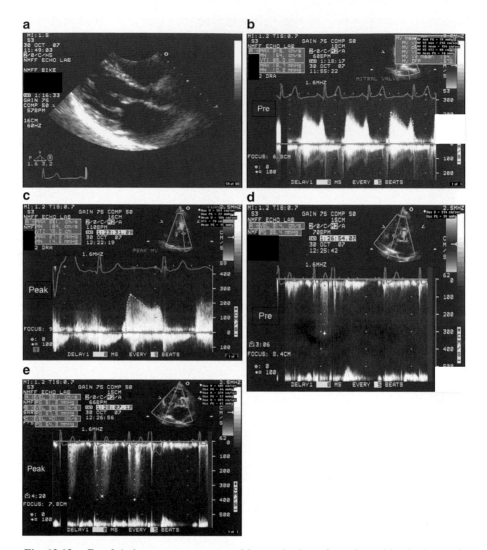

**Fig. 13.13** **Panel A** demonstrates parasternal long axis view of a patient with mitral stenosis. **Panels B and C** demonstrate mitral valve gradients at rest and peak exercise. Note the increase in the mean transmitral gradient from 10.2 to 14.6 mmHg. **Panels D and E** show the spectral Doppler of tricuspid regurgitation pre and peak exercise. The right ventricular systolic pressure increased from 49 to 74 mmHg

pump activity remains.[81,82] A critical mass of viable cells is needed for contractile reserve (>50% in a given segment) in order for wall motion to improve following revascularization.[83] Thallium and PET are thus able to detect a small mass of viable cells that may be insufficient to result in improved function following revascularization.

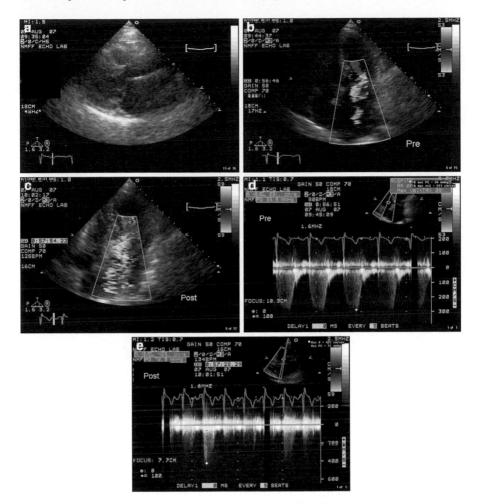

**Fig. 13.14   Panel A** shows the parasternal long axis view of a patient with mitral valve prolapse and a flail P2 segment. **Panels B and C** show the apical four-chamber view demonstrating the increase in the severity of mitral regurgitation pre and post-exercise. **Panels D and E** show the spectral Doppler of tricuspid regurgitation pre and post-exercise. The right ventricular systolic pressure increased from 44 to 82 mmHg post-exercise, assuming a right atrial pressure of 10 mmHg

## The Use of Stress Echo for the Assessment of Valvular Heart Disease

Stress echocardiography can be extremely useful for the assessment of valvular heart disease, particularly in situations where symptoms may be present and valve lesion severity is borderline. Specific clinical scenarios where stress echo has been found to be useful include mitral stenosis, mitral regurgitation, aortic stenosis,

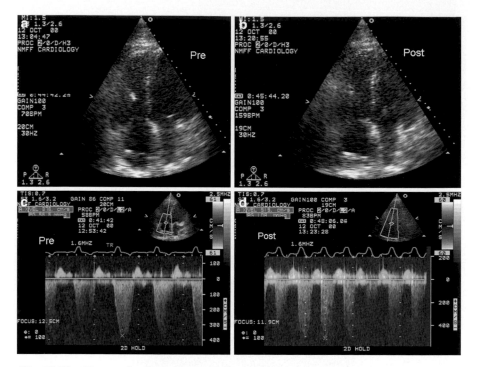

**Fig. 13.15** These series of figures are from a patient with Tetralogy of Fallot and pulmonic stenosis. At rest, right ventricular function is normal. The right atrial–right ventricular pressure gradient was 67 mmHg. After exercise, there is an increase in the size of the right atrium and the right ventricle. The right atrial–right ventricular pressure gradient increases to 108 mmHg

prosthetic valve dysfunction, and congenital heart disease. The interpretation of stress echo for non-coronary artery disease relies heavily on the interpretation of Doppler findings. In addition, however, the assessment of the left and right ventricles to stress also provides a clue to the hemodynamic significance of the valve lesion. Figures 13.12, 13.13, 13.14, and 13.15 demonstrate the utility of stress echo in patients with various valvular lesions.

## Summary

Stress echocardiography has been well validated as a sensitive and specific test for the diagnosis, assessment, and prognosis of coronary artery disease. Over the past decade, numerous studies have documented its role in a wide variety of patient populations. The interpretation of stress echo imaging is dependent on image quality, rapid image acquisition, and expertise of the interpreter. The future of this technique will be determined by the development of more precise quantification methods and other technical developments to improve image quality, interpretation, and reproducibility.

# References

1. Stratmann HG, Kennedy HL. Evaluation of coronary artery disease in the patient unable to exercise: alternatives to exercise stress testing. *Am Heart J*. 1989;June:117(6):1344–65.
2. Peteiro J, Garrido I, Monserrat L, et al. Comparison of peak and postexercise treadmill echocardiography with the use of continuous harmonic imaging acquisition. *J Am Soc Echocardiogr*. 2004;17:1044–1049.
3. Modesto K, Rainbird A, Klarich K, et al. Comparison of supine bicycle exercise and treadmill exercise Doppler echocardiography in evaluation of patients with coronary artery disease. *Am J Cardiol*. 2003; 91:1245–1248.
4. Barasch E, Wilansky S. Dobutamine stress echocardiography in clinical practice with a review of the recent literature. *Tex Heart Inst J*. 1994;21(3):202–210.
5. Chaudhry FA, Tauke JT, Alessandrini RS, Greenfield SA, Tommasso CL, Bonow RO. Enhanced detection of ischemic myocardium by transesophageal dobutamine stress echocardiography: comparison with simultaneous transthoracic echocardiography. Echocardiography. 2000 April;17(3):241–253.
6. Hoffmann R, Marwick TH, Poldermans D, et al. Refinements in stress echocardiographic techniques improve inter-institutional agreement in interpretation of dobutamine stress echocardiograms. *Eur Heart J*. 2002;23:821–829.
7. Mälder CF, Payne N, Wilkenshoff U, et al. Non-invasive diagnosis of coronary artery disease by quantitative stress echocardiography. *Eur Heart J*. 2003;24:1584–1594.
8. Rainbird AJ, Mulvagh SL, McCully OJK, et al. Contrast dobutamine stress echocardiography: clinical practice assessment in 300 consecutive patients. *J Am Soc Echocardiogr*. 2001;14:378–385.
9. Picano E, Lattanzi F, Orlandini A, et al. Stress echocardiography and the human factor: the importance of being expert. *J Am Coll Cardiol*. 1991;17:666–669.
10. Quinones MA, Douglas PS, Foster E et al. ACC/AHA clinical competence statement on echocardiography a report of the American College of Cardiology/American Heart Association/American College of Physicians/American Society of Internal Medicine Task Force on Clinical Competence, *J Am Coll Cardiol*. 2003;41:687–708.
11. Pellikka PA, Nagueh SF, Elhendy AA, et al. American Society of Echocardiography recommendations for performance, interpretation, and application of stress echocardiography. *J Am Soc Echocardiogr*. 2007 September;20(9):1021–1041
12. Hoffmann R, Lethen H, Marwick T, et al. Analysis of interinstitutional observer agreement in interpretation of dobutamine stress echocardiograms. *J Am Coll Cardiol*. 1996;27:330–336.
13. Chuah S, Pellikka P, Roger V, et al. Role of dobutamine stress echocardiography in predicting outcome in 860 patients with known or suspected coronary artery disease. Circulation. 1998; 97:1474–1480.
14. Arruda A, Das M, Roger V, et al. Prognostic value of exercise echocardiography in 2,632 patients >=65 years of age. *J Am Coll Cardiol*. 2001;37:1036–1041.
15. Lang R., Bierig M, Devereux R, Flachskampf F, Foster E, Pellikka P, et al: Recommendations for chamber quantification: a report from the American Society of Echocardiography's guidelines and standards committee and the chamber quantification writing group, developed in conjunction with the European Association of Echocardiography, a branch of the European Society of Cardiology. *J Am Soc Echocardiogr*. 2005;18:1440–1463.
16. Feigenbaum H, Armstrong W, Ryan T. Stress echocardiography. In: Feigenbaum H, Armstrong W, Ryan T, eds. *Echocardiography*. Philadelphia: Lippincott Williams and Wilkins; 2005:488–522.

17. Feigenbaum H, Armstrong W, Ryan T. Coronary artery disease. In: Feigenbaum H, Armstrong W, Ryan T, eds. *Echocardiography*. Philadelphia: Lippincott Williams and Wilkins; 2005:437–487.
18. Ahmad M, Tianrong X, McCulloch M, et al. Real-time three-dimensional dobutamine stress echocardiography in assessment of ischemia: comparison with two-dimensional dobutamine stress echocardiography. *J Am Coll Cardiol*. 2001;37:1303–1308.
19. Elhendy A, O'Leary E, Xie F, et al. TR P: comparative accuracy of real-time myocardial contrast perfusion imaging and wall motion analysis during dobutamine stress echocardiography for the diagnosis of coronary artery disease. *J Am Coll Cardiol*. 2004;44:2185–2191.
20. Moir S, Haluska B, Jenkins C, et al. Incremental benefit of myocardial contrast to combine dipyridamole-exercise stress echocardiography for the assessment of coronary artery disease. *Circulation*, 2004;110:1108–1113.
21. Ling L, Pellikka P, Mahoney D, et al. Atropine augmentation in dobutamine stress echocardiography: role and incremental value in a clinical practice setting. *J Am Coll Cardiol*. 1996;28:551–557.
22. Mor-Avi V, Vignon P, Koch R, et al. Segmental analysis of color kinesis images: new method for quantification of the magnitude and timing of endocardial motion during left ventricular systole and diastole. *Circulation*. 1997;95:2082–2097.
23. Smiseth O, Stoylen A, Halfdan I. Tissue Doppler imaging for the diagnosis of coronary artery disease. *Curr Opin Cardiol*. 2004;19:421–429.
24. Marwick TH. Stress echocardiography. *Heart*. 2003;89:113–118.
25. Quinones M, Verani M, Haichin R, et al. Exercise echocardiography versus 201T1 single-photon emission computed tomography in evaluation of coronary artery disease: analysis of 292 patients. *Circulation*. 1992;85:1217–1218.
26. Fleischmann K, Hunink M, Kuntz K, et al. Exercise echocardiography or exercise SPECT imaging? A meta-analysis of diagnostic test performance. *JAMA*. 1998;280:913–920.
27. Schinkel A, Bax J, Geleijnse M, et al. Noninvasive evaluation of ischemic heart disease: myocardial perfusion imaging or stress echocardiography? *Eur Heart J*. 2003;24: 789–800.
28. Smart S, Bhatia A, Hellman R, et al. Dobutamine-atropine stress echocardiography and dipyridamole sestamibi scintigraphy for the detection of coronary artery disease: limitations and concordance. *J Am Coll Cardiol*. 2000;36:1265–1273.
29. Marwick T, D'Hondt A, Baudhuin T, et al. Optimal use of dobutamine stress for the detection and evaluation of coronary artery disease: combination with echocardiography or scintigraphy, or both? *J Am Coll Cardiol*. 1993;22:159–167.
30. Geleijnse ML, Elhendy A. Can stress echocardiography compete with perfusion scintigraphy in the detection of coronary artery disease and cardiac risk assessment? *Eur J Echocardiogr*. 2000;1:12–21.
31. Senior R, Monaghan M, Becher H et al. Stress echocardiography for the diagnosis and risk stratification of patients with suspected or known coronary artery disease: a critical appraisal. Supported by the British Society of Echocardiography.
32. Bach D, Muller D, Gros B, et al. False positive dobutamine stress echocardiograms: characterization of clinical, echocardiographic and angiographic findings. *J Am Coll Cardiol*. 1994;24:928–933.
33. Ha J, Juracan E, Mahoney D, et al. Hypertensive response to exercise: a potential cause for new wall motion abnormality in the absence of coronary artery disease. *J Am Coll Cardiol*. 2002;39:323–327.
34. Okeie K, Shimizu M, Yoshio H, et al. Left ventricular systolic dysfunction during exercise and dobutamine stress in patients with hypertrophic cardiomyopathy. *J Am Coll Cardiol*. 2000;36:856–863.
35. Miller D, Ruddy T, Zusman R, et al. Left ventricular ejection fraction response during exercise in asymptomatic systemic hypertension. *Am J Cardiol*. 1987;59:409–413.

36. Mottram P, Haluska B, Yuda S, et al. Patients with a hypertensive response to exercise have impaired systolic function without diastolic dysfunction or left ventricular hypertrophy. *J Am Coll Cardiol*. 2004;43:848–853.

37. Geleijnse M, Vigna C, Kasprzak J, et al. Usefulness and limitations of dobutamine-atropine stress echocardiography for the diagnosis of coronary artery disease in patients with left bundle branch block. *Eur Heart J*. 2000;21:1666–1673.

38. Waters DD, Gordon D, Rossouw JE, et al. National Heart, Lung and Blood Institute; American College of Cardiology Foundation. Women's Ischemic Syndrome Evaluation: current status and future research directions: report of the National Heart, Lung and Blood Institute workshop: October 2–4, 2005: Section 4 lessons from hormone replacement trials. *Circulation*. 2004;109:e53–e55.

39. Morise AP, Dala JN, Duval RD. Value of a simple measure of estrogen status for improving the diagnosis of coronary artery disease in women. *Am J Med*. 1993;94:491–496.

40. Kawano H, Motoyama T, Ohgushi K, et al. Menstrual cyclic variation of myocardial ischemia in premenopausal women with variant angina. *Ann Intern Med*. 2001;135:977–981. [Erratum in: *Ann Intern Med*. 2002;136:253.]

41. Kawano H, Motoyama T, Hirai N, et al. Estradiol supplementation supplementation suppresses hyperventilation-induced attacks in postmenopausal women with variant angina. *J Am Cardiol*. 2001;37:735–740.

42. Schulman SP, Theimann DR, Ouyang P, et al. Effects of acute hormone therapy on recurrent ischemia on postmeopausal women with unstable angina. *J Am Coll Cardiol*. 2002;39:231–237.

43. Rosano GM, Webb CM, Chierchia S, et al. Natural progesterone, but not medroxyprogesterone acetate, enhances the beneficial effect of estrogen on exercise – induced myocardial ischemia in postmenopausal women. *J Am Coll Cardiol*. 2000;36:2154–2159.

44. Morise AP, Dalal JN, Duval RD. Frequency of oralestrogen replacement therapy in women with normal and abnormal exercise electrocardiograms and normal coronary arteries by angiogram. *Am J Cardiol*. 1993;72:1197–1199.

45. Morise AP, Haddad WJ. Validation of estrogen status as an independent predictor of coronary artery disease presence and extent in women. *J Cardiovasc Risk*. 1996;3:507–511.

46. Hlatky MA, Pryor DB Harrell FE Jr, et al. Factors affecting sensitivity and specificity of exercise electrocardiography:multivariable analysis. *Am J Med*. 1984;77:64–71.

47. Weiner DA, McGabe C, et al. Exercuse testing for the diagnosis of coronary aretery disease. *Am Heart J*. 1980;99:811–812.

48. Guiteras VP, Chaitman BR, Waters DD, et al. Diagnostic accuracy of exercise ECG lead systems in clinical subsets of women. *Circulation*. 1982;65:1465–1474.

49. Linhart JW, Laws JG, Satinsky JD. Maximum treadmill exercise electrocardiography in female patients. *Circulation*. 1974;50:1173–1178.

50. Sketch MH, Mohiuddin SM, Lynch JD, et al. Significant sex differences in the correlation of electrocardiographic exercise testing and coronary arteriograms. *Am J Cardiol*. 1975;36:169–173.

51. Barolsky SM, Gilbert CA, Faruqui A, et al. Differences in electrocardiographic response to exercise of women and men: a non Bayesian factor. *Circulation*. 1979;60:1021–1027.

52. Hung J, Chaitman BR, Lam J, et al. Nonivasive diagnostic test choices for the evaluation of coronary aretery disease in women: a multivariate comparison of cardiac fluoroscopy, exercise electrocardiography and exercise thallium myocardial perfusion scintigraphy. *J Am Coll Cardiol*. 1984;4:8–16.

53. Robert AR, Melin JA, Detry JM. Logistic discriminant analysis improves diagnostic accuracy of exercise testing for coronary artery disease in women. *Circulation*. 1991;83:1202–1209.

54. Kwok Y, Kim C, Grady D, Segal M, Redberg R. Meta-analysis of exercise testing to detect coronary aretery disease in women. *Am J Cardiol*. 1999;83:660–666.

55. Marwick TH, Anderson T, Williams MJ, et al.: Exercise echocardiography is an accurate and cost-efficient technique for detection of coronary artery disease in women. *J Am Coll Cardiol.* 1995;26:335–341.

56. Grundy SM, Pasternak R, Greenland P, et al. Assessment of cardiovascular risk by use of multiple risk-factor assessment equations: a statement for healthcare professionals from the American Heart Association and the American College of Cardiology. *Circlulation.* 1990;100:1481–1492.

57. Roger VL, Pellikka PA, Bell MR, et al. Sex and test verification bias: impact on the diagnostic value of exercise echocardiography. *Circulation.* 1997;95:405–410.

58. Mieres JH, Shaw LJ, Arai A, et al. Role of noninvasive testing in the clinical evaluation of women with suspected coronary artery disease consensus statement from the Cardiac Imaging Committee, Council on Clinical Cardiology, and the Cardiovascular Imaging and Intervention Committee, Council on Cardiovascular Radiology and Intervention, American Heart Association. *Circulation.* 2005;111:682–696.

59. Kim C, Kwok YS, Heagerty P, et al. Pharmacologic stress testing for coronary artery disease: a meta-analysis. *Am Heart J.* 2001;142:934–944.

60. Lewis JF, Lin L, McGorray S, et al. Dobutamine stress echocardiography in women with chest pain. Pilot phase data from the National Heart, Lung and Blood Institute Women's Ischemia Syndrome Evaluation (WISE). *J Am Coll Cardiol.* 1999;33:1462–1468.

61. Heupler S, Mehta R, Lobo A, et al. Prognostic implications of exercise echocardiography in women with known or suspected coronary artery disease. *J Am Coll Cardiol.* 1997;30: 414–420.

62. Sawada SG, Ryan T, Fineberg NS, et al. Exercise echocardiographic detection of coronary artery disease in women. *J Am Coll Cardiol.* 1989;14:1440–1447.

63. Dionosopoulos PN, Collins JD, Smart SC, et al. The value of dobutamine stress echocardiography for the detection of coronary artery disease in women. *J Am Soc Echocardiogr.* 1997;10:811–817.

64. Elhendy A, Geleijnese ML, van Domburg RT, et al. Gender differences in the accuracy of dobutamine stress echocardiography for the diagnosis of coronary artery disease. *Am J Cardiol.* 1997;80:1414–1418.

65. Masini M, Picano E, Lattanzi F, et al. High dose dipyridamole-echocardiography test in women: correlation with exercise-electrocardiography test and coronary arteriography. *J Am Coll Cardiol.* 1988;12:682–685.

66. Severi S, Picano E, Michelassi C, et al. Diagnostic and prognostic value of dipyridamole echocardiography in patients with suspected coronary artery disease. Comparison with exercise electrocardiography. *Circulation.* 1994;89:1160–1173.

67. Ho YL, Wu CC, Huang PJ, et al. Assessment of coronary artery disease in women by dobutamine stress echocardiography: comparison with stress thallium-201 single-photon emission computed tomography and exercise electrocardiography. *Am Heart J.* 1998;135: 655–662.

68. Williams MJ, Marwick TH, O'Gorman D, et al. Comparison of exercise echocardiography with an exercise score to diagnose coronary artery disease in women. *Am J Cardiol.* 1994;74:435–438.

69. Senior R, Lahiri A. Enhanced detection of myocardial ischemia by stress dobutamine echocardiography utilizing the "biphasic" response of wall thickening during low and high dose dobutamine infusion. *J Am Coll Cardiol* 1995;26:26–32.

70. Perrone-Filardi P, Pace L, Prastaro M et al. Assessment of myocardial viability in patients with chronic coronary artery disease: Rest-4 hour-24 hour 201Tl tomography versus dobutamine echocardiography. *Circulation.* 1996;94:2712–2719.

71. Arnese M, Cornel JH, Salustri A et al. Prediction of improvement of regional left ventricular function after surgical revascularization: a comparison of low dose dobutamine echocardiography with 201Tl single photon emission computed tomography. *Circulation.* 1995;91: 2748–2752.

72. Haque T, Furukawa T, Takahashi M, et al. Identification of hybernating myocardium by dobu-
    tamine stress echocardiography: comparison with thallium-201 reinjection imaging. *Am Heart
    J*. 1995;130:553–563.
73. Skopicki HA, Weissman NJ, Rose GA et al. Thallium imaging, dobutamine echocardiography,
    and photon emission tomography for the detection of myocardial viability. *J Am Coll Cardiol*.
    1996;27:162A abstract.
74. Vanoverschelde JJ, D'Hondt AM, Marwick T et al. Head to head comparison of exercise
    redistribution-reinjection thallium single photon emission tomography and low dose dobu-
    tamine echocardiography for prediction of reversibility of chronic left ventricular ischemic
    dysfunction. *J Am Coll Cardiol*. 1996;28:432–442.
75. Bax JJ, Cornel JH, Vissner FC, et al. Prediction of recovery or regional left ventricu-
    lar dysfunction following revascularization: comparison of F18-fluorodeoxyglucose SPECT,
    thallium stress-reinjection SPECT and dobutamine echocardiography. *J Am Coll Cardiol*.
    1996;28:558–564.
76. Charney R, Schwinger ME, Chung J, et al. Dobutamine echocardiography and resting-
    redistribution thallium-201 scintigraphy predicts recovery of hibernating myocardium after
    coronary revascularization. *Am Heart J*. 1994;128:864–869.
77. Perrone-Filardi P, Pace L, Prastaro M, et al. Dobutamine stress echocardiography predicts
    improvement of hyoperfused dysfunctional myocardium after revascularization in patients
    with coronary artery disease. *Circulation*. 1995;91:2556–2565.
78. Cigarroa CG, deFilippi CR, Brickner E, et al. Dobutamine stress echocardiography identi-
    fies hibernating myocardium and predicts recovery of left ventricular function after coronary
    revascularization. *Circulation*. 1993;88:430–436.
79. Marzullo P, Parodi O, Reisenhofer B et al. Value of rest thallium-201/technetium-99m ses-
    tamibi scans and dobutamine echocardiography for detecting myocardial viability. *Am J Car-
    diol*. 1993;71:166–172.
80. La Canna G, Alfieri O, Giubbini R, et al. Echocardiography during infusion of dobutamine
    for identification of reversible dysfunction in patients with chronic coronary artery disease. *J
    Am Coll Cardiol*. 1994;23:617–626.
81. Seghal R, Lambert KL, Saham GM, et al. Prediction of viable myocardium by dobu-
    tamine echocardiography in patients with chronic left ventricular dysfunction. *Clin Res*.
    1994;42:160A. Abstract.
82. Afridi I, Kleiman NS, Raizner AE, et al. Dobutamine echocardiography in myocardial hiber-
    nation: optimal dose and accuracy in predicting recovery of ventricular function after coronary
    revascularization. *Circulation*. 1995;91:663–670.
83. deFillipe CR, Willet DR, Irani WN et al. Comparison of myocardial contrast echocardiogra-
    phy and low dose dobutamine stress echocardiography in predicting recovery of left ventricu-
    lar function after revascularization after coronary revascularization in chronic ischemic heart
    disease. *Circulation*. 1995;91:990–998.
84. Bonow RO. Identification of viable myocardium. *Circulation*. 1996 December
    1;94(11):2674–2680.
85. Bax JJ, Wijns W, Cornel JH, et al. Accuracy of currently available techniques for predic-
    tion of functional recovery after revascularization in patients with left ventricular dysfunction
    due to chronic coronary artery disease: comparison of pooled data. *J Am Coll Cardiol*. 1997
    November 15;30(6):1451–1460.

# Chapter 14
# Pathway for the Management of Patients Based on Stress Echo Results

Sripal Bangalore and Farooq A. Chaudhry

## Introduction

The objective of an ideal stress testing modality is to effectively risk stratify patients with known or suspected coronary artery disease (CAD) for future cardiovascular events. This is crucial as treatment options and the benefits of treatment vary with the risk category of patients. Surgical literature suggests that the morbidity and mortality benefits of surgical revascularization for CAD is highest in the intermediate to high-risk subgroups, whereas there is a trend toward increased mortality in the low-risk cohort compared to medical therapy alone.[1] In the recently concluded Clinical Outcomes Utilizing Revascularization and Aggressive Drug Evaluation (COURAGE) trial of 2287 patients with stable CAD, an initial revascularization strategy using percutaneous coronary intervention (PCI) did not reduce the risk of death, myocardial infarction, or other major cardiovascular events when added to optimal medical therapy,[2] thus creating an intense debate among physicians, media, and the public on the utility of PCI in patients with abnormal stress test and CAD. Before we throw out PCI, it is better to critically analyze these results. Though this was a well-conducted study, the risk profile of the patients in this trial suggests that this was a relatively low-risk cohort – the mean ejection fraction at the beginning of the study was normal (60.8%). The cardiac death rate (%/year) in the PCI group and the medical group was only 0.43 and 0.48%/year, respectively, implying a low-risk cohort. Clearly, there is a need to better risk stratify patients so as to tailor management strategies to better suit the risk groups.

Moreover, identifying patients at high risk for ischemic events versus high risk for sudden cardiac death is also important in deciding on the appropriate treatment modality. Proper risk stratification is critical for the management of patients with known or suspected coronary artery disease. Informed choices regarding revascularization procedures or medical therapy can only be made after accurately identifying the patients who may benefit most with a given treatment strategy. In a meta-analysis

S. Bangalore (✉)
Cardiology, Brigham and Women's Hospital, Harvard Medical School, Boston, MA, USA
e-mail: sbangalore@partners.org

E. Herzog, F.A. Chaudhry (eds.), *Echocardiography in Acute Coronary Syndrome*,     193
DOI 10.1007/978-1-84882-027-2_14, © Springer-Verlag London Limited 2009

of randomized trials of coronary artery bypass surgery versus medical management, Yusuf et al.[1] examined the value of a strategy of early bypass surgery versus initial medical therapy with delayed surgery for advanced symptoms and showed a beneficial effect on survival for early bypass surgery over a 10-year follow-up. This beneficial effect was more pronounced in the subgroup of patients at intermediate risk or high risk of cardiac death. However, in low-risk patients, a non-significant trend toward greater mortality with bypass surgery was evident. Other large-scale studies have shown similar mortality benefits of early surgical revascularization in patients with intermediate or high risk of cardiac death.[3,4] In low-risk patient groups the rate of ischemic events and cardiac death has been low with aggressive medical therapy. Pitt et al.[5] showed that aggressive lipid lowering significantly reduces the ischemic event rate and delays the time for the first ischemic event. Large trials[5–7] which evaluated the long-term survival and prevention of nonfatal MI were unable to prove any beneficial effect for an initial invasive strategy over medical therapy for these selected patient groups. In the Coronary Angioplasty Versus Medical Therapy for Angina (RITA-2) trial a significant excess in mortality and nonfatal MI was seen in the group on an initial coronary angioplasty strategy compared with conventional medical therapy.[6] Thus in the low-risk groups, initial medical therapy and delayed revascularization would be more beneficial than an early angioplasty strategy.

Stress echocardiography is routinely used for the diagnosis, risk stratification, and prognosis of patients with known or suspected coronary artery disease (CAD).[8–10] Traditionally, stress echocardiography results are interpreted as binary (normal or abnormal). Previous studies have shown that risk stratification and prognosis using such an approach indicate that a normal study has a benign prognosis (low risk) and an abnormal study has a high risk for future cardiac events (myocardial infarction or cardiac death).[10–12] The drawback of such a "binary" approach is oversimplification of patients who fall in the "gray" zone (intermediate group) to either the low-risk group resulting in false reassurance or the high-risk group resulting in subjecting patients to unnecessary invasive procedures. Among stress echocardiography variables, left ventricular ejection fraction and peak wall motion score index have shown to be independent and significant predictors of cardiovascular morbidity and mortality.[6,10–13]

## Prognostic Value of Peak Wall Motion Score Index

Conventionally, stress echocardiography studies are interpreted based on wall motion abnormalities of the left ventricle. For this purpose, the left ventricle is divided into 16 segments (Fig. 14.1) based on the recommendation by the American Society of Echocardiography and a score is assigned to each segment at baseline, with each stage of stress and during the recovery phase.[14] Each segment is scored as follows: 1 = normal; 2 = mild to moderate hypokinesis (reduced wall thickening and excursion); 3 = severe hypokinesis (marked reduced wall thickening and excursion); 4 = akinesis (no wall thickening and excursion); 5 = dyskinesis (paradoxical wall motion away from the center of the left ventricle during systole).[15] The peak

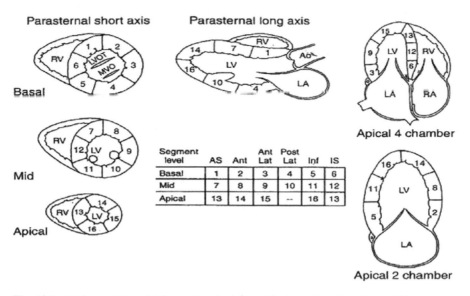

**Fig. 14.1**  A 16-segment model for scoring the left ventricular wall motion abnormalities

wall motion score index following stress is derived from the cumulative sum score of 16 left ventricular wall segments divided by the number of visualized segments. Abnormal stress echocardiography study is defined as those with either infarction or ischemia (peak WMSI >1.0).

Prior studies have shown the importance of peak wall motion score index as a predictor of cardiovascular events.[6,10,13,16–18] Peak wall motion score index incorporates both extent and severity of CAD and hence is a very powerful predictor of cardiac events. Arruda et al.[16] in an analysis of 5798 patients with known or suspected CAD undergoing exercise echocardiography showed that exercise WMSI was a significant predictor of cardiovascular events (MI or cardiac death) for both men (RR = 1.53; 95% CI = 1.32–1.77; p = 0.0001) and women (RR = 1.49; 95% CI = 1.14–1.94; p = 0.003) even after controlling for baseline clinical, exercise, and echocardiographic variables. In an analysis of 1323 patients with known or suspected CAD undergoing dobutamine echocardiography, we have shown that peak WMSI was a significant univariate and multivariate (RR = 1.92; 95% CI – 1.07–3.33; p = 0.03) predictor of cardiovascular events (MI or cardiac death).[19] Prior attempts at risk stratification using peak wall motion score index have interpreted the outcome as binary (normal or abnormal). Very few studies have risk stratified patients into low-, intermediate-, and high-risk subgroups.[10,20] We have shown that stress echocardiography is an effective technique for diagnosis, risk stratification, and prognosis of patients and that the peak WMSI was able to risk stratify patients not just into a normal or abnormal group but into low (peak WMSI = 1.0; hard event rate <1%/year), intermediate (peak WMSI = 1.0–1.7; hard event rate 1–4%/year), and high-risk (peak WMSI >1.7; hard event rate >4%/year) groups for future cardiovascular events (Fig. 14.2).[10]

**Fig. 14.2** Cardiac event rate per year as a function of wall motion score index (WMSI). The number of patients within each WMSI category is shown below each column. Statistical significance increases as a function of the WMSI result[10]

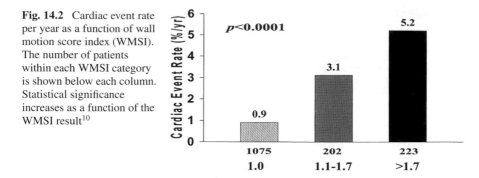

## Prognostic Value of Resting Ejection Fraction

Previous studies have shown the importance of resting ejection fraction as a predictor of cardiovascular events.[10,11,20,21] Ejection fraction is a measure of the physiology/functional status of the heart and has been shown to be better than the anatomically determined coronary artery stenosis for prediction of future events.[22] In an analysis of 1500 patients undergoing stress echocardiography, we have shown that an EF $\leq$ 45% further risk stratified the results of stress echocardiography based on WMSI. An EF $\leq$ 45% and peak WMSI of 1.1–1.7 (6.2%/year) or >1.7 (5.6%/year) were associated with high cardiac event rates, whereas an EF > 45% demonstrated an intermediate cardiac event rate, even in patients with a peak WMSI of 1.1–1.7 (2.0%/year) or >1.7 (2.3%/year) (Fig. 14.3).[10] In an analysis of 2705 patients referred for stress echocardiography, we showed that for every 1% decrease in resting ejection fraction, the risk of cardiovascular events (MI or cardiac death) increased by 4%.[23]

**Fig. 14.3** Cardiac event rate per year as a function of wall motion score index and ejection fraction (EF). The number of patients within each category is indicated below each column. *Shaded columns* = EF > 45%; *solid columns* = EF $\leq$ 45%[10]

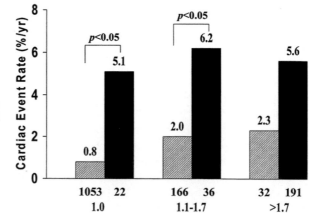

## Prognostic Value of Resting Ejection Fraction and Peak WMSI

The risk of cardiovascular events thus increases with decreasing ejection fraction and increasing peak WMSI. This risk has been shown independently for ejection fraction and peak WMSI. However, the combination of EF and WMSI can further effectively risk stratify patients referred for stress echocardiography (Fig. 14.4). Using a combination of resting EF and peak WMSI, patients can be risk stratified into low (event rate <1%/year), intermediate (event rate 1–4%/year), or high-risk (event rate >4%/year) groups for cardiovascular events (Fig. 14.4).[24] We have shown that using a ratio of peak WMSI to resting ejection fraction (stress function index – SFI), patients can be risk stratified into low (SFI < 1.9), intermediate (SFI = 1.9–3.1), and high-risk (SFI > 3.1) groups with an event rate of <1, 1–4, and >4%/year, respectively. Risk stratification based on stress function index (global $\chi^2$ = 106.05; p <0.0001) provided incremental value beyond that provided by risk stratification by peak WMSI (global $\chi^2$ = 79.23; p <0.0001) or risk stratification by EF alone (global $\chi^2$ = 87.12; p <0.0001) (Fig. 14.5).[24] For each 0.10 U increase in stress function index the risk of cardiac event increases by 10%.[24] Hence

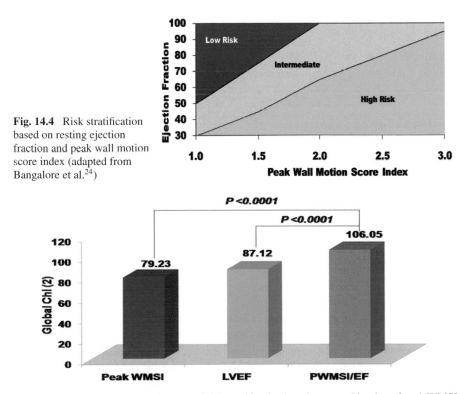

**Fig. 14.4**  Risk stratification based on resting ejection fraction and peak wall motion score index (adapted from Bangalore et al.[24])

**Fig. 14.5**  Incremental prognostic value of risk stratification based on a combination of peak WMSI and EF when compared to either alone (adapted from Bangalore et al.[24])

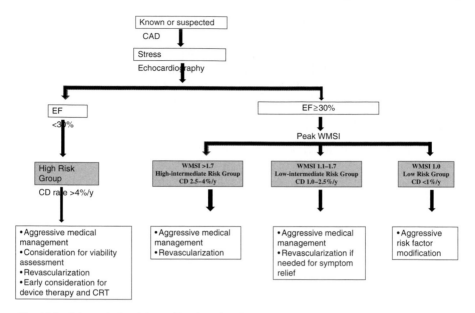

**Fig. 14.6** Schematic for risk stratification of patients undergoing stress echocardiography

an effective risk stratification strategy should not only include data from the peak WMSI but also take into consideration the resting ejection fraction.

## Pathway for Management

Based on the data presented above, any effective risk stratification of patients undergoing stress echocardiography should thus be based both on peak WMSI (which includes both extent and severity of ischemia/infarction) and on left ventricular ejection fraction (resting). Figure 14.6 represents a schematic for the risk stratification of patients with known or suspected CAD referred for stress echocardiography. These data for risk stratification are based on an analysis of 3259 patients (59 ± 13 years; 48% males) followed for up to 4 years in our laboratory.

The first step in the risk stratification process is evaluation of ejection fraction. Patients with EF < 30% are a high-risk group with a cardiac death (CD) rate of >4%/year regardless of the peak WMSI. Such patients should be aggressively managed. These patients may also benefit from viability assessment (Chapter 22) and consideration for revascularization as deemed necessary. They should also be considered for early device therapy (ICD/CRT) and for cardiac transplant evaluation.

In patients with EF ≥ 30%, peak WMSI can further risk stratify the patient subgroup into low (peak WMSI = 1.0; CD < 1%/year), low-intermediate (peak WMSI = 1.1–1.7; CD 1–2.5%/year), and high-intermediate-risk (peak WMSI >1.7; CD 2.5–4.0%/year) groups. Patients in the low-risk category will benefit from aggressive risk factor modification. Those in the low-intermediate-risk group may benefit from aggressive medical management and consideration of revascularization for symptom relief only. Patients in the high-intermediate-risk group may benefit from aggressive medical management and revascularization therapy. Such a risk stratification approach would potentially avoid unnecessary revascularization procedures for low-risk individuals and at the same time give a framework for the management of intermediate and high-risk subgroups.

# References

1. Yusuf S, Zucker D, Peduzzi P, et al. Effect of coronary artery bypass graft surgery on survival: overview of 10-year results from randomised trials by the Coronary Artery Bypass Graft Surgery Trialists Collaboration. *Lancet*. 1994;344(8922):563–70.
2. Boden WE, O'Rourke RA, Teo KK, et al. Optimal medical therapy with or without PCI for stable coronary disease. *N Engl J Med*. 2007;356(15):1503–1516.
3. Eleven-year survival in the Veterans Administration randomized trial of coronary bypass surgery for stable angina. The Veterans Administration Coronary Artery Bypass Surgery Cooperative Study Group. *N Engl J Med*. 1984;311(21):1333–1339.
4. Varnauskas E. Twelve-year follow-up of survival in the randomized European Coronary Surgery Study. *N Engl J Med*. 1988;319(6):332–337.
5. Pitt B, Waters D, Brown WV, et al. Aggressive lipid-lowering therapy compared with angioplasty in stable coronary artery disease. Atorvastatin versus Revascularization Treatment Investigators. *N Engl J Med*. 1999;341(2):70–76.
6. Steinberg EH, Madmon L, Patel CP, Sedlis SP, Kronzon I, Cohen JL. Long term prognostic significance of dobutamine echocardiography in patients with suspected coronary artery disease: results of a 5-year follow-up study. *J Am Coll Cardiol*. 1997;29(5):969–73.
7. Parisi AF, Folland ED, Hartigan P. A comparison of angioplasty with medical therapy in the treatment of single-vessel coronary artery disease. Veterans Affairs ACME Investigators. *N Engl J Med*. 1992;326(1):10–16.
8. Bangalore S, Gopinath D, Yao SS, Chaudhry FA. Risk stratification using stress echocardiography: incremental prognostic value over historic, clinical, and stress electrocardiographic variables across a wide spectrum of bayesian pretest probabilities for coronary artery disease. *J Am Soc Echocardiogr*. 2007;20(3):244–252.
9. Bangalore S, Yao SS, Puthumana J, Chaudhry FA. Incremental prognostic value of stress echocardiography over clinical and stress electrocardiographic variables in patients with prior myocardial infarction: "warranty time" of a normal stress echocardiogram. *Echocardiography*. 2006;23(6):455–464.
10. Yao SS, Qureshi E, Sherrid MV, Chaudhry FA. Practical applications in stress echocardiography: risk stratification and prognosis in patients with known or suspected ischemic heart disease. *J Am Coll Cardiol*. 2003;42(6):1084–1090.
11. Krivokapich J, Child JS, Walter DO, Garfinkel A. Prognostic value of dobutamine stress echocardiography in predicting cardiac events in patients with known or suspected coronary artery disease. *J Am Coll Cardiol*. 1999;33(3):708–716.
12. Marwick TH, Case C, Sawada S, et al. Prediction of mortality using dobutamine echocardiography. *J Am Coll Cardiol*. 2001;37(3):754–760.
13. Pingitore A, Picano E, Varga A, et al. Prognostic value of pharmacological stress echocardiography in patients with known or suspected coronary artery disease: a prospective, large-scale, multicenter, head-to-head comparison between dipyridamole and dobutamine test. Echo-Persantine International Cooperative (EPIC) and Echo-Dobutamine International Cooperative (EDIC) Study Groups. *J Am Coll Cardiol*. 1999;34(6):1769–1777.

14. Schiller NB, Shah PM, Crawford M, et al. Recommendations for quantitation of the left ven-tricle by two-dimensional echocardiography. American Society of Echocardiography Com-mittee on Standards, Subcommittee on Quantitation of Two-Dimensional Echocardiograms. *J Am Soc Echocardiogr*. 1989;2(5):358–367.

15. Chaudhry FA, Tauke JT, Alessandrini RS, Vardi G, Parker MA, Bonow RO. Prognostic impli-cations of myocardial contractile reserve in patients with coronary artery disease and left ventricular dysfunction. *J Am Coll Cardiol*. 1999;34(3):730–738.

16. Arruda-Olson AM, Juracan EM, Mahoney DW, McCully RB, Roger VL, Pellikka PA. Prog-nostic value of exercise echocardiography in 5,798 patients: is there a gender difference? *J Am Coll Cardiol*. 2002;39(4):625–631.

17. Elhendy A, Mahoney DW, McCully RB, Seward JB, Burger KN, Pellikka PA. Use of a scor-ing model combining clinical, exercise test, and echocardiographic data to predict mortality in patients with known or suspected coronary artery disease. *Am J Cardiol*. 2004;93(10): 1223–1228.

18. Elhendy A, Shub C, McCully RB, Mahoney DW, Burger KN, Pellikka PA. Exercise echocar-diography for the prognostic stratification of patients with low pretest probability of coronary artery disease. *Am J Med*. 2001;111(1):18–23.

19. Bangalore S, Yao SS, Chaudhry FA. Comparison of heart rate reserve versus 85% of age-predicted maximum heart rate as a measure of chronotropic response in patients undergoing dobutamine stress echocardiography. *Am J Cardiol*. 2006;97(5):742–747.

20. Arruda AM, Das MK, Roger VL, Klarich KW, Mahoney DW, Pellikka PA. Prognostic value of exercise echocardiography in 2,632 patients > or = 65 years of age. *J Am Coll Cardiol*. 2001;37(4):1036–1041.

21. Elhendy A, Mahoney DW, Khandheria BK, Paterick TE, Burger KN, Pellikka PA. Prognostic significance of the location of wall motion abnormalities during exercise echocardiography. *J Am Coll Cardiol*. 2002;40(9):1623–1629.

22. Mock MB, Ringqvist I, Fisher LD, et al. Survival of medically treated patients in the coronary artery surgery study (CASS) registry. *Circulation*. 1982;66(3):562–568.

23. Bangalore S, Yao SS, Chaudhry FA. Role of left atrial size in risk stratification and prognosis of patients undergoing stress echocardiography. *J Am Coll Cardiol*. 2007;50(13):1254–1262.

24. Bangalore S, Yao SS, Chaudhry FA. Stress function index, a novel index for risk stratifi-cation and prognosis using stress echocardiography. *J Am Soc Echocardiogr*. 2005;18(12): 1335–1342.

# Chapter 15
# Echocardiography in Identifying Subclinical Disease

Merle Myerson and Ajay Shah

## Introduction

There are two possible approaches to preventing manifest cardiovascular disease (CVD). One involves prompt treatment of the earliest possible symptoms such as angina. The other is an attempt to detect disease in asymptomatic, apparently healthy individuals, known as screening.

With screening, a major concern is the appropriate selection of asymptomatic persons who should be placed on drugs, perhaps for a lifetime to prevent conditions that they might never develop in the first place. Ultrasound imaging holds great promise to identify patients in whom lifestyle, drug, and invasive intervention for primary prevention is appropriate.

This chapter will review the role of assessing preclinical atherosclerosis and the particular role ultrasound plays in this assessment. Two methods will be discussed, carotid intimal-medial thickness and brachial artery flow-mediated dilation.

## Emerging Role of Assessment of Preclinical Atherosclerosis

### How Risk Has Traditionally Been Assessed

At present the most widely used method to estimate absolute risk for major CVD events are algorithms that combine the major risk factors. Most commonly used is the Framingham risk score[1] or in Europe, the Systemic Coronary Risk Evaluation (SCORE).[2]

While risk-assessment algorithms have been very useful they are not without their limitations. For example, the Framingham score is not able to accurately predict events beyond 10 years and is not useful for younger persons.

M. Myerson (✉)
Director, Cardiovascular Disease Prevention Program, Division of Cardiology, St. Luke's-Roosevelt Hospital Center, New York, NY, USA
e-mail: myersonm@optonline.net

E. Herzog, F.A. Chaudhry (eds.), *Echocardiography in Acute Coronary Syndrome*,
DOI 10.1007/978-1-84882-027-2_15, © Springer-Verlag London Limited 2009

## *Considerations for Testing Asymptomatic Persons*

Screening tests yield surrogate markers for atherosclerosis. As such, when testing asymptomatic persons for presence of subclinical atherosclerosis there are several considerations[3]:

1. Does the test provide additive information to conventional risk factors?
2. Is the use of the test associated with improved outcomes?
3. Is there evidence that the test is cost-effective in asymptomatic persons?

An NIH Task Force (NIH) was convened in 2004 to examine the role of sub-clinical disease testing. They concluded that these tests are most likely to benefit persons at "intermediate risk" based on the Framingham risk score—a 10-year risk for coronary artery disease of 6–20%.[1]

## *Advantages of Ultrasound Imaging for Testing*

Ultrasound imaging provides reliable documentation of the presence of atherosclerotic plaques. Compared with other methods of evaluating preclinical disease, ultrasound is relatively inexpensive, non-invasive, and does not require radiation. The test can be completed within 30 min with no discomfort to the patient.

Change can be assessed after short intervals, ideal to see response to intervention. Both cIMT and FMD focus only on the intended target and therefore do not have the problem of incidental findings.

## Indications for Ultrasound Assessment of Preclinical Atherosclerosis

At present there are no single, comprehensive guidelines for assessment of preclinical atherosclerosis.

The National Cholesterol Education Program Adult Treatment Panel III (NCEP ATP III) issued in 2001 states that there are "a large body of data indicates that persons with advanced subclinical coronary atherosclerosis are at greater risk for major coronary events than are persons with less severe atherosclerosis."

The report suggests that cIMT could be used as an adjunct in CHD risk assessment. An elevated reading (greater than the 75th percentile for age and sex) could elevate a person with multiple risk factors to a higher risk category. "If carried out under proper conditions, carotid IMT could be used to identify persons at higher risk than that revealed by the major risk factors alone".[4]

The European guidelines on cardiovascular disease prevention in clinical practice states that "One of the major objectives of a CVD detection program should be to identify those apparently healthy individuals who have asymptomatic arterial disease …". They mention several methods including carotid ultrasound.[5]

The Screening for Heart Attack Prevention and Education (SHAPE) Task Force issued a report in 2006. The task force realized the limitations of existing risk scores such as Framingham, especially in the intermediate-risk group. They proposed an algorithm that included either coronary artery calcium or cIMT. All asymptomatic men 45–75 years old and women 55–75 years old who do not have very-low-risk characteristics or have known cardiovascular disease would undergo screening.

Individuals who test negative (coronary artery calcium score = 0 or cIMT < 50th percentile without carotid plaque) would be classified as either *lower risk* (no conventional risk factors) or *moderate risk* (with established risk factors) and treated according to NCEP ATP III guidelines.

Those who test positive (coronary artery calcium score ≥1, cIMT ≥ 50th percentile, or presence of carotid plaque) would be stratified:

- *Moderately high risk:* coronary calcium score >0 and <100, cIMT < 1 mm and ≥50th but <75th percentile without discernible carotid plaque
- *High risk:* coronary calcium score 100–399 and cIMT ≥ 1 mm or >75th percentile or a carotid plaque causing <50% stenosis
- *Very high risk:* coronary calcium score ≥400 or carotid plaque causing ≥50% stenosis.[6]

## Alternative Methods to Identify Subclinical Atherosclerosis: Coronary Calcium

In addition to ultrasound methods, computed tomography scanning can determine presence of calcium in coronary arteries. The measurement, expressed as a calcium score, is associated with presence of atherosclerosis and has been found to predict risk for CAD events independent of traditional risk factors.[7–9]

Not all calcium deposits in the coronary arteries represent a significant (flow-limiting) blockage and not all blocked arteries contain calcium. The earliest form of coronary artery disease, soft plaque, cannot be detected by cardiac CT.

In a study by Rozanski et al., 1,153 patients with no known coronary artery disease undergoing both exercise myocardial perfusion scintigraphy and CT coronary calcium screening within 6 months were followed for 32 months. Among the 1,089 patients with non-ischemic myocardial perfusion testing, the annualized cardiac event rate was <1% in all calcium score groups including those with calcium scores over 1,000 (N = 112) and between 400 and 999 (N = 212).[10]

The test is not covered by Medicare or by the majority of private insurers and costs approximately $400 in most centers. There is radiation involved, equivalent to that from 7–10 chest x-rays (one view) or about 10–20% of that involved in a standard diagnostic cardiac catheterization. There is no requirement for contrast material.

Although progression of coronary calcium can be detected, serial measurements of coronary calcium are of unclear benefit and involve cost and radiation exposure and are not recommended at this time.[11]

The CT scan of the heart will also include images of other structures, in particular portions of the lungs, mediastinum, aorta, and bone. Pathology in all of these structures can potentially be identified and is the responsibility of the physician requesting and interpreting the scan.

The 2007 ACCF/AHA expert consensus document on coronary artery calcium scoring concluded that "it may be reasonable to consider use of coronary artery calcium measurement in asymptomatic patients with intermediate risk based on available evidence that demonstrates incremental risk prediction information in this selected patient group." The committee felt that available data could not answer the question which method of assessing subclinical atherosclerosis was superior.[11]

## Carotid Intimal-Medial Thickness

### Background

The benefits of measuring carotid artery intimal-medial thickness (cIMT) have been known for some time with initial studies coming from the late 1980s. Carotid imaging has traditionally been used in the setting of symptomatic cerebrovascular disease or asymptomatic carotid bruit to identify significant obstructive disease. Subsequently, large observational studies have shown that cIMT correlates with levels of CVD risk factors and is an independent marker for risk.

In a study of 13,870 black and white middle-aged adults in the Atherosclerosis Risk in Communities (ARIC) study, the mean carotid far wall IMT was consistently greater in participants with prevalent clinical cardiovascular disease.[12] In the Rotterdam study, 7,983 adults 55 years or older had baseline cIMT and were followed for a mean of 2.7 years. Stroke risk increased gradually with increasing IMT. The odds ratio per standard deviation increase (0.163 mm) was 1.41 (95% CI, 1.25–1.82). For MI, an OR of 1.43 (95% CI, 1.16–1.78) was found.[13] A meta-analysis designed to examine the association of cIMT and its ability to predict future cardiovascular end points found that it is a strong predictor with the relative risk per IMT difference slightly higher for stroke than myocardial infarction.[14]

### Methodology

cIMT is measured with B-mode images using transducers in the frequencies between 7.5 and 10 MHz. Another approach is to use two-dimensionally guided M-mode images that provide comparable spatial resolution but better temporal resolution. Both methods should have electrocardiographic gating to determine the minimum end-diastolic diameter (Figs. 15.1, 15.2, 15.3, 15.4, 15.5, 15.6, and 15.7).

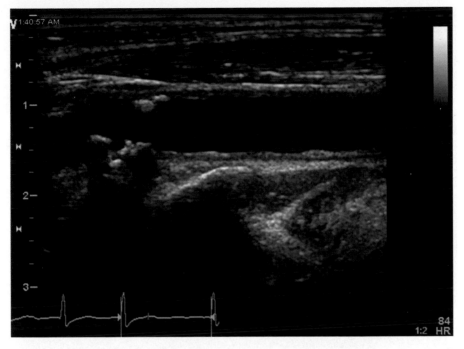

**Fig. 15.1** Irregular heterogenous plaque in carotid artery with calcification causing acoustic shadowing

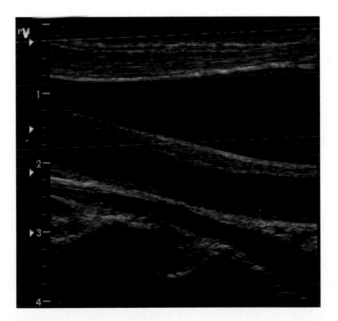

**Fig. 15.2** Smooth long heterogenous plaque

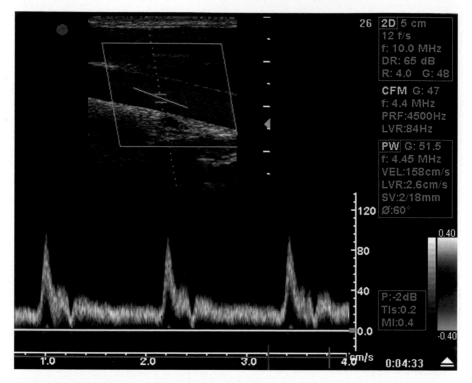

**Fig. 15.3** Normal spectral doppler in common carotid artery

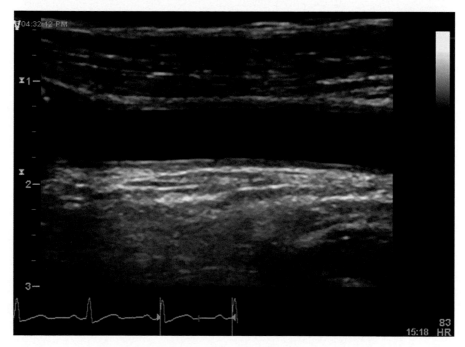

**Fig. 15.4** Abnormal Carotid intimal medial thickness

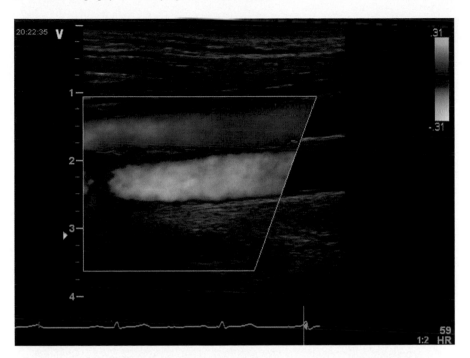

**Fig. 15.5** Normal color doppler in carotid artery (bottom) and internal jugular vein (top)

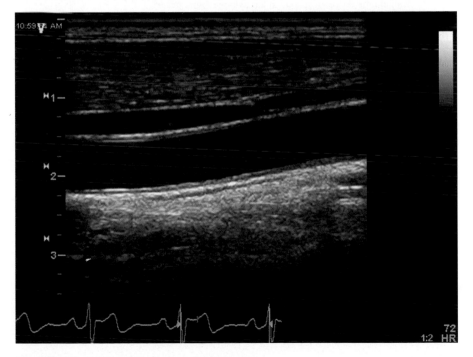

**Fig. 15.6** Normal Carotid intimal medial thickness

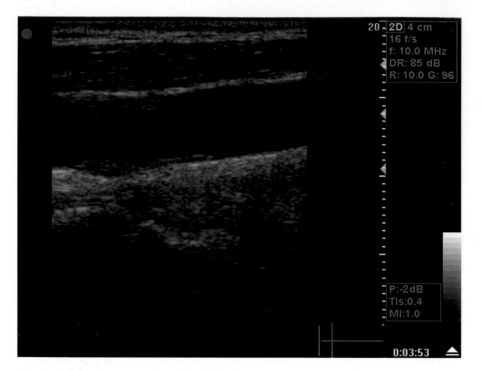

**Fig. 15.7** Irregular heterogeous plaque in the bulb with ann ulcer

The preferred site for measurement is the far wall rather than the near wall as acoustic reflection of the echo-dense intima into the lumen and/or to high gain setting in near-wall measurements may lead to overestimation of IMT. The reproducibility of the common carotid artery is superior to that of the internal carotid artery or the carotid bulb as the common carotid is tubular and can be aligned perpendicular to the transducer beam. Patients do not have to be in a fasted state.[15]

There is no defined "upper limit of normal" for cIMT; however, age-based nomograms and 75th percentiles can determine risk level. The SHAPE Task Force has suggested a treatment algorithm based on percentile and presence or absence of plaque.[6]

Serial measurements and measurements before and after interventions are practical with cIMT. Most studies have an interval of 1–2 years but change may be seen after 6 months. Because the study focuses on the carotid artery, there are no incidental findings. Reproducibility studies have shown that intrareader differences in the common carotid are in the range of 0.04 mm.[15]

Carotid IMT can differentiate between soft, fibrocalcific, and calcific plaque. Echographic evaluation of carotid plaques has been shown to be very close to the histological findings and to be better than angiographic imaging.[16] Inclusion of the echographic characteristics of carotid plaques improves the risk stratification for stroke.[17]

In comparison to carotid IMT, relatively fewer studies have evaluated the relationship between coronary and carotid artery and disease as reflected by plaque morphology. The majority of studies performed have focused on acute coronary syndromes or high-risk patients.

In 125 patients with acute coronary syndromes, carotid plaques were assessed. Plaques were identified as a distinct area with an IMT 50% thicker than the neighboring site. Plaques were divided into soft (low echoic or isoechoic structures without any high echoic region indicating calcification) or hard (high echoic areas of atherosclerotic calcification). The frequency of soft plaques and carotid calcification was higher in the group that had multiple plaques on cardiac angiography.[18]

Rossi and colleagues examined 64 patients with recent acute MI and gender-matched controls. Carotid ultrasound was performed and plaques were divided into two different types according to the echographic characteristics: stable or unstable. Atherosclerotic plaque was defined as stable when characterized by homogeneous aspect (moderate or high echogenicity). Plaque was considered unstable because of low echogenicity or a herterogeneous aspect due to the coexistence, within the same plaque, of areas with markedly different echogenicity. In MI patients, 19% of the total number of plaques were unstable vs. 8% in the controls ($p = 0.005$).[19]

A total of 144 patients undergoing angiography had carotid ultrasound. Positive predictive values for coronary artery disease were 45, 48, and 75% in patients with increased IMT, fibrous plaque, and calcific plaque, respectively. Compared to the normal group, risk for CAD increased by 4.3-fold with the existence of fibrous plaque ($p = 0.02$) and by 9.9-fold with the existence of calcific plaque ($p < 0.001$). The presence of calcific plaque is a better predictor for CAD than that of fibrous plaque and increased IMT.[20]

## Brachial Artery Flow-Mediated Dilation

### Background

Many studies have demonstrated the importance of endothelial cell function in both healthy and disease states. An important function of endothelium is to release factors that control vascular tone. Endothelial dysfunction is characterized by an imbalance between endothelium-dependent vasodilator and vasoconstrictor activity and impaired anti-inflammatory and anticoagulant functions. A compromised vasodilation due to endothelial dysfunction is often associated with diseases such as atherosclerosis, hypertension, and congestive heart failure.[21,22]

The method most commonly used to assess endothelial function is ultrasound measurement of flow-mediated brachial artery dilation.

## Cut-Points for FMD

While definitive cut-points defining level of risk have not been established, research has suggested FMD values that correlate to risk. In a study of 205 consecutive outpatients with chest pain syndromes followed for 24 months, those who developed cardiovascular events had lower FMD than those without, $3.5 \pm 2.1$ vs. $5.0 \pm 3.0\%$. Patients were also divided into three groups based on FMD, $>6$, $3–6$, and $<3\%$. Patients with lower FMD ($\leq 6\%$) had more combined events than those with FMD $> 6\%$.[23]

Time frame in which to expect changes in FMD

Change in FMD can be seen within several weeks; studies have used varying time periods of 8 weeks,[24] and 4 months.[25]

## *Methodology*

Subjects should be fasted overnight, refrain from smoking, ingesting alcohol or caffeine on the day of testing and to hold any vasoactive medications for 12 h before the imaging studies. Vascular ultrasound scans should be performed with subjects positioned supine or erect with arm resting with the temperature of the room maintained between 20 and 25°C (Figs. 15.8, 15.9, 15.10, and 15.11).

# The genesis of FMD

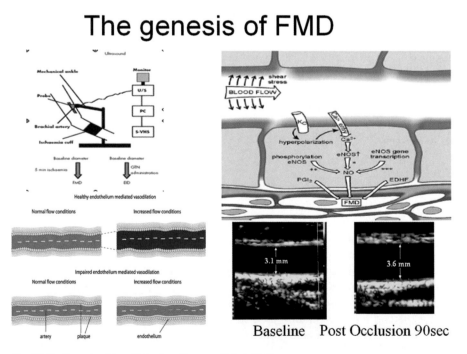

**Fig. 15.8** Genesis of brachial artery flow-mediated dilation

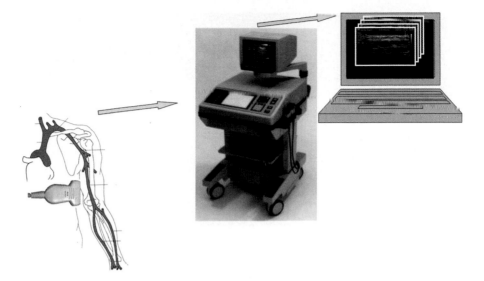

**Fig. 15.9**  Imaging method of brachial artery flow-mediated dilation

The patient is attached to a three-lead ECG, which is demonstrated on the ultrasound monitor. A gray scale (B-scan) of the right brachial artery is obtained in the cross-sectional plane between 5 and 10 cm above the elbow using the *VIVID 7 compound imaging vascular* transducer. The region of interest is marked with indelible ink. Baseline images are obtained and digitized online.

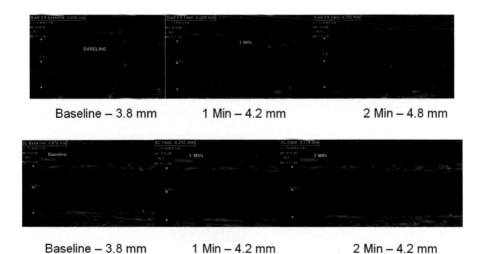

Baseline – 3.8 mm          1 Min – 4.2 mm          2 Min – 4.8 mm

Baseline – 3.8 mm          1 Min – 4.2 mm          2 Min – 4.2 mm

**Fig. 15.10**  (top) Normal flow mediated dilatation of brachial artery (cross section); (bottom) Normal flow mediated dilatation of brachial artery (longitudinal)

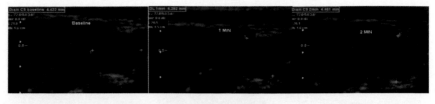

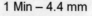

Baseline – 4.4 mm        1 Min – 4.4 mm        2 Min – 4.5 mm

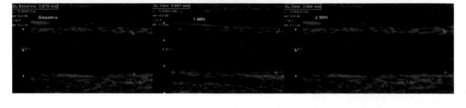

Baseline – 3.9 mm        1 Min – 3.9 mm        2 Min – 3.9 mm

**Fig. 15.11** (top) Abnormal flow mediated dilatation of brachial artery (cross section); (bottom) Abnormal flow mediated dilatation of brachial artery (longitudinal)

The brachial artery is occluded for 5 min using a standard adult pressure cuff (size 24–32 cm). Post-occlusion images are obtained. After 15 min of rest the above imaging procedure is repeated with the transducer oriented longitudinally to the length of the brachial artery.

The approach is based on the hypothesis that if the images are acquired at a high frame rate, the coordinates of the arterial wall in an image are in close proximity to the coordinates of the vessel wall in the previous frame. That is, the coordinates of an arterial lumen wall boundary in any given frame can be "propagated" to the next consecutive frame in a search for the arterial boundary. This process, if repeated in sequence from one frame to the next, can be used to detect boundaries in a series of acquired images.

The above analysis will provide data on the change in area and diameter as a function of flow-mediated dilation. The "area" vs. "diameter" changes will be compared to evaluate the performance of cross-sectional imaging relative to longitudinal imaging.

To minimize intra-individual variation, the same technicians should perform all studies.

In our laboratory, intraobserver and interobserver variability was acceptable. Using analyses on fixed images (i.e., when same images were analyzed) the intraobserver and interobserver percentage coefficient variation using cross-sectional area was $0.2 \pm 0.2$ and $0.4 \pm 0.6$, respectively. For longitudinal plane imaging the intraobserver and interobserver percentage coefficient of variation was much greater, i.e., $1.4 \pm 0.6$ and $1.9 \pm 0.6$, respectively. Given that the largest variation occurs during selection of images and this variation is greater in longitudinal plane imaging than cross-sectional imaging, it can be, therefore, hypothesized that the above difference in intraobserver and interobserver variability between the two techniques would be much greater.

## When to Use FMD or cIMT

As mentioned earlier, there are no established guidelines on testing asymptomatic persons for subclinical atherosclerosis and what treatment paradigms correspond to values derived from testing.

There is a consensus that these tests are most helpful and appropriate in persons deemed to be at intermediate risk by traditional risk factors. Testing may then help to place a person at higher or lower risk and help guide intensity of pharmacologic, lifestyle, and interventional therapy.

No study to date has compared cIMT and FMD in their prediction for CVD events. Carotid IMT has been more extensively studied, both in epidemiologic and clinical studies and is currently more widely used. cIMT gives thickness of the carotid intima but also provides information on plaque characteristics.

## Summary

As advances have been made in treating acute coronary syndromes, we have also made remarkable advances in *preventing* those at risk from developing manifest disease. Assessing preclinical atherosclerosis in asymptomatic persons has helped us to better risk stratify our patients and identify in whom lifestyle, drug, or invasive intervention is appropriate.

Ultrasound imaging, in particular cIMT and FMD, has been shown to accurately and specifically assist in the prediction of cardiovascular risk. Given the relative low cost and that it is non-invasive and does not require contrast material or radiation, ultrasound is a valuable component of risk assessment.

## Case Studies

### *Case #1: Use of Carotid Intimal-Medial Thickness to Risk Stratify a Patient*

A 66-year-old Asian woman presented to her primary provider for an annual physical examination. She has no known cardiovascular disease and denies any chest pain or pressure, dyspnea, dyspnea on exertion. Her primary provider refers her to the Cardiovascular Disease Prevention Program for evaluation.

*Past Medical History*
She is postmenopausal, never on hormone replacement therapy. Hypertension was diagnosed 2 years ago and is well controlled on medication. She has not had a recent fasting lipid panel. Childbirth, normal, twice.

*Social History*

She is a retired librarian and lives with her husband. She does not smoke and has four to five glasses of wine a week. She does no regular exercise but is "active" in her daily life. She follows no regular diet but "tries" to eat well. She was never instructed on a heart-healthy diet. Her family history is notable for a brother who underwent elective PCI with a stent at age 48 years.

*Medications*

Angiotensin receptor blocker, Fosamax 5 mg daily, multivitamin, calcium + vitamin D.

*Examination*

BP 140/78, HR 72 and regular. Height 62 in., weight 145 lbs, waist circumference 36 in., BMI 26.5. HEENT: no JVD, normal carotid upstroke, no bruit heard over carotid arteries. Chest: clear, no crackles or wheezes. CV: S1, S2, no S3 or S4, no murmurs heard. Abdomen: no organomegaly. Extremities: warm, no edema, good pulses.

*Pertinent Test Results*

Lab values: total cholesterol 257 mg/dL, LDL cholesterol 154 mg/dL, HDL cholesterol 65 mg/dL, triglycerides 190 mg/dL, serum creatinine 0.7 mg/dL, AST 20 U/L, ALT 22 U/L, TSH normal, fasting glucose 90 mg/dL.

EKG: NSR, mild LVH.

*Indication for Carotid IMT*

This patient has several risk factors for cardiovascular disease: age, hypertension, dyslipidemia, sedentary lifestyle, and she is overweight. She also has a brother with premature coronary artery disease. Her Framingham risk score is 11% (estimated 10-year risk of MI/CHD death), in the intermediate range.

According to NCEP guidelines, her LDL cholesterol should be less than 130 mg/dL. The question would be whether she should be treated more aggressively? In this patient, the results of a non-invasive test to detect presence and extent of subclinical atherosclerosis would be very helpful.

*Carotid IMT*

The patient underwent ultrasound assessment of her carotid intimal-medial thickness. The results showed far-wall left side thickness 1.20 mm and right side thickness 1.15 mm, both greater than the 75th percentile for age and presence of plaque but less than 50% stenosis.

*Assessment and Plan*

This is a 66-year-old woman with multiple risk factors for coronary artery disease. Her Framingham risk score places her at intermediate risk; however, the results of cIMT suggest that she is at higher risk. Based on this assessment, a clinician could reasonably choose to be more aggressive with management of her risk factors.

1. *Dyslipidemia*: Although her NCEP goal for LDL is <130 mg/dL, the carotid IMT shows that she has significant atherosclerosis. A goal based on this could be

considered similar to a patient with known cardiovascular disease, <100 mg/dL. Her HDL is at goal; her triglycerides are elevated and would be expected to come down with treatment of her LDL and lifestyle changes. Would start a low dose of a statin.

2. *Hypertension*: She is being treated although her systolic reading is high. Lifestyle changes may bring her to goal but would also consider increasing her medication to bring systolic readings under 130 mmHg.

3. *Lifestyle modification*: Her BMI of 26.5 indicates that she is overweight. She will benefit from nutritional counseling, for a heart-healthy diet and weight loss, and initiation of an exercise program.

4. *Indication for stress testing?* She is not complaining of angina or possible anginal equivalents. Her exercise program will consist of walking and she will start slowly and build up. At this time there is no indication for stress testing.

## Case #2: Use of Brachial Artery Flow-Mediated Dilation to Guide Risk Factor Management

A 61-year-old white man was referred to the Cardiovascular Disease Prevention Program for evaluation. He is reluctant to be on lipid-lowering medication and wants to know if the dose can be reduced or discontinued. He has no known cardiovascular disease but has hypertension and dyslipidemia, both treated. He denies chest pain, pressure, dyspnea, and dyspnea on exertion.

*Past Medical History*
Hypertension and dyslipidemia.

*Social History*
Does not drink or smoke. He swims ½ mile once a week and tries to walk 30 min several times a week. He does not follow any specific diet. He is a music teacher and lives with his wife; children are grown and healthy. Family history is noncontributory.

*Medications*
Enalapril 2.5 mg daily, aspirin 81 mg daily, Atorvastatin 20 mg daily, MVI.

*Examination*
Weight 186 lbs; height 5 ft 5½ in.; BMI 31; blood pressure 135/75; heart rate 66, regular. HEENT: no JVD, normal carotid upstroke, no bruit heard over carotid arteries. Chest: clear, no crackles or wheezes. CVL: S1, S2, no S3 or S4, no murmurs. Abdomen: no organomegaly. Extremities: warm, no edema, good pulses.

*Pertinent Test Results*
Lab tests (on Lipitor 20 mg daily): total cholesterol 148 mg/dL, LDL cholesterol 76 mg/dL, HDL cholesterol 56 mg/dL, triglycerides 80 mg/dL, AST 20 U/L, ALT 25 U/L, serum creatinine 0.9 mg/dL.

EKG: NSR.

*Indication for FMD*

This patient has several risk factors for coronary heart disease including age, hypertension, dyslipidemia, and being overweight. His Framingham risk score is 12 representing a 10% risk of MI/CHD death over the next 10 years, an intermediate-risk category. He is taking Atorvastatin 20 mg daily with an LDL of 76 mg/dL. He would like to reduce or stop taking lipid-lowering medication. Brachial artery flow-mediated dilation can help risk stratify this patient.

*Brachial Artery FMD*

The patient underwent measurement of his brachial artery flow-mediated dilation. The result was 3%. While there is no universally accepted scoring system, research has shown that lower values, in particular values less than 6%, indicated greater risk for coronary events.

*Assessment and Plan*

This is a 61-year-old patient with several risk factors for coronary heart disease and an intermediate Framingham risk score. He would like to lower his dose or stop taking lipid-lowering medication. His FMD indicates that he has endothelial dysfunction, a risk for cardiovascular disease. Based on this it would be reasonable to keep his LDL cholesterol lower than the NCEP guidelines (<130 mg/dL); in this case <100 mg/dL. A statin drug would be recommended as one of the non-LDL lowering benefits is improvement in endothelial function. In addition to lifestyle modifications including diet, weight loss, and increased exercise, the clinician may want to consider increasing the statin dose and repeating the FMD to see if there is improvement.

# References

1. US Department of Health and Human Services/National Heart, Lung, and Blood Institute. Framingham Heart Study. Available at: http://www.nhlbi.nih.gov/about/framingham
2. Conroy RM, Pyorala K, Fitzgerald AP, et al. Estimation of ten year risk of fatal cardiovascular disease in Europe: the SCORE project. *Eur Heart J.* 2003;24:987–1003.
3. Lauer M, Froelicher ES, Williams M, Kligfield P. Exercise testing in asymptomatic adults. AHA Scientific Statement. *Circulation.* 2005;112:771–776.
4. Expert Panel on Detection, Evaluation, and Treatment of High Blood Cholesterol in Adults: Executive summary of the third report of the National Cholesterol Education (NCEP) Expert Panel on Detection, Evaluation, and Treatment of High Blood Cholesterol in Adults (ATP III). *JAMA.* 2001;285:2486–2497.
5. Graham I, Atar D, Borch-Johnsen K, et al. European guidelines on cardiovascular disease prevention in clinical practice: executive summary. *Eur Heart J.* 2007;28:2375–2414.
6. Naghavi M, Falk E, Hecht HS, et al. From vulnerable plaque to vulnerable patient: Part III: executive summary of the Screening for Heart Attack Prevention and Education (SHAPE) Task Force Report. *Am J Cardiol.* 2006;98:2H–15H.
7. Arad Y, Spadaro LA, Roth M, Newstein D, Guerci AD. Coronary calcification, coronary disease risk factors, C-reactive protein, and atherosclerotic cardiovascular disease events: the St. Francis Heart Study. *J Am Coll Cardiol.* 2005;46:158–165.

8. LaMonte MJ, Fitzgerald SJ, Church TS, et al. Coronary artery calcium score and coronary heart disease events in a large cohort of asymptomatic men and women. *Am J Epidemiol.* 2005;162:421–429.

9. Taylor AJ, Bindeman J, Feuerstein J, Cao F, Brazaitis M, O'Malley PG. Coronary calcium independently predicts incident premature coronary heart disease over measured cardiovascular risk factors. *J Am Coll Cardiol.* 2005;46:807–814.

10. Rozanski A, Gransar H, Wong ND, et al. Clinical outcomes after both coronary calcium scanning and exercise myocardial perfusion scintigraphy. *J Am Coll Cardiol.* 2007;49:1352–1361.

11. ACCF/AHA 2007 Clinical expert consensus document on coronary artery calcium scoring by computed tomography in global cardiovascular risk assessment and in evaluation of patients with chest pain. *J Am Coll Cardiol.* 2007;49:377–402.

12. Burke GL, Evans G, Riley WA, et al. Arterial wall thickness is associated with prevalent cardiovascular disease in middle-aged adults: The Atherosclerosis Risk in Communities (ARIC) Study. *Stroke.* 1995;26:386–391.

13. Bots ML, Hoes A, Koudstaal PJ, HOfman A, Grobbee DE. Common carotid intima-media thickness and risk of stroke and myocardial infarction the Rotterdam Study. *Circulation.* 1997;96:1432–1437.

14. Lorenz MW, Markus HS, Bots ML, Rosvall M, Sitzer M. Prediction of clinical cardiovascular events with carotid intima-media thickness. *Circulation.* 2007;115:459–467.

15. Redberg RF, Vogel RA, Criqui MH, Herrington DM, Lima JAC, Roman MJ. Task Force #3, 34th Bethesda Conference: Can atherosclerosis imaging techniques improve the detection of patients at risk for ischemic heart disease? *J Am Coll Cardiol.* 2003;41:1886–1898.

16. Kagawa R, Kouzou M, Takeshi S, Yohikazu O. Validity of B-mode ultrasonographic findings in patients undergoing carotid endarterectomy in comparison with angiographic and clinico-pahtologic features. *Stroke.* 1996;27:700–705.

17. Geroulakos G, Hobson RW, Ricolaides A. Ultrasonographic carotid plaque morphology in predicting stroke risk. *Br J Surg.* 1996;83:582–587

18. Kato M, Dote K, Habara S, Takemoto H, Goto K, Nakaoka K. Clinical implications of carotid artery remodeling in acute coronary syndromes. *J Am Coll Cardiol.* 2003;42:1026–1032.

19. Rossi A, Franceschini L, Fusaro M, et al. Carotid atherosclerotic plaque instability in patients with acute myocardial infarction. *Int J Cardiol.* 2006;111:263–266.

20. Kanadasi M, Cayli M, San M, et al. The presence of a calcific plaque in the common carotid artery as a predictor of coronary atherosclerosis. *Angiology.* 2006;57:585–592.

21. Schachinger V, Britten MB, Zeiher AM. Prognostic impact of coronary vasodilator dysfunction on adverse long-term outcome of coronary heart disease. *Circulation.* 2000;101: 1899–1906.

22. Suwaidi JA, Hamasaki S, HIgano ST, Nishimura RA, Holoomes DR, Jr., Lerman A. Long-term follow-up of patients with mild coronary artery disease and endothelial dysfunction. *Circulation.* 2000;101:948–954

23. Huang, P-O, Chen J-W, Lu T M, ding P Y-A, Lin S-J. Combined use of endothelial function assessed by brachial ultrasound and high-sensitive C-reactive protein in predicting cardiovascular events. *Clin Cardiol,* 2007;30:135–140.

24. Guven GS, Atalar E, Yavuz B, et al. Simvastatin treatment improves endothelial function and increases fibrinolysis in patients with hypercholesterolemia. *J Natl Med Assoc.* 2006;98: 627–630.

25. Dupuis J, Tardiff JC, Rouleau JL, et al. Intensity of lipid lowering with statins and brachial artery vascular endothelium reactivity after acute coronary syndromes (from the BRAVER trial). *Am J Cardiol.* 2005;96:1207–1213.

# Chapter 16
# Diagnosis of Acute Coronary Syndrome

Gurusher Singh Panjrath and Eyal Herzog

Acute coronary syndrome, a spectrum extending from unstable angina to acute myocardial infarction, is a key manifestation of coronary artery disease. With coronary artery disease being the leading cause of death in the United States, it is essential to understand the basic pathophysiology and spectrum of presentation prior to making an effort to identify it.

In this chapter we review the various presentations of ACS and the clinical as well as the biochemical tools available to aid diagnosis and management of these patients. Our recommendations are based on previously published pathways to guide management appropriately.

Initial assessment of patients with suspected ACS should include two key goals. First, accurate and timely identification of the patient having an acute coronary syndrome, entertain a different diagnosis and institute appropriate management. Second goal is to address outcomes and prognosis within the hospital and post-hospital stay. This goal in particular plays an important role with advances in reperfusion strategies and decreased mortality from the primary event. Those at higher risk may need more aggressive management strategies and follow-up.

## Pathophysiology

The proportion of unstable angina (UA) and non-ST-elevation myocardial infarction (NSTEMI) as compared to ST-elevation myocardial infarction (STEMI) has been increasing over the last couple of years. As a result this has brought greater attention toward risk stratification. Various modalities including biomarkers and echocardiographic assessment of left ventricular function are the mainstay in accurately identifying high-risk patients. While the basic principle of ACS is an imbalance or mismatch between myocardial oxygen supply and demand, the specific mechanism by which this imbalance occurs varies in NSTEMI and STEMI. With advent of

G.S. Panjrath (✉)
The Johns Hopkins Hospital, Division of Cardiology, Baltimore, MD, USA
e-mail: gpanjra1@jhmi.edu

E. Herzog, F.A. Chaudhry (eds.), *Echocardiography in Acute Coronary Syndrome*,
DOI 10.1007/978-1-84882-027-2_16, © Springer-Verlag London Limited 2009

intravascular ultrasound and angiographic methods comes a better understanding of fundamental differences in the pathophysiology of NSTEMI and STEMI.

NSTEMI results from several plausible mechanisms, of which a disrupted plaque and resulting thromboemboli are the most discussed.[1] A thrombus forms at the site of an atherosclerotic plaque, thus causing an incomplete vessel occlusion or a transient total occlusion. Disruption of the fibrous cap, which overlies the lipid core and cellular debris, leads to exposure of the lipid core to the arterial lumen. This forms the basis of platelet aggregation and activation at the disrupted endothelial surface. Fibrinogen, by binding to glycoprotein IIb/IIIa receptors, forms a bridge between the activated platelets and thus results in a platelet–fibrin hemostatic plug. This plug can further propagate into either an occlusive or a non-occlusive thrombus. NSTEMI is associated with subtotal occlusion and preserved forward flow. However, microemboli, which are clumps of activated platelets or constituents from the disrupted lipid core, can get disseminated further downstream resulting in myocardial injury. The ensuing necrosis results in release of biomarkers which aid in diagnosis. Other mechanisms which contribute to NSTEMI are transient obstruction secondary to vasospasm or emboli from outside the coronary vasculature (myxoma, atrial fibrillation, vegetations, paradoxical emboli, etc.), vasculitis resulting from inflammation of vessel wall thus causing intimal thickening and arterial narrowing, and conditions causing increase in myocardial oxygen demand (anemia) resulting in mismatch in the setting of advanced atherosclerosis of the coronary vessels.

In contrast to NSTEMI, pathophysiology of STEMI involves the progression of a stable plaque to an ulcerated or disrupted prothrombotic plaque. This erosion facilitates the process of thrombus formation at the site of the erosion. The process involves interaction between vascular endothelium, platelets, and circulating coagulation factors. Occlusion is frequently total with obstruction of forward flow and resultant myocardial necrosis.

## Diagnosis and Risk Assessment

Early diagnosis and identification of patient at risk is fundamental in management of patients with chest pain. While diagnosis is paramount, initiating appropriate therapy at the earliest is the key. Additionally, initial assessment should aid in identification of patients at risk of future events or at high risk of death or poor outcomes.

## History and Physical Examination

In brief, patients presenting with chest pain should be considered candidates for serial electrocardiogram or placed on continuous monitoring. A careful history addressing all potential risk factors and a thorough physical exam should be part of the initial assessment. History and physical exam should consider other serious life-threatening causes of chest pain. Having a high index of suspicion will allow the operator to evaluate for other differential diagnosis during the study. While taking history, in addition to traditional risk factors and characteristics of pain, special attention should be paid to chest pain equivalents such as dyspnea, jaw/neck pain, or discomfort in the epigastrium and upper extremity. Key components of history that strongly support likelihood of ischemia due to coronary artery disease include characteristics of anginal symptoms, prior history of CAD, sex, age, and number of risk factors present.[2–6] However, some of the traditional risk factors such as hypertension, hypercholesterolemia, and cigarette smoking are only weak predictors of acute ischemia in patients with symptoms.[7,8] Therefore, absence of risk factors in patients with characteristic symptoms should not be used to guide the decision to initiate management of ACS. However, presence of traditional risk factors does relate to poor outcomes in patients with confirmed ACS. Diabetes, history of extracardiac vascular disease, and renal dysfunction in particular are associated with poor outcomes including higher mortality and risk of acute heart failure.[9–11] Renal dysfunction is associated with, in addition to higher rates of heart failure, increased bleeding risks and arrhythmias.[11,12]

Physical exam should be aimed to assess the hemodynamic status of the patient and findings which may support a diagnosis of ischemia or other non-ischemic diagnosis. Exam should also look for comorbid conditions which may be the precipitating cause of ischemia and conditions which may interfere with management and therapeutic strategy (gastrointestinal bleeding, uncontrolled hypertension, malignancy, or pulmonary disease).[13] Special attention should be paid to physical findings which may increase the likelihood of the patient having an ischemic event. This will be of additional importance for patients with non-diagnostic electrocardiograms. Physical findings which may suggest an acute coronary event and a high short-term risk of death include pulmonary edema, new or worsening mitral regurgitation, S3 gallop, hypotension, or bradycardia/tachycardia.

## Electrocardiogram

An initial electrocardiogram should be obtained on all patients within 10 min of presentation with chest pain.[13–15] While abnormal electrocardiogram provides powerful information for diagnosis and risk stratification,[16] an initial normal electrocardiogram does not exclude acute coronary syndrome.[17] Normal electrocardiogram should not allow the reader to be misled into excluding ACS. A significant number of such patients may result in having a true ischemic event.[17–19] Valuable prognostic information is obtained based on pattern and magnitude of electrocardiographic changes.[15–17,20] Subsequently, serial ECGs should be performed at 5- to 10-min intervals or patients should be considered for continuous 12-lead ST-segment monitoring. Close observation and monitoring is suggested for patients with ongoing symptoms and strong clinical suspicion with an initial non-diagnostic ECG. Recommendations are made on basis of evolving or dynamic changes of the ST segment during ischemia. Risk of long-term complications are lower in patients with non-diagnostic electrocardiogram compared to patients with dynamic electrocardiographic changes.[21,22] While ST-segment elevation is related to a high risk of early death, ST-segment depression and its magnitude is associated with poor outcomes at 6 months.[23]

## Cardiac Biomarkers

Serum biomarkers are an important component of initial management of a patient with chest pain. Not only do the biomarkers help in conforming diagnosis, the level of biomarker release also helps in estimation of infarct size and provides useful prognostic information and identifies patients at high risk for poor outcomes. The extent of biomarker elevation or release depicts myocardial necrosis and damage. The kinetics of release of biomarkers serves as a surrogate marker or assessment of successful reperfusion.[24]

Advances in biomarkers include point of care assays and improved sensitivity and precision. In clinical practice, panel of biomarkers are utilized to overcome sensitivity- and specificity-related concerns of individual markers and provide substantial information.

Current biomarkers of choice are troponin (I and T) and CK-MB. Cardiac troponin I (cTnI) is very specific for myocardial injury. Levels of cTnI are detectable after 4–6 h after initial event and usually peak at 12–18 h. However, they may remain detectable until 1–2 weeks after an ischemic event. Unfortunately, unstable angina cannot be excluded based on negative biomarker assays. In those patients echocardiography plays a key role at peak stress or symptom. Interpretation of elevated troponin I levels requires caution in patients with sepsis, congestive heart failure, pulmonary embolism, arrhythmias, myocarditis, renal failure, trauma, and cerebrovascular accidents to name a few in the absence of chest pain or supportive ECG findings.[25] The list of conditions where an elevation of troponin level can be seen is exhaustive. Nevertheless, any elevation in troponin I in those patients portends a poor long-term prognosis.[26] ST-elevation myocardial infarction patients with an elevated level of troponin T within 6 h of chest pain onset have higher mortality.[27] As mentioned earlier, troponin elevation provides prognostic information beyond that provided by patient characteristics and admission electrocardiogram. In addition a strong relationship exists between the level of troponin elevation and risk of death. [28–30]

CK-MB is among the three creatine kinase isoenzymes. Even though CK-MB constitutes 15% of the cardiac creatine kinase, cardiac tissue is the most abundant source of CK-MB. CK-MB levels are useful in estimating the size and extent of infarct. In addition, due to near normalization of its level within 2–3 days after an acute coronary syndrome, CK-MB is useful in detection of reinfarction. As with troponin, elevation of CK-MB can be associated with non-ACS conditions including exercise, trauma, muscular dystrophies, muscle inflammation, and breakdown.[31,32]

B-type natriuretic peptide has been predominantly used in heart failure, but it has found its use in ACS as well. Elevation of BNP and N-terminal (NT)-pro BNP has a strong association with mortality in ACS and portends poor prognosis.[33] Currently, the role of BNP in ACS is limited to being an adjunct marker to those discussed above. A biphasic peak has been observed in levels of NT-pro BNP in association with anterior myocardial infarction. In that case, the second peak has a better correlation with poor outcome.

Myoglobin, found both in cardiac and in skeletal muscles, can be found as early as 1–4 h after an acute event. Due to its rapid rise and fall, myoglobin allows for early detection of myocardial injury (sensitivity 95%). However, its use is limited as it is not cardiac specific. High concentrations are found in skeletal muscles and it depends on renal function for clearance. The rapid release of myoglobin, however, makes it an attractive biomarker for early diagnosis of reperfusion after STEMI. This approach may be useful in early exclusion of ACS when combined with clinical characteristics of the patients and electrocardiographic presentation.[34,35]

Finally, an alternate proposed methodology has been to measure changes in serum levels of biomarkers over shorter time periods. [36–41] Rationale behind this approach is to be able to detect high-risk patients with positive delta values to undergo aggressive anti-ischemic therapy. Low-risk patients with negative delta values may be considered for early stress testing. The sensitivity for identifying myocardial ischemia with this approach ranges around 93% with a specificity of 94%.[38,41]

Many more biomarkers are under investigation for potential use in acute coronary syndrome.[42,13] They are not discussed in this chapter as none have matched the sensitivity and specificity and clinical applicability of the markers in current use. It is important though to interpret cautiously absence of any detectable biomarkers within first 6 h of onset of chest pain.[44] Serial testing should be performed at baseline, at 6–9, and at 12–24 h to detect or exclude myocardial injury. At our center we perform biomarker testing at 6- to 9-h intervals as mentioned in the PAIN algorithm (Chapter 2).

# Echocardiography

As will be discussed in subsequent chapters, echocardiography plays an important role in diagnosis and management of acute coronary syndrome. Role of echocardiography is maximal in patients with high clinical suspicion but non-diagnostic ECG. Stress echocardiography may play a significant role in triage of patients from emergency room. Pitfalls include false-negative patients getting discharged or missed subendocardial infarctions.

Role of echocardiography in acute coronary syndrome is two-fold. It aids in diagnosis of acute coronary syndrome by detection of regional or global ventricular wall motion abnormalities and ejection fraction. It is useful in assessment of hemodynamic instability. Its role in evaluating other potential life-threatening diagnosis presenting as chest pain (e.g., aortic dissection) is well established. In addition, echocardiography plays a key role in identification of complications of acute coronary syndrome such as left ventricular aneurysm, papillary muscle rupture, ventricular wall rupture, pseudoaneurysm, and mitral regurgitation.

## Conclusion

Application of a multipronged approach is fundamental in evaluating patients with chest pain. An approach inclusive of biomarkers and echocardiography, in addition to a good history and physical examination, aids in defining the patients who truly have an acute coronary syndrome or who are at risk of poor outcomes. An evidence-based algorithm may be developed at institutions to aid multidisciplinary teams in identification and management approaches in patients with suspicion of ACS.[45,46] Other goal of assessment is to identify patients who are at low risk and can be safely discharged home. The impact on health-care resources with this approach may be immense. However, caution should be exercised with this approach due to potential false negatives in the early stage after presentation to the hospital. Hospitals should institute chest pain pathway involving a multidisciplinary approach to assess and manage these patients. A rational use of echocardiography in this schema would be to assess for wall motion abnormalities in patients with equivocal history and negative biomarkers. Those with no wall motion abnormalities may be considered for discharge while others may be considered for early stress testing and discharge.

## References

1. Davies MJ. The pathophysiology of acute coronary syndromes. *Heart*. 2000 March;83(3):361–366.
2. Ho KT, Miller TD, Hodge DO, Bailey KR, Gibbons RJ. Use of a simple clinical score to predict prognosis of patients with normal or mildly abnormal resting electrocardiographic findings undergoing evaluation for coronary artery disease. *Mayo Clin Proc*. 2002 June;77(6):515–521.
3. Morise AP, Haddad WJ, Beckner D. Development and validation of a clinical score to estimate the probability of coronary artery disease in men and women presenting with suspected coronary disease. *Am J Med*. 1997 April;102(4):350–356.
4. Pryor DB, Harrell FE, Jr., Lee KL, Califf RM, Rosati RA. Estimating the likelihood of significant coronary artery disease. *Am J Med*. 1983 November;75(5):771–780.
5. Pryor DB, Shaw L, McCants CB, et al. Value of the history and physical in identifying patients at increased risk for coronary artery disease. *Ann Intern Med*. 1993 January 15;118(2):81–90.
6. Chaitman BR, Bourassa MG, Davis K, et al. Angiographic prevalence of high-risk coronary artery disease in patient subsets (CASS). *Circulation*. 1981 August;64(2):360–367.
7. Jayes RL, Jr., Beshansky JR, D'Agostino RB, Selker HP. Do patients' coronary risk factor reports predict acute cardiac ischemia in the emergency department? A multicenter study. *J Clin Epidemiol*. 1992 June;45(6):621–626.
8. Selker HP, Griffith JL, D'Agostino RB. A time-insensitive predictive instrument for acute myocardial infarction mortality: a multicenter study. *Med Care*. 1991 December;29(12): 1196–1211.

9.  Inhibition of platelet glycoprotein IIb/IIIa with eptifibatide in patients with acute coronary syndromes. The PURSUIT Trial Investigators. Platelet Glycoprotein IIb/IIIa in Unstable Angina: Receptor Suppression Using Integrilin Therapy. *N Engl J Med*. 1998 August 13;339(7):436–443.

10. Mak KH, Moliterno DJ, Granger CB, et al. Influence of diabetes mellitus on clinical outcome in the thrombolytic era of acute myocardial infarction. GUSTO-I Investigators. Global Utilization of Streptokinase and Tissue Plasminogen Activator for Occluded Coronary Arteries. *J Am Coll Cardiol*. 1997 July;30(1):171–179.

11. Coca SG, Krumholz HM, Garg AX, Parikh CR. Underrepresentation of renal disease in randomized controlled trials of cardiovascular disease. *Jama*. 2006 September 20;296(11): 1377–1384.

12. Das M, Aronow WS, McClung JA, Belkin RN. Increased prevalence of coronary artery disease, silent myocardial ischemia, complex ventricular arrhythmias, atrial fibrillation, left ventricular hypertrophy, mitral annular calcium, and aortic valve calcium in patients with chronic renal insufficiency. *Cardiol Rev*. 2006 January-February;14(1):14–17.

13. Anderson JL, Adams CD, Antman EM, et al. ACC/AHA 2007 guidelines for the management of patients with unstable angina/non ST-elevation myocardial infarction: a report of the American College of Cardiology/American Heart Association Task Force on Practice Guidelines (Writing Committee to Revise the 2002 Guidelines for the Management of Patients With Unstable Angina/Non ST-Elevation Myocardial Infarction): developed in collaboration with the American College of Emergency Physicians, the Society for Cardiovascular Angiography and Interventions, and the Society of Thoracic Surgeons: endorsed by the American Association of Cardiovascular and Pulmonary Rehabilitation and the Society for Academic Emergency Medicine. *Circulation*. 2007 August 14;116(7):e148–e304.

14. Antman EM, Anbe DT, Armstrong PW, et al. ACC/AHA guidelines for the management of patients with ST-elevation myocardial infarction–executive summary: a report of the American College of Cardiology/American Heart Association Task Force on Practice Guidelines (Writing Committee to Revise the 1999 Guidelines for the Management of Patients With Acute Myocardial Infarction). *Circulation*. 2004 August 3;110(5):588–636.

15. Selker HP, Zalenski RJ, Antman EM, et al. An evaluation of technologies for identifying acute cardiac ischemia in the emergency department: a report from a National Heart Attack Alert Program Working Group. *Ann Emerg Med*. 1997 January;29(1):13–87.

16. Savonitto S, Ardissino D, Granger CB, et al. Prognostic value of the admission electrocardiogram in acute coronary syndromes. *Jama*. 1999 February 24;281(8):707–713.

17. Rouan GW, Lee TH, Cook EF, Brand DA, Weisberg MC, Goldman L. Clinical characteristics and outcome of acute myocardial infarction in patients with initially normal or nonspecific electrocardiograms (a report from the Multicenter Chest Pain Study). *Am J Cardiol*. 1989 November 15;64(18):1087–1092.

18. Slater DK, Hlatky MA, Mark DB, Harrell FE, Jr., Pryor DB, Califf RM. Outcome in suspected acute myocardial infarction with normal or minimally abnormal admission electrocardiographic findings. *Am J Cardiol*. 1987 October 1;60(10):766–770.

19. McCarthy BD, Wong JB, Selker HP. Detecting acute cardiac ischemia in the emergency department: a review of the literature. *J Gen Intern Med*. 1990 July-August;5(4):365–373.

20. Zaacks SM, Liebson PR, Calvin JE, Parrillo JE, Klein LW. Unstable angina and non-Q wave myocardial infarction: does the clinical diagnosis have therapeutic implications? *J Am Coll Cardiol*. 1999 January;33(1):107–118.

21. Cannon CP, McCabe CH, Stone PH, et al. The electrocardiogram predicts one-year outcome of patients with unstable angina and non-Q wave myocardial infarction: results of the TIMI III Registry ECG Ancillary Study. Thrombolysis in Myocardial Ischemia. *J Am Coll Cardiol*. 1997 July;30(1):133–140.

22. Welch RD, Zalenski RJ, Frederick PD, et al. Prognostic value of a normal or nonspecific initial electrocardiogram in acute myocardial infarction. *Jama*. 2001 October 24–31;286(16): 1977–1984.

23. Savonitto S, Cohen MG, Politi A, et al. Extent of ST-segment depression and cardiac events in non-ST-segment elevation acute coronary syndromes. *Eur Heart J.* 2005 October;26(20):2106–2113.

24. Alpert JS, Thygesen K, Antman E, Bassand JP. Myocardial infarction redefined–a consensus document of The Joint European Society of Cardiology/American College of Cardiology Committee for the redefinition of myocardial infarction. *J Am Coll Cardiol.* 2000 September;36(3):959–969.

25. Jaffe AS. Elevations in cardiac troponin measurements: false false-positives: the real truth. *Cardiovasc Toxicol.* 2001;1(2):87–92.

26. Aviles RJ, Askari AT, Lindahl B, et al. Troponin T levels in patients with acute coronary syndromes, with or without renal dysfunction. *N Engl J Med.* 2002 June 27;346(26): 2047–2052.

27. Ohman EM, Armstrong PW, White HD, et al. Risk stratification with a point-of-care cardiac troponin T test in acute myocardial infarction. GUSTOIII Investigators. Global Use of Strategies To Open Occluded Coronary Arteries. *Am J Cardiol.* 1999 December 1;84(11): 1281–1286.

28. Hamm CW, Goldmann BU, Heeschen C, Kreymann G, Berger J, Meinertz T. Emergency room triage of patients with acute chest pain by means of rapid testing for cardiac troponin T or troponin I. *N Engl J Med.* 1997 December 4;337(23):1648–1653.

29. Galvani M, Ottani F, Ferrini D, et al. Prognostic influence of elevated values of cardiac troponin I in patients with unstable angina. *Circulation.* 1997 April 15;95(8):2053–2059.

30. Ohman EM, Armstrong PW, Christenson RH, et al. Cardiac troponin T levels for risk stratification in acute myocardial ischemia. GUSTO IIA Investigators. *N Engl J Med.* 1996 October 31;335(18):1333–1341.

31. Tsung SH. Several conditions causing elevation of serum CK-MB and CK-BB. *Am J Clin Pathol.* 1981 May;75(5):711–715.

32. Eggers KM, Oldgren J, Nordenskjold A, Lindahl B. Diagnostic value of serial measurement of cardiac markers in patients with chest pain: limited value of adding myoglobin to troponin I for exclusion of myocardial infarction. *Am Heart J.* 2004 October;148(4):574–581.

33. de Lemos JA, Morrow DA, Bentley JH, et al. The prognostic value of B-type natriuretic peptide in patients with acute coronary syndromes. *N Engl J Med.* 2001 October 4;345(14): 1014–1021.

34. McCord J, Nowak RM, McCullough PA, et al. Ninety-minute exclusion of acute myocardial infarction by use of quantitative point-of-care testing of myoglobin and troponin I. *Circulation.* 2001 September 25;104(13):1483–1488.

35. Ng SM, Krishnaswamy P, Morissey R, Clopton P, Fitzgerald R, Maisel AS. Ninety-minute accelerated critical pathway for chest pain evaluation. *Am J Cardiol.* 2001 September 15;88(6):611–617.

36. Fesmire FM, Percy RF, Bardoner JB, Wharton DR, Calhoun FB. Serial creatinine kinase (CK) MB testing during the emergency department evaluation of chest pain: utility of a 2-hour deltaCK-MB of +1.6 ng/ml. *Am Heart J.* 1998 August;136(2):237–244.

37. Apple FS, Christenson RH, Valdes R, Jr., et al. Simultaneous rapid measurement of whole blood myoglobin, creatine kinase MB, and cardiac troponin I by the triage cardiac panel for detection of myocardial infarction. *Clin Chem.* 1999 February;45(2):199–205.

38. Young GP, Gibler WB, Hedges JR, et al. Serial creatine kinase-MB results are a sensitive indicator of acute myocardial infarction in chest pain patients with nondiagnostic electrocardiograms: the second Emergency Medicine Cardiac Research Group Study. *Acad Emerg Med.* 1997 September;4(9):869–877.

39. Marin MM, Teichman SL. Use of rapid serial sampling of creatine kinase MB for very early detection of myocardial infarction in patients with acute chest pain. *Am Heart J.* 1992 February;123(2):354–361.

40. Fesmire FM. Delta CK-MB outperforms delta troponin I at 2 hours during the ED rule out of acute myocardial infarction. *Am J Emerg Med.* 2000 January;18(1):1–8.

41. Fesmire FM, Hughes AD, Fody EP, et al. The Erlanger chest pain evaluation protocol: a one-year experience with serial 12-lead ECG monitoring, two-hour delta serum marker measurements, and selective nuclear stress testing to identify and exclude acute coronary syndromes. *Ann Emerg Med*. 2002 December;40(6):584–594.

42. Morrow DA, Braunwald E. Future of biomarkers in acute coronary syndromes: moving toward a multimarker strategy. *Circulation*. 2003 July 22;108(3):250–252.

43. Maisel AS, Bhalla V, Braunwald E. Cardiac biomarkers: a contemporary status report. *Nat Clin Pract Cardiovasc Med*. 2006 January;3(1):24–34.

44. Newby LK, Christenson RH, Ohman EM, et al. Value of serial troponin T measures for early and late risk stratification in patients with acute coronary syndromes. The GUSTO-IIa Investigators. *Circulation*. 1998 November 3;98(18):1853–1859.

45. Herzog E, Aziz E, Hong M. The PAIN pathway for the management of acute coronary syndrome. In: Hong M, Herzog E, eds. *Acute Coronary Syndrome Multidisciplinary and Pathway-Based Approach*. Berlin: Springer; 2008:9–19.

46. Herzog E, Saint-Jacques H, Rozanski A. The PAIN pathway as a tool to bridge the gap between evidence and management of acute coronary syndrome. *Crit Pathw Cardiol: J Evid Based Med*. 2004;3(1):20–24.

# Chapter 17
# Comprehensive Evaluation of Cardiac Hemodynamics – "Echocardiography-Guided Cardiac Catheterization"

Itzhak Kronzon

While most echocardiographers are familiar with the use of Doppler echocardiography in the evaluation of transvalvular gradients, valvular regurgitation, and evaluation of certain clinically important values such as pulmonary artery pressure, they rarely use the echocardiographic examination for a comprehensive detailed evaluation of intracardiac pressures and flows as it is done during cardiac catheterization. In this chapter, the practical aspects of such an examination will be described with the demonstration of a comprehensive hemodynamic evaluation in a patient. The information in this chapter is based on known and accepted hemodynamic and Doppler echocardiographic information and common practice. More data and references can be found in larger, detailed texts.[1]

The simplified Bernoulli equation is the basis for the calculation of all intracardiac pressures.[2]

$$\Delta P = 4V^2$$

where $\Delta P$ = pressure gradient in mmHg and $V$ = velocity in m/s.

## Evaluation of Right Atrial Pressure

This may be the first stage in the hemodynamic evaluation. It is performed with the transducer in the subxiphoid position. At this point, one can evaluate the inferior vena cava as it travels through the liver into the right atrium. During its course, the inferior vena cava will be perpendicular to the interrogating beam and therefore its size and the changes of its diameter during the respiratory cycle can be recorded by M-mode echocardiography. The normal diameter of the inferior vena cava in the adult is 1.5–2.5 cm measured just proximal to its entrance into the right atrium. Normally, with inspiration, there is a decrease of 50% or more in the diameter of the

I. Kronzon (✉)
Department of Medicine (Cardiology), NYU Medical Center, New York, NY, USA
e-mail: itzhak.kronzon@med.nyu.edu

E. Herzog, F.A. Chaudhry (eds.), *Echocardiography in Acute Coronary Syndrome*, DOI 10.1007/978-1-84882-027-2_17, © Springer-Verlag London Limited 2009

**Table 17.1** Evaluation of right atrial pressure

| IVC (cm) | Δ with resp (%) | RA pressure (mmHg) |
|---|---|---|
| <1.5 | Collapse | 0–5 |
| Nl (1.5–2.5) | >50 | 5–10 |
| Nl | <50 | 11–15 |
| >2.5 | <50 | 16–20 |
| >2.5 | No change | >20 |

inferior vena cava. Failure to collapse with respiration and a dilated inferior vena cava are markers of elevated right atrial pressures. Table 17.1 correlates inferior vena cava characteristics (diameter and respiratory changes) and right atrial pressure.[3] Figure 17.1 shows a two-dimensional image and M-mode echocardiogram of a patient with a markedly elevated right atrial pressure (more than 20 mmHg). The inferior vena cava is markedly dilated near its entrance into the right atrium (2.8 cm). The M-mode recorded at low paper speed demonstrates the lack of respiratory variation.

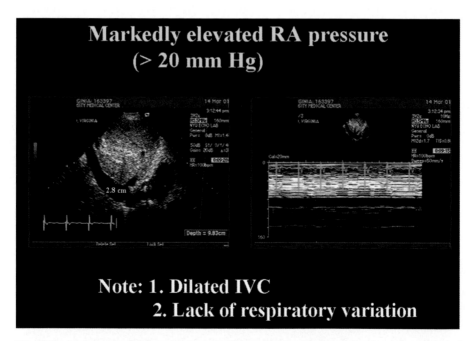

**Fig. 17.1** Assessment of right atrial pressure. Note markedly dilated inferior vena cava (IVC) and lack of respiratory variations in diameter (M-mode)

## Evaluation of Right Ventricular Systolic Pressure

Figure 17.2 shows the right heart pressures with the right atrial pressure, right ventricular pressure, and pulmonary artery pressure superimposed on each other. During diastole there is only a very small gradient across the tricuspid valve and during systole there is only a small gradient across the pulmonic valve. Those gradients are so small that their measurement is beyond the sensitivity of cardiac catheterization, which usually reports no gradients across the normal pulmonic or tricuspid valve. Figure 17.2 also shows that during systole, with the tricuspid valve closed, there is a pressure gradient between the right ventricle and the right atrium. About 90% of normal adults have some degree (usually trace or mild) of tricuspid regurgitation. The velocity of the tricuspid regurgitant jet (as measured by continuous wave Doppler) is related to the pressure gradient between the right ventricle and right atrium. Using the simplified Bernoulli equation, the tricuspid regurgitation gradient can be calculated. The right ventricular systolic pressure (RVSP) is the tricuspid regurgitant (TR) gradient plus the right atrial pressure (RAP).

$$RVSP = TR \text{ gradient} + RAP$$

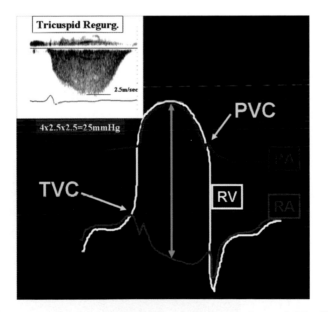

**Fig. 17.2**   Assessment of right ventricular (RV) systolic pressure (see text). The diagram shows normal right-sided pressures with no significant systolic gradient across the pulmonic valve and no significant diastolic gradient across the tricuspid valve. The gradient across the tricuspid valve in systole is marked by the *arrow* and is responsible for the tricuspid regurgitation velocity seen in the *upper left corner*. Other abbreviations: PA = pulmonary artery pressure, PVC = pulmonic valve closure, RA = right atrial pressure, TVC = tricuspid valve closure

In patients who have ventricular septal defects with a left to right shunt, the ventricular septal defect jet velocity is related to the pressure gradient between the left ventricle and the right ventricle. If there is no aortic stenosis, the systolic pressure in the left ventricle equals the systolic blood pressure measured by a blood pressure cuff (or by other invasive or noninvasive methods). Thus, the right ventricular systolic pressure (RVSP) equals systolic blood pressure (SBP) minus the systolic VSD (SVSD) gradient.

$$RVSP = SBP - SVSD \text{ gradient}$$

The lower the blood pressure and the higher the right ventricular systolic pressure, the smaller the gradient. Ventricular septal defects that are associated with lower blood pressure and with high right ventricular systolic pressure (as may be the case in ventricular septal defect during acute myocardial infarction) will have a lower VSD systolic flow velocity and lower systolic VSD gradient.

## Evaluation of Right Ventricular Diastolic Pressure

In the absence of tricuspid stenosis, there is only a small gradient between the right atrial diastolic pressure and the right ventricular diastolic pressure. This gradient can be ignored, and therefore, it can be said that right ventricular diastolic pressure (RVDP) equals right atrial pressure (RAP).

$$RVDP = RAP$$

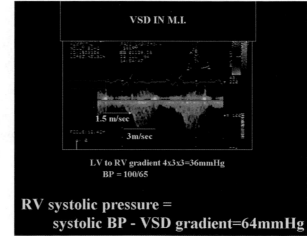

**Fig. 17.3** Assessment of RV systolic pressure in a patient with ventricular septal defect (VSD) after myocardial infarction (MI). Note that VSD flow persists during both systole (*horizontal line*) and diastole (*horizontal arrow*). See text for details

In the presence of ventricular septal defects with left to right shunts, the left ventricular diastolic pressure is usually higher than the right ventricular diastolic pressure. Therefore, there is flow between the left ventricle and right ventricle that continues throughout diastole. When compared to the velocity of the jet across the ventricular septal defect during systole, the diastolic jet velocity is significantly smaller (Fig. 17.3). However, if the left ventricular diastolic pressure is known, then the right ventricular diastolic pressure (RVDP) can be calculated as the left ventricular diastolic pressure (LVDP) minus the diastolic ventricular septal defect (DVSD) gradient.

$$RVDP = LVDP - DVSD \text{ gradient}$$

## Evaluation of Pulmonary Artery Systolic Pressure

In the absence of pulmonic stenosis, the pressure gradient between the right ventricle and the pulmonary artery can be ignored and it can be assumed that the pulmonary artery systolic pressure equals the right ventricular systolic pressure. Therefore, the pulmonary artery systolic pressure (PASP) equals the tricuspid regurgitation gradient plus the right atrial pressure (RAP).

$$PASP = TV \text{ gradient} + RAP$$

In the presence of pulmonic stenosis, the flow velocity across the stenotic pulmonic valve can be evaluated and the pulmonic stenosis gradient can be calculated. In these patients, the pulmonary artery systolic pressure (PASP) equals the right ventricular systolic pressure (RVSP) minus the pulmonic stenosis gradient.

$$PASP = RVSP - PS \text{ gradient}$$

## Evaluation of Pulmonary Artery Diastolic Pressure

The majority of patients have some degree (trace to mild) of pulmonic regurgitation. The velocity of the pulmonic regurgitation is defined by the diastolic pressure gradient between the pulmonary artery and the right ventricle. Thus, the pulmonary artery diastolic pressure (PADP) equals the pulmonary regurgitation gradient plus the right ventricular diastolic pressure (RVDP).

$$PADP = PR \text{ gradient} + RVDP$$

Since the right atrial pressure (in the absence of tricuspid stenosis) is approximately equal to the right ventricular diastolic pressure, pulmonary artery diastolic pressure (PADP) equals the pulmonic regurgitation gradient plus right atrial pressure (RAP).

$$PADP = PR\ gradient + RAP$$

The ability to measure the pulmonic regurgitation velocity may be helpful in the evaluation of the pulmonary artery pressure in patients who do not have tricuspid regurgitation. Figure 17.4 shows a continuous wave Doppler tracing of pulmonic valve flow in a patient evaluated for significant pulmonary hypertension who did not have tricuspid regurgitation. The velocity of the pulmonic regurgitant flow is 2.5 m/s at end diastole, which indicates an end-diastolic gradient of 25 mmHg across the pulmonic valve. The diastolic pulmonary artery pressure is therefore at least 25 mmHg, a markedly elevated value.

**Fig. 17.4** Assessment of pulmonary artery diastolic pressure in a patient with pulmonary hypertension

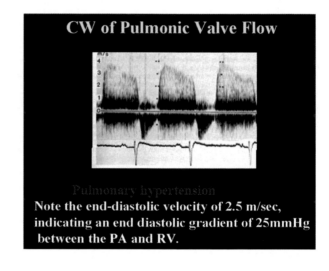

## Evaluation of Pulmonary Artery Pressure in the Absence of Tricuspid or Pulmonic Regurgitation

Rough, indirect estimation of PA pressure can be obtained by M-mode echocardiography. Characteristic M-mode pattern of the pulmonic valve in patients with severe pulmonary HTN (>70 mmHg) includes absence of "a" deflection during atrial contraction (in spite of normal sinus rhythm), "flying W" appearance of the systolic opening, and lack of backward motion of the diastolic closure line (Fig. 17.5).

Better estimation can be obtained by measuring the systolic acceleration time of the antegrade flow velocity measured by pulse wave Doppler just proximal to the pulmonic valve.[4] Mean PA pressure is inversely related to the acceleration time. The equation used is

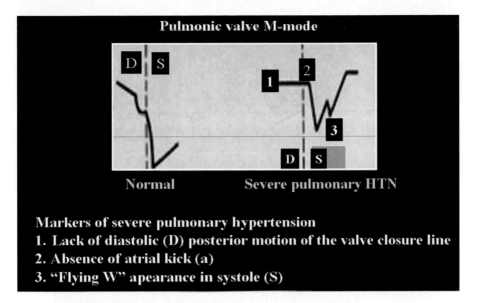

**Fig. 17.5** M-mode echocardiography in severe pulmonary hypertension

$$PAMP = 79 - (0.45 \times AcT)$$

where PAMP is mean PA pressure in mmHg and AcT is acceleration time in milliseconds.

Normal AcT is >120 ms. Values less than 90 ms are associated with PA mean pressure of 40 mmHg or more.

## Evaluation of Left Ventricular Systolic Pressure

In patients without valve disease, there is only a minimal gradient between the left ventricle and the aorta during systole. This small gradient can be ignored, and thus left ventricular systolic pressure (LVSP) equals the systolic blood pressure (SBP).

$$LVSP = SBP$$

In patients with aortic valve (or subvalvular or supravalvular) stenosis, there is a gradient between the left ventricle and the ascending aorta. Since the systolic ascending aortic pressure equals the systolic blood pressure, the left ventricular systolic pressure (LVSP) equals the systolic blood pressure (SBP) plus the systolic pressure gradient across the aortic valve (or other subvalvular or supravalvular sites).

$$LVSP = SBP + \text{aortic stenosis gradient}$$

The maximal gradient measured by the Doppler examination is the maximum instantaneous gradient across the aortic valve. This gradient is usually higher than the peak-to-peak gradient (between peak aortic systolic pressure and peak left ventricular systolic pressure) that is frequently measured and reported during cardiac catheterization. In most cases of severe aortic stenosis, the peak-to-peak gradient is approximately 70% of the maximum instantaneous gradient. The mean gradient across the aortic valve can also be calculated (both by Doppler echo and by pressure measurement during invasive procedures) (Fig. 17.6). When Doppler is used for the evaluation of left ventricular pressure, the value for measurement should be the peak-to-peak gradient (peak left ventricular systolic to peak systolic blood pressure obtained by cuff). Therefore

$$LVSP = SBP + 70\% \text{ aortic stenosis gradient}$$

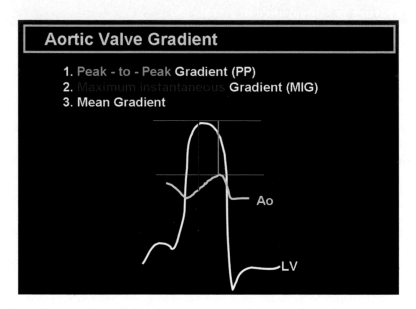

**Fig. 17.6**   Diagram of left-sided pressure in aortic stenosis (see text for details)

## Evaluation of Left Ventricular Diastolic Pressure

In the absence of mitral stenosis, the gradient between the left atrium and the left ventricle during diastole is small and can be ignored. Therefore, in these patients, the left atrial pressure is very close to the left ventricular diastolic pressure. The left atrial pressure can be estimated and this will give a good idea about left ventricular diastolic pressure as well.

In patients who have aortic regurgitation, the regurgitant jet velocity is a function of the diastolic gradient between the aorta and the left ventricle. If the aortic diastolic pressure is known, then the left ventricular diastolic pressure equals the aortic diastolic pressure minus the aortic regurgitation gradient. In most patients, the aortic pressure equals the cuff pressure in the arm. Therefore, the left ventricular end-diastolic pressure (LVEDP) equals the diastolic blood pressure (DBP) minus the aortic (AR) gradient at end diastole.

$$LVEDP = DBP - AR \text{ gradient (end diastolic)}$$

In patients with VSD and left to right shunt, the LVEDP can be calculated if the RA pressure (RAP) (and therefore RV diastolic pressure) is known. In these patients

$$LVEDP = RAP + VSD \text{ end-diastolic gradient}$$

Figure 17.7 is a continuous wave tracing taken from a patient with aortic valve disease. The aortic stenosis and aortic regurgitation jets are readily identified. The

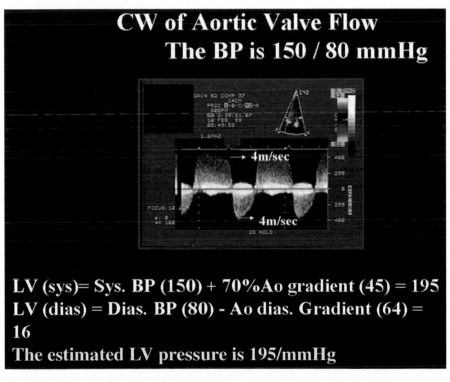

CW of Aortic Valve Flow
The BP is 150 / 80 mmHg

4m/sec

4m/sec

LV (sys)= Sys. BP (150) + 70%Ao gradient (45) = 195
LV (dias) = Dias. BP (80) - Ao dias. Gradient (64) =
16
The estimated LV pressure is 195/mmHg

**Fig. 17.7** Continuous wave Doppler (CW) in the calculation of left ventricular (LV) pressures in a patient with aortic stenosis and insufficiency (see text). Other abbreviations: Ao = aorta, BP = blood pressure, Dias = diastolic, Sys = systolic

peak aortic stenosis velocity is 4 m/s and the aortic regurgitation jet end-diastolic velocity is also 4 m/s. This patient had a blood pressure of 150/80 mmHg. Therefore, the left ventricular systolic pressure equals the systolic blood pressure (150 mmHg) plus 70% of the aortic systolic gradient. Since the peak instantaneous aortic gradient is 64, the peak-to-peak gradient is 70% of 64, which is 45 mmHg. The left ventricular systolic pressure is therefore 150 + 45 = 195 mmHg. The left ventricular diastolic pressure equals the diastolic blood pressure (80 mmHg) minus the aortic diastolic gradient (64 mmHg), which equals 16 mmHg. Therefore, this patient's left ventricular pressure is 195/16 mmHg.

## Evaluation of Left Atrial Pressure

The evaluation of left atrial pressure and its clinical importance has been discussed in prior chapters in this book. Noninvasively the left atrial pressure can be estimated from the transmitral and pulmonary venous flow measured by pulsed Doppler. When these flow patterns are normal, the pressure in the left atrium is normal (6–12 mmHg). When there is a decreased relaxation flow pattern across the mitral valve (low E, high A) the left atrial pressure is normal or minimally elevated (8–14 mmHg). With pseudonormalization of transmitral flow, the left atrial pressure is high, usually 15–22 mmHg. Finally, with a restrictive pattern (high E, low A, and a rapid transmitral flow deceleration of 160 ms or less), the left atrial pressure is usually 23 mmHg or more. Another simple method of calculation of left atrial pressure (LAP) uses the transmitral flow E-wave velocity and the tissue Doppler (E'). The higher the left atrial pressure, the higher the E and lower the E'.

An E/E' ratio of <9 is associated with normal LAP. An E/E' ratio of more than 14 is associated with elevated LAP (>14 mmHg).

The equation reported by Nagueh et al.[5] describes the relation between LAP and E/E'

$$LAP = 1.24[(E/E') + 1.9]$$

A simpler equation is used at our laboratory:

$$LAP = E/E' + 4\,mmHg$$

As was noted before, the estimation of left atrial pressure in the absence of mitral stenosis can give a good idea about the left ventricular diastolic pressure.

In patients with mitral regurgitation, the left atrial pressure during ventricular systole (LAS) equals the systolic blood pressure (SBP) (which in the absence of aortic stenosis equals the left ventricular systolic pressure) minus the mitral regurgitation (MR) gradient.

$$LAS = SBP - MR\ gradient$$

In patients with mitral stenosis (MS), the left atrial pressure during ventricular diastole (LAD) equals the left ventricular end-diastolic pressure (LVDP) plus the mean transmitral gradient.

$$LAD = LVDP + transmitral\ gradient$$

## Calculation of Cardiac Output

A calculation of the cardiac output can be performed using the left heart (systemic blood flow) or the right heart (pulmonary blood flow). In the absence of shunts, the pulmonary blood flow is equal to the systemic blood flow. The calculation of the systemic blood flow (SBF) is best done at the left ventricular outflow tract (LVOT). The diameter of the LVOT can be measured and the cross-sectional area (CSA) calculated. The multiplication of the LVOT cross-sectional area by the velocity time integral (VTI) at that site will provide the value of the stroke volume (SV). Stroke volume times heart rate (HR) equals cardiac output (CO) (Fig. 17.8).

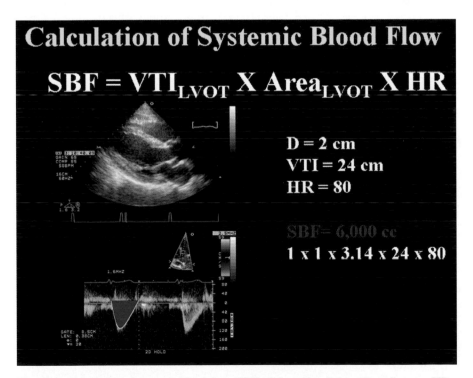

**Fig. 17.8** Calculation of systemic blood flow (SBF). Other abbreviations: D = diameter, HR = heart rate, LVOT = left ventricular outflow tract, VTI = velocity time integral

$$SV = CSA_{LVOT} \times VTI_{LVOT}$$

$$CO = SV \times HR$$

Similarly, calculation of pulmonary blood flow can be done at the right ventricular outflow tract just proximal to the pulmonic valve.

## Calculation of Shunt Flow

The evaluation of shunt flow in patients with an atrial septal defect or ventricular septal defect with a left to right shunt can be performed by the calculation of pulmonary blood flow (PBF) minus systemic blood flow (SBF).

$$\text{Shunt flow} = PBF - SBF$$

Another approach is the evaluation of the atrial septal defect or ventricular septal defect orifice area (DOA) and multiplying it by the shunt velocity time integral (VTI) and by the heart rate (HR).

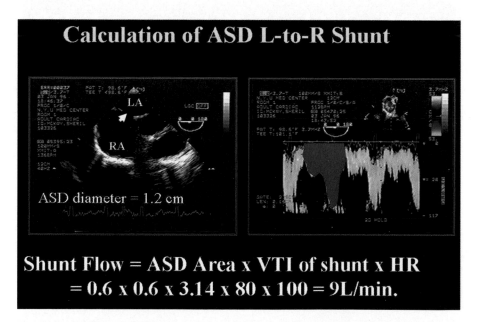

**Fig. 17.9** Calculation of atrial septal defect (ASD) left to right (L-to-R) shunt flow. The images were obtained by transesophageal echocardiography. The ASD is marked by an *arrowhead*

$$\text{Shunt flow} = \text{DOA} \times \text{VTI}_{shunt} \times \text{HR}$$

Figure 17.9 is an example of the calculation of atrial septal defect flow with a left to right shunt. The shunt flow equals the orifice area multiplied by the velocity time integral of the shunt and multiplied by the heart rate. In this case, the atrial septal diameter was 1.2 cm; therefore, the radius was 0.6 cm. With a VTI$_{shunt}$ of 80 cm and HR of 100/min, the shunt flow is

$$3.14 \times 0.6 \times 0.6 \times 80 \times 100 = 9000\,\text{cc/min} = 9\,\text{L/min}$$

## Estimation of Pulmonary Vascular Resistance (PVR)

This important hemodynamic parameter is the ratio between the pressure gradient and the blood flow across the pulmonary vascular tree. Invasively, PVR can be calculated using the equation

$$\text{PVR} = (\text{PAMP} - \text{LAMP})/\text{PBF}$$

where PVR is measured in Wood's units, PAMP = pulmonary artery mean pressure in mmHg, LAMP = left atrial mean pressure in mmHg, and PBF = pulmonary blood flow in L/min. Example: with normal PAMP (15 mmHg), normal LAMP (5 mmHg), and normal PBF (5 L/min) the calculated PVR is approximately 2 units.

The PVR is directly related to the PA pressure (and therefore to the maximal TR jet velocity); on the other hand, the PVR is inversely related to the stroke volume in the RVOT (which can be measured noninvasively by pulsed Doppler, using the velocity time integral (VTI) at the right ventricular outflow tract, just proximal to the pulmonic valve).

PVR can therefore be calculated by Doppler using the following equation:[6]

$$\text{PVR} = 10(\text{TR jet V} - \text{VTI}_{RVOT}) + 0.16)$$

where PVR is expressed in Wood's units, TR jet V = tricuspid regurgitation jet velocity in m/s, and VTI$_{RVOT}$ = velocity time integral at the right ventricular outflow tract in cm (Fig. 17.10)

## Clinical Case

### Comprehensive Hemodynamic Evaluation

The echocardiographic examination can provide many hemodynamic details. Sometimes the hemodynamic information is not less comprehensive than which is

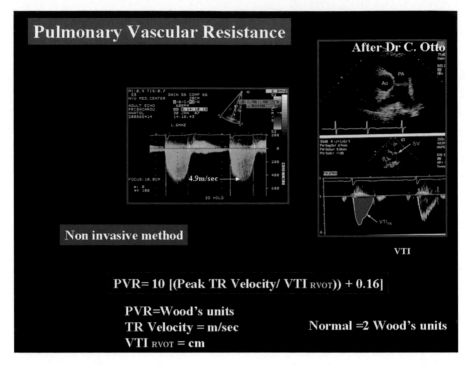

**Fig. 17.10** Noninvasive calculation of pulmonary vascular resistance (PVR). Other abbreviations: VTI_RVOT = Velocity time integral at the right ventricular outflow tract

available from invasive examinations (cardiac catheterization). In the next few paragraphs, we will evaluate noninvasively a 53–year-old male and acute shortness of breath. The blood pressure was 100/65 mmHg, heart rate 70/min and regular, and there was no jugular venous distention. There was an apical diastolic rumble (mitral stenosis) and a basal systolic ejection murmur radiating to the carotids (aortic stenosis). In the reporting of this patient's hemodynamics we used the form that is used in our cardiac catheterization laboratory. Figure 17.11 shows the hemodynamic information that was available at this stage. With a blood pressure of 100/65 mmHg, we assume that the aortic pressure is the same.

The first stage of our evaluation was subxiphoid echocardiography for the evaluation of the inferior vena cava. As can be seen in Fig. 17.12 A, the inferior vena cava has a normal size (1.6 cm) and there was more than 50% respiratory collapse. Therefore, the inferior vena cava and the right atrial pressure (and also the superior vena cava) are normal (5–10 mmHg) and for the sake of simplicity we picked the value of 6 mmHg. At this point, what is known is presented in the diagram on the right (Fig. 17.12B). The patient also had mild tricuspid regurgitation (Fig. 17.13 A). The jet velocity of the tricuspid regurgitation was 3.2 m/s and therefore the tricuspid regurgitation gradient (between the right ventricle and the right atrium) was 40 mmHg. With a right atrial pressure of 6 mmHg, the right ventric-

**Fig. 17.11** Patient history and physical findings (JVD = jugular venous distension)

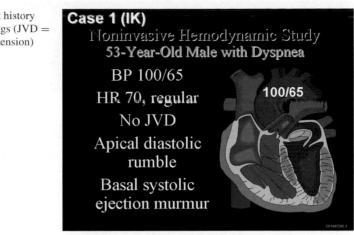

ular systolic pressure equals the right atrial diastolic pressure (6 mmHg) plus the tricuspid regurgitation gradient (40 mmHg) or 46 mmHg. In the absence of tricuspid stenosis, the right ventricular diastolic pressure equals the right atrial pressure and therefore the pressure in the right ventricle is 46/6 mmHg. The diagram on the right represents these new findings (Fig. 17.13B). Now we can calculate the pul-

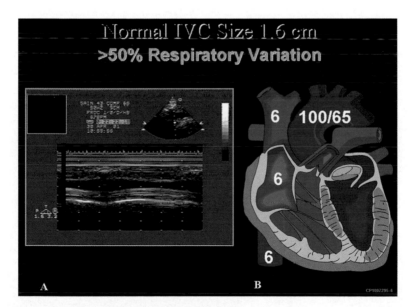

**Fig. 17.12** (**A**) M-mode echo in the evaluation of RA pressure. Normal diameter and more than 50% respiratory collapse are suggestive of normal (5–10 mmHg) right atrial (RA) pressure. (**B**) The hemodynamic diagram now shows normal RA pressure (6 mmHg)

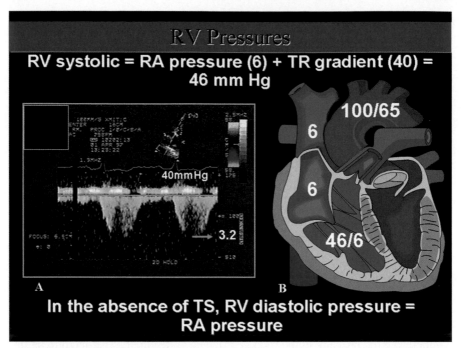

**Fig. 17.13** (**A**) Calculation of right ventricular (RV) pressures. (**B**) The hemodynamic diagram now shows the RV pressures

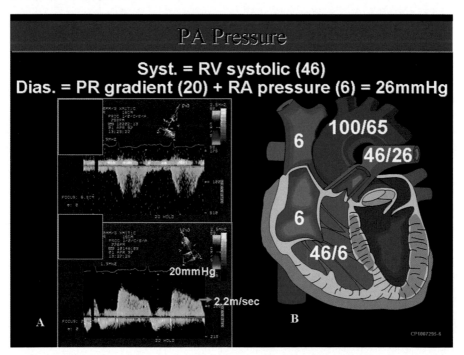

**Fig. 17.14** (**A**) Calculation of pulmonary artery (PA) pressures. (**B**) The hemodynamic diagram now shows the PA pressures

monary artery pressure. In the absence of pulmonic stenosis, the right ventricular systolic pressure (46 mmHg) practically equals pulmonary arterial systolic pressure. This patient also has pulmonic regurgitation (Fig. 17.14 A). At end diastole, the velocity of the pulmonic regurgitation jet is 2.2 m/s, which indicated a pulmonic regurgitant gradient of 20 mmHg. The pulmonary artery diastolic pressure is therefore the pulmonary regurgitation gradient (20 mmHg) plus right atrial pressure (6 mmHg), or 26 mmHg. The diagram on the right represents the information known so far (Fig. 17.14B). The patient also has mild aortic regurgitation (Fig. 17.15 A). The end-diastolic velocity of the aortic regurgitation jet is 3.7 m/s and therefore the aortic end-diastolic gradient is 55 mmHg. Therefore, the left ventricular end-diastolic pressure equals the aortic diastolic pressure (65 mmHg) minus the aortic regurgitation gradient (55 mmHg) or 10 mmHg. The diagram on the right again shows what is available so far (Fig. 17.15B). In addition, this patient has aortic stenosis (Fig. 17.16A). The peak instantaneous aortic flow velocity is 4.8 m/s, which is the equivalent of a transaortic peak instantaneous gradient of 92 mmHg. Since the peak-to-peak gradient is only 70% of the peak instantaneous gradient, the peak-to-peak gradient is 64 mmHg. The left ventricular systolic pressure is therefore the aortic systolic pressure (100 mmHg) plus 70% of the aortic valve gradient (64 mmHg), or 164 mmHg. The diagram on the right shows what we know so far (Fig. 17.16B). Finally, this patient also has mitral stenosis (Fig. 17.17 A). The

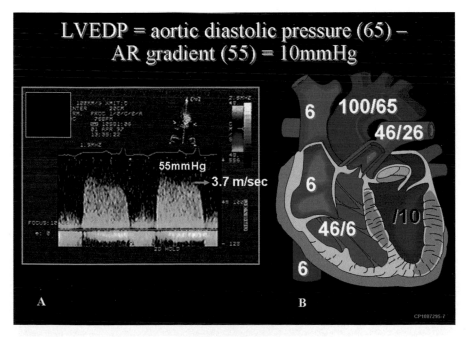

**Fig. 17.15** (**A**) Calculation of LV end-diastolic pressure (LVEDP). (**B**) The hemodynamic diagram now includes LVEDP (AR = aortic regurgitation)

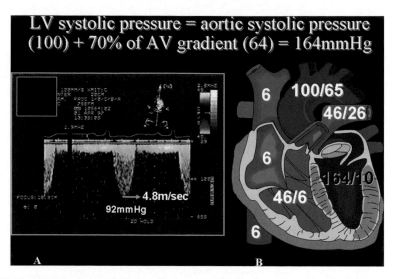

**Fig. 17.16** (**A**) Calculation of LV systolic pressure. (**B**) The hemodynamic diagram now includes LV systolic pressure (AV = aortic valve)

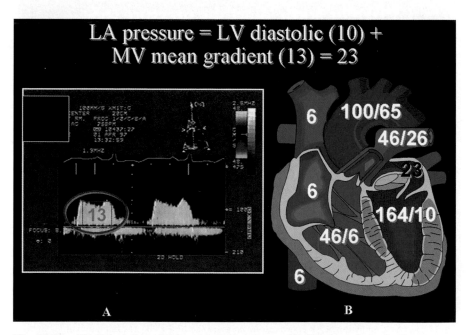

**Fig. 17.17** (**A**) Calculation of left atrial (LA) pressure. (**B**) The hemodynamic diagram now includes all intracardiac pressures (MV = mitral valve)

mean mitral gradient was calculated to be 13 mmHg. The left atrial pressure, therefore, equals the left ventricular diastolic pressure (10 mmHg) plus the mitral valve mean gradient (13 mmHg), or 23 mmHg. The diagram on the right indicates all the pressures (Fig. 17.17B). Thus, without the use of catheters, punctures, or blood we obtained all the pressures in the cardiac chambers, the great arteries, and the veins.

# References

1. Oh JK, Seward JB, Tajik JA, eds. *The Echo Manual. Doppler Echocardiography and Color Flow Imaging: Comprehensive Non Invasive Hemodynamic Assessment.* 3rd ed., Chapter 4. Philadelphia, PA: Lippinkot, Williams and Wilkins; 2007:59–79.
2. Hatle L, Angelsen B. *Doppler Ultrasound in Cardiology.* 2nd ed. Philadelphia, PA: Lea & Febiger; 1985.
3. Otto C ed. *Textbook of Clinical Echocardiography.* 3rd ed. Philadelphia, PA: Elsevier–Saundres; 2007:157.
4. Mahan G, Dabestani A, Gardin J, et al. Estimation of pulmonary artery pressure by pulsed Doppler echocardiography. *Circulation.* 1983;68(suppl III):III-367.
5. Nagueh SF, Middleton KJ, Kopelen HA, et al. Doppler tissue imaging: a noninvasive technique for evaluation of LV filling pressure. *J Am Coll Cardiol.* 1997; 30:1527–1533.
6. Scapellato F, Temporrelli PL, Eleuteri E, et al. Accurate noninvasive assessment of pulmonary vascular resistance in patients with chronic heart failure. *Am J Cardiol.* 2001; 37:1813–1819.

# Chapter 18
# Echocardiography During Angina Pectoris and Acute Myocardial Infarction in the Emergency Room

**Emad Aziz and Eyal Herzog**

## Background

The evaluation of patients presenting to the emergency department (ED) with chest pain can be very challenging for the clinician. The early identification of patients with coronary artery disease from those who have other causes of chest pain is critical to delivering appropriate medical care. It is estimated that 8 million patients present annually to the emergency department with chest pain[1] and that only a small subset of then will ultimately be diagnosed as having acute coronary syndrome (ACS).

Current guidelines stress the importance of identifying patients who have increased likelihood of acute myocardial infarction (AMI) and thus likely to benefit from early prompt diagnosis and delivery of evidence-based medical therapies.[2–4] Failure to identify and provide early treatment to these high-risk patients will have important negative implications on their outcomes.

Surprisingly, Lee et al. reported that despite the low threshold for unnecessary admission of patients with chest pain, 8% of patients with AMI are erroneously sent home, 75% had less typical symptoms and were less likely to have electrocardiographic evidence of ischemia.[5]

ECG interpretation in the ED is central in the assessment of patients with possible cardiac ischemia; however, discrepancies have been reported on triage and treatment decisions have been debated.[6–9]

In addition, a recent report from the Emergency Department Quality in Myocardial Infarction (EDQMI) study reported that one in eight AMI patients had high-risk ECG findings that were not identified and that, among these patients, the delivery

E. Aziz (✉)
Cardiology, St Luke's Roosevelt Hospital Center, New York, NY, USA
e-mail: Eaziz@chpnet.org

E. Herzog, F.A. Chaudhry (eds.), *Echocardiography in Acute Coronary Syndrome*,
DOI 10.1007/978-1-84882-027-2_18, © Springer-Verlag London Limited 2009

of evidence-based therapies in the ED, including aspirin, β-blockers, and acute reperfusion, was markedly lower. There was also a trend toward higher in-hospital mortality rates in patients with missed high-risk ECG findings.[10]

Thus, a diagnostic dilemma exists for a subset of patients which accounts for 20–45% who present to the ED with typical or atypical chest pain and nondiagnostic electrocardiogram; subsequently, a significant proportion of these patients might show signs of myocardial injury.[11]

Acute coronary syndrome spans a broad classification, including ST-elevation myocardial infarction (STEMI), non-ST-elevation myocardial infarction (NSTEMI), and unstable angina. Traditional ways for diagnosing ACS on the basis of ECG and initial troponin levels can only be designated in a small percentage of these patients. Cardiac enzymes are extremely sensitive to myocardial infarction; however, these assays do not detect unstable angina.[12] Furthermore, it might take 4–12 h after presentation before cardiac enzymes are definitive.

Acute ischemia results in a cascade of biochemical physiologic changes in the myocardial tissues.[13] These biochemical changes are followed by abnormalities in diastolic and then systolic function, which produce regional wall motion abnormalities (RWMAs) that can be visualized echocardiographically within seconds of coronary artery occlusion.[14] In many cases these changes precede any ECG changes or even the development of symptoms.[15] The RWMAs reflect a localized decrease in the amplitude and rate of myocardial excursion, as well as a blunted degree of myocardial thickening. Transthoracic echocardiography (TTE) has the advantages of being readily accessible, portable, noninvasive, and fast; it may detect significant findings that are misdiagnosed or not detected on initial clinical evaluation.

Hence, in 2003, a task force of the American College of Cardiology (ACC), the American Heart Association (AHA), and the American Society of Echocardiography (ASE) gave a class I recommendation to the use of echocardiography for evaluation of patients with chest pain in the following settings:[16]

1. For diagnosis of underlying cardiac disease in patients with chest pain and clinical evidence of valvular, pericardial, or myocardial disease.
2. For evaluation of chest pain in patients with suspected acute myocardial ischemia, when baseline ECG and other laboratory markers are nondiagnostic and when the study can be obtained during pain or within minutes after its abatement.
3. For evaluation of chest pain in patients with suspected aortic dissection.
4. For evaluation of patients with chest pain and hemodynamic instability unresponsive to simple therapeutic measures.

The task force recommended against the routine use of echocardiography for diagnosis of chest pain in patients with electrocardiographic changes diagnostic of myocardial ischemia or infarction.

## Role of Echocardiography in the Emergency Department

Several studies have examined the feasibility and efficacy of echocardiography in emergency department (ED) patients with chest pain. Most of these studies were performed on patients with chest pain hoping to identify those with AMI. Early use of echocardiography can be essential in providing crucial information about wall motion abnormalities and also diagnose other non-ischemic causes of chest pain like pulmonary embolism, hypertrophic cardiomyopathy, pericarditis, and aortic dissection. It can provide incremental prognostic information to identify patients at risk of early clinical, historical, and electrocardiographic variables. The event rates within 48 h of ED admission are different for patients with and without left ventricular systolic dysfunction (LVSD); a significantly greater event rate exists for patients with LVSD as a group and for those with even mild-to-moderate wall motion abnormalities, compared with patients without LVSD.[17]

In a prospective study involving 466 visits to a large urban ED by patients with acute chest pain, Sabia et al.[18] examined echocardiographic predicators of serious predischarge complications in patients with chest pain. Regional wall motion was assessed using a wall motion index on the basis of a 16-segment model. The composite complications end point included significant recurrent myocardial ischemia, heart failure, or arrhythmia. In a univariate analysis, the following variables predicated complications: left ventricular function (OR, 2.9; 95% CI, 1.6–5.1), right ventricular function (OR, 2.7; 95% CI, 1.2–6.2), left ventricular end-diastolic dimension (OR, 1.6/cm; 95% CI, 1.1–2.3), left ventricular end-systolic function (OR, 1.4/cm; 95% CI, 1.1–1.9), and wall motion index (OR, 3.0; 95% CI, 1.8–4.8). Left ventricular ejection fraction,[19] end-systolic volume,[19] WMSI,[20] and the presence of even mild MR[21] are all early predictors of adverse outcome.

Thus, one strategy for screening chest pain patients for RWMAs with echocardiography would be as follows:

1. If an adequate echocardiogram can be obtained and there are no RWMAs, it is relatively safe to discharge the patient from the emergency department.
2. Patients with RWMAs should be admitted for further observation and treatment. Those patients with a suspicious chest pain syndrome in whom an adequate echocardiogram cannot be obtained would also warrant observation.

This scheme could provide a screening mechanism to reduce the number of admissions that use ECG and clinical criteria alone and would also identify acute mechanical complications of a myocardial infarction.[22] However, using RWMA to screen for ischemia rather than waiting for cardiac enzymes is not perfect; there are limitations to screening with echocardiography. It is reasonable only if a high-quality echocardiogram can be obtained and an experienced echocardiographer available to interpret the echocardiogram 24 h a day. Furthermore, even if the echocardiographic procedure is technically feasible, some patients with a small myocardial infarction who spontaneously reperfused, but may still have an unstable lesion, could potentially be discharged under this protocol. Despite these limitations, the 2003 ACC/AHA/ASE task force gave a class I recommendation to the use of echocardiography for evaluation of chest pain in patients with suspected acute myocardial ischemia, when baseline ECG and other laboratory markers are nondiagnostic and when the study can be obtained during pain or within minutes after its abatement.

## Different Modalities of Echocardiography that is Feasible in the Emergency Department

Echocardiography must be performed by a trained operator and interpreted by physicians experienced in wall motion analysis. Adequate images are obtainable in about 90% of cases. Its utility in the evaluation of chest pain appears high with sensitivity of 93% and specificity of 71% as seen in 16 published studies including more than 1300 patients. Wall motion may be normal in patients with small infarctions; however, these patients have a low risk of complications. Previous MI can make it difficult to identify new wall motion abnormalities. The severity of ischemia, its duration, and the extent of the ischemic zone may affect the persistence of wall motion abnormalities in patients with unstable angina; performing echocardiography during the symptomatic episode or within 1 h will make findings more reliable.[11]

## Clinical Applications

As mentioned above the main function for echocardiography in the ED is early detection of wall motion abnormalities and risk stratification for patients with possible myocardial ischemia. In our PAIN pathway for management of patients admitted with ACS, echocardiography plays an important role in recognizing patients with advanced risk from patients with intermediate and low risk.[23]

## Early Detection of Acute Myocardial Infarction Complications in the Emergency Department

Echocardiography is the mainstay of diagnosis of mechanical complications of myocardial infarction (MI),[24] and patients with unexplained hemodynamic deterioration should be immediately evaluated.

The following are some of the most common complications diagnosed:

1. *Right ventricular infarction*: Recognition of right ventricular (RV) infarction is important, as it requires specific hemodynamic management. This syndrome occurs in more than 30% of patients with inferior MI but is rare in anterior infarction. Many right coronary artery occlusions do not result in significant RV infarction due to the lower RV oxygen demand, higher oxygen extraction ration, greater systolic/diastolic flow ratio, and collateral supply. Right ventricular infarction may be diagnosed clinically and from right-sided

ECG leads, but echocardiography provides better assessment of the extent and severity.[25]

2. *Ventricular septal rupture*: The diagnosis can usually be made by TTE; experience is essential as the most useful views depend on the location of defect. Subcostal views are particularly useful in the critically ill, supine patient with inferior infarction. Small defects may not be visible but color Doppler is very sensitive. A large left–right shunt is characterized by hypercontractility of non-infarcted LV segments with a low LV stroke volume, high pulmonary artery flow velocities, and pulmonary hypertension. Posterior septal ruptures in particular tend to be complex and often associated with right ventricular infarction, which has an adverse prognosis.

3. *Papillary muscle rupture*: Papillary muscle rupture is the most serious mechanism of MR in acute infarction. It usually involves the posteromedial muscle, which is perfused from the posterior descending artery, whereas the anterolateral muscle has blood supply from both diagonal and circumflex arteries. Rupture of a papillary muscle head causes severe MR; rupture of the entire trunk is generally fatal. Transthoracic echocardiography can be suboptimal and the views of the papillary muscles are often limited, the MR jet is eccentric, and color Doppler is influenced by the low LV/LA gradient in acute severe MR.

4. *Aneurysm formation and left ventricular thrombus*: True aneurysms complicate transmural infarction and are caused by dilatation of an area of scar. An aneurysm is defined as deformation of both the diastolic and systolic LV contours with dyskinesis in systole. TTE is a sensitive tool for the diagnosis; aneurysm formation is a poor prognostic sign and is associated with congestive cardiac failure, arrhythmias, and thrombus formation. Left ventricular thrombi form in regions of stasis; they most commonly occur in the apex but may also be seen in lateral and inferior aneurysms.

5. *Pericarditis*: Echocardiography is a sensitive technique for the diagnosis of pericardial effusion; however, the absence of fluid does not exclude pericarditis. In patients who are anticoagulated, intrapericardial thrombus may be recognized. Echocardiography can identify a site for percutaneous drainage if required and be used to monitor the procedure.

6. *Cardiac rupture*: Many LV ruptures cause sudden death. However, rupture may be subacute, allowing time for intervention. Direct visualization of the rupture is often difficult as it may be only a "slit" in the myocardium and the location of pericardial fluid may not correlate with the area of rupture.

# Clinical Cases

## *Case 1*

A 41-year-old male with a history of hypertension presented to the ED with severe substernal chest pain, sharp, radiating to the left arm, that started while climbing upstairs and lifting his bags of grocery. The pain lasted 30 min until his wife called emergency medical services (EMS). On EMS arrival, they found the patient to be diaphoretic, still complaining of severe chest pain. He was given oxygen via nasal cannula and two sublingual nitroglycerin and the pain subsided. On initial triage in the ED, he again reported severe chest pain. He was found to have severe hypertension and tachycardia. His initial ECG showed 2 mm ST-segment elevation in leads V1–V2. He was given sublingual nitroglycerin, aspirin, metoprolol, and heparin drip was started. The emergency "cardiac myocardial infarction" team was activated. Cardiology fellow rushed to assess the patient, while the cardiac catheterization laboratory was getting ready to accept the patient. The fellow performed emergent 2D echo while the patient was still having severe chest pain. Echocardiography showed normal LV systolic and diastolic function, mild LVH, no wall motion abnormalities, and no Doppler evidence of any valvular disease. On further evaluation, the patient stated that the pain was actually reproducible by pressing the chest. The care of the patient was then changed and he was further risk stratified using an exercise stress echocardiography, which revealed no evidence of ischemia (Figs. 18.1, 18.2, 18.3, and 18.4).

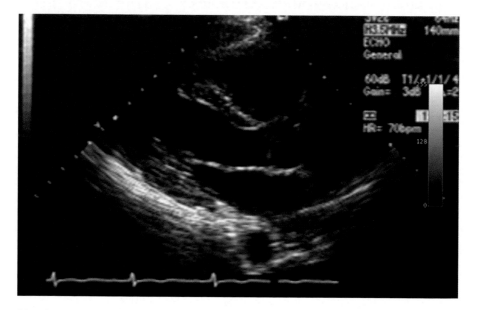

**Fig. 18.1** Parasternal long axis (diastolic frame) showing normal wall motion

## Case 2

A 77-year-old female with a history of mild early dementia, hypertension, dyslipidemia, non-insulin-dependent diabetes mellitus, and smoking presented to the ED with epigastric discomfort for 3 days. The pain was not associated with food. She

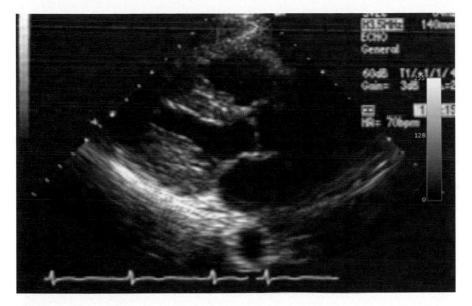

**Fig. 18.2**  Parasternal long axis (systolic frame) showing normal wall motion

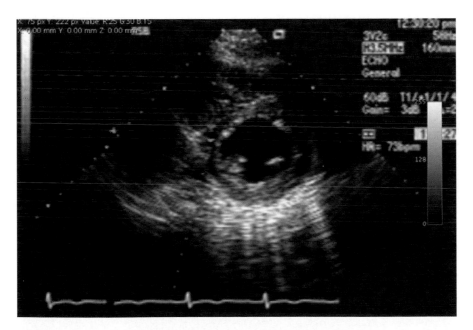

**Fig. 18.3**  Parasternal short axis (diastolic frame) showing normal wall motion

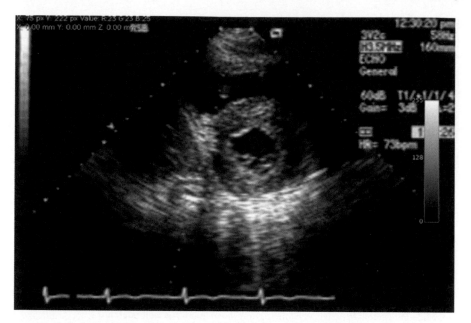

**Fig. 18.4** Parasternal short axis (systolic frame) showing normal wall motion

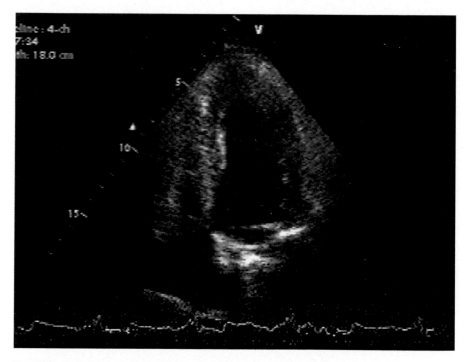

**Fig. 18.5** Apical four (systolic frame) showing apical akinesis

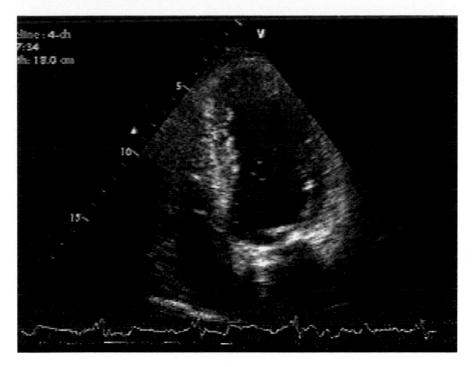

**Fig. 18.6**  Apical four (diastolic frame) showing apical akinesis

also reported some vague back pain. Vital signs on presentation were unremarkable; however, initial ECG showed normal sinus rhythm with normal axis, but with T-wave inversions in the anterior leads (V2–V4). Initial troponin was negative, and the cardiology team was consulted to evaluate the patient. Bedside echocardiography was performed by the cardiology fellow which showed anterio and antero-septal hypokinesis with apical akinesis (Figs. 18.5 and 18.6). The patient was rushed to the cardiac catheterization laboratory and was found to have critical left anterior descending artery (LAD) lesion. An urgent PCI was performed using drug-eluted stent (DES) to the proximal LAD.

## References

1. Burt C. Summary statistics for acute cardiac ischemia and chest pain visits to united states EDs, 1995–1996. *Am J Emerg Med*. 1999;17:552–559
2. Antman EM, Anbe DT, Armstrong PW, et al. ACC/AHA guidelines for the management of patients with ST-elevation myocardial infarction: executive summary. A report of the American College of Cardiology/American Heart Association Task Force on Practice Guidelines (Writing Committee to Revise the 1999 Guidelines for the Management of Patients with Acute Myocardial Infarction). *Circulation*. 2004;110:588–636
3. Braunwald E, Antman EM, Beasley JW, et al. ACC/AHA guideline update for the management of patients with unstable angina and non-St-segment elevation myocardial infarction –

2002: summary article. A report of the American College of Cardiology/American Heart Association Task Force on Practice Guidelines (Committee on the Management of Patients with Unstable Angina). *Circulation.* 2002;106:1893–1900

4. Pollack CV Jr, Roe MT, Peterson ED. 2002 Update to the ACC/AHA guidelines for the management of patients with unstable angina and non-ST-segment elevation myocardial infarction: implications for emergency department practice. *Ann Emerg Med.* 2003;41: 355–369

5. Lee TH, Rouan GW, Weisberg MC, et al. Clinical characteristics and natural history of patients with acute myocardial infarction sent home from the emergency room. *Am J Cardiol.* 1987;60:219–224

6. Todd KH, Hoffman JR, Morgan MT. Effect of cardiologist ECG review on emergency department practice. *Ann Emerg Med.* 1996;27:16–21

7. Westdrop EJ, Gratton MC, Watson WA. Emergency department interpretation of electrocardiograms. *Ann Emerg Med.* 1992;21:541–544

8. Erling BF, Perron AD, Brady WJ. Disagreement in the interpretation of electrocardiographic ST segment elevation: a source of error for emergency physicians? *Am J Emerg Med.* 2004;22:65–70

9. Jayes RL Jr, Larsen GC, Beshansky JR, D'Agostino RB, Selker HP. Physician electrocardiogram reading in the emergency department – accuracy and effect on triage decisions: findings from a multicenter study. *J Gen Intern Med.* 1992;7:387–392

10. Tandberg D, Kastendieck KD, Meskin S. Observer variation in measured ST-segment elevation. *Ann Emerg Med.* 1999;34:448–452

11. Masoudi FA, Magid DJ, Vinson DR, et al. Implications of the failure to identify high-risk electrocardiogram findings for the quality of care of patients with acute myocardial infarction: results of the emergency department quality in myocardial infarction (EDQMI) study. *Circulation.* 2006;114:1565–1571

12. Autore C, Agati L, Picininno M, Lino S, Musaro S. Role of echocardiography in acute chest pain syndrome. *Am J Cardiol.* 2000;86(4A):41G–42G.

13. Storrow AB, Gibler WB. Chest pain centers: diagnosis of acute coronary syndromes. *Ann Emerg Med.* 2000;35:449–461

14. Tennant R, Wiggers CJ. The effect of coronary artery occlusion on myocardial contraction. *Am J Physiol.* 1935;112:351–361

15. Hauser AM, Gangadhara V, Ramos RG, et al. Sequence of mechanical, electrocardiographic and clinical effects of repeated coronary artery occlusion in human beings: echocardiographic observations during coronary angioplasty. *J Am Coll Cardiol.* 1985;5(2pt1):193–197.

16. Cheitlin MD, Armstrong WF, Aurigemma GP, et al. ACC/AHA/ASE 2003 guideline for the clinical application of echocardiography. Available at: www.acc.org/qualityandscience/clinical/statements.htm. Accessed August 24, 2006.

17. Fleischmann KE, Lee TH, Come PC, et al. Echocardiographic prediction of complications in patients with chest pain. *Am J Cardiol.* 1997;79:292–298

18. Sabia P, Afrookteh A, Touchstone DA, Keller MW, Esquivel L, Kaul S. Value of regional wall motion abnormality in the emergency room diagnosis of acute myocardial infarction: a prospective study using two-dimensional echocardiography. *Circulation.* 1991;84(suppl I):85–92.

19. Romano S, Dagianti A, Penco M, et al. Usefulness of echocardiography in the prognostic evaluation of non-Q-wave myocardial infarction. *Am J Cardiol.* 2000;86(suppl 4A): 43G–45G.

20. Peels KH, Visser CA, Dambrink JHE, et al. on behalf of the CATS Investigators Group. Left ventricular wall motion score as an early predictor of left ventricular dilation and mortality after first anterior infarction treated with thrombolysis. The CATS investigators group. *Am J Cardiol.* 1996;77:1149–1154

21. Feinberg MS, Schwammenthal E, Shllzerman L, et al. Prognostic significance of mild mitral regurgitation by color Doppler echocardiography in acute myocardial infarction. *Am J Cardiol.* 2000;86:903–907

22. Kontos MC. Role of echocardiography in the emergency department for identifying patients with myocardial infarction and ischemia. *Echocardiography.* 1999;16:193–205

23. Herzog E., Aziz E, Hong MK. The pain pathway for the management of acute coronary syndrome. *Acute Coronary Syndrome: Multidisciplinary and Pathway Based Approach.* Chapter 2. New York: Springer; 2008:9–19.

24. Greaves S. Role of echocardiography in acute coronary syndromes. *Heart.* October 2002;88(4):419–425.

25. Goldberger JJ, Himelman RB, Wolfe CL, et al. Right ventricular infarction: recognition and assessment of its hemodynamic significance by two-dimensional echocardiography. *J Am Soc Echocardiogr.* 1991;4:140–146

# Chapter 19
# Handheld and Miniature Echocardiography in Acute Coronary Syndrome

Sandeep Joshi and Eyal Herzog

In the United States millions of patients present to the emergency department (ED) annually with signs and symptoms suggestive of acute coronary syndrome (ACS). The electrocardiogram (ECG) is often the first diagnostic tool used by physicians in the triage of patients with chest pain and is an invaluable tool that can guide clinical management decisions including potential reperfusion therapy. Albeit quite useful, the ECG has certain limitations, such as the presence of a paced rhythm, an underlying left bundle branch block, or nonspecific ST-segment changes, which may result in the ECG becoming an indeterminate factor. In this instance, physicians are faced with a daunting challenge and often have to rely on other diagnostic modalities such as a standardized transthoracic two-dimensional echocardiogram (SE) for assessing possible wall motion abnormalities (WMA). It can aid in risk stratification, guide therapy, increase the sensitivity and predictive values of chest pain algorithms, and expedite chest pain triage especially in the setting of a nondiagnostic ECG, indeterminate serum cardiac markers, and/or vague signs and symptoms. Regional WMA occurs within seconds following acute coronary occlusion and thus rapid assessment is an integral aspect of the treatment as viable myocardium deteriorates every second until coronary reperfusion is restored and as a result, SE is often the first test ordered when clinicians are facing the possibility of ACS.

SE has proven to be more accurate in assessing WMA, valvular disease, effusions, and overall left ventricular (LV) function than any existing imaging technique. SE has surpassed virtually every other diagnostic modality for the sole purpose of regional or global WMA detection in the presence of ACS. Its inherent noninvasiveness, portability, and rapid interpretation of myocardial disease pathology has made it a vital asset in providing crucial information about cardiac morphology, physiology, and pathophysiology. However, due to constraints in size and maneuverability of conventional echocardiographic machines (Fig. 19.1), newer smaller (Fig. 19.2) and handheld echocardiographic (HHE) devices (Fig. 19.3) have been developed. These miniature devices are lightweight and portable and are simpler to

S. Joshi (✉)
Cardiology, St Luke's Roosevelt Hospital Center, 1111 Amsterdam Ave, New York, NY, USA
e-mail: sjoshi@chpnet.org

E. Herzog, F.A. Chaudhry (eds.), *Echocardiography in Acute Coronary Syndrome*,
DOI 10.1007/978-1-84882-027-2_19, © Springer-Verlag London Limited 2009

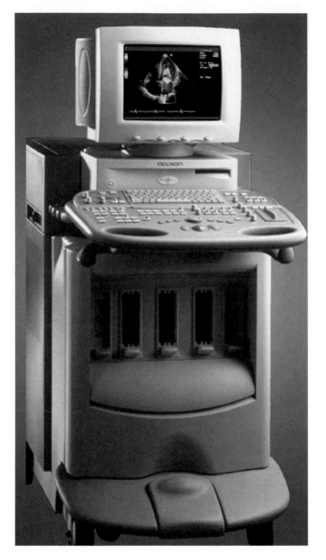

**Fig. 19.1** Standard transthoracic echocardiographic machine

use in a unit setting, ED, and for bedside rounds. These newer generation devices can reduce the overall volume of SE performed, thereby reducing the financial burden incurred from costly diagnostic testing. These "ultrasound stethoscopes" have emerged as useful tools in an overwhelmed global healthcare phenomenon. Many newer generation devices are equipped with color Doppler capabilities and may be used to assess valvular disease as well. They can be used to assess for left ventricular hypertrophy, the presence of an abdominal aneurysm, LV function, and pericardial effusion analysis. Moreover, their effectiveness has been proven during cardiology

**Fig. 19.2** Portable
echocardiographic machine

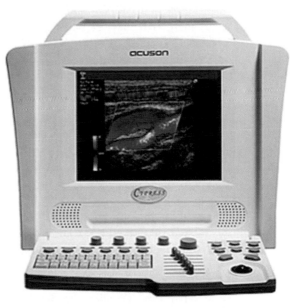

**Fig. 19.3** Miniature
handheld echocardiographic
machine

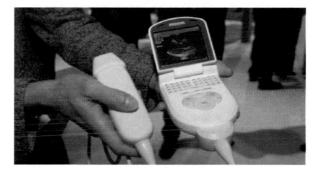

rounds, inpatient and outpatient settings, and ED settings. Also contributing is the fact that over the past decades the decline of the physician's auscultatory and examination skills, experience, presumably due to limited exposure in training and more reliance on sophisticated imaging techniques, has become the cornerstone of practiced medicine. Faced against an overwhelmed healthcare system and limited reimbursements and managed care, physicians have less time availability and increased time pressure constraints imposed resulting in an increased reliance on rapid and accurate diagnostic testing for immediate patient turnover and triage.

The first HHE devices were introduced in the late 1970s; however, due to poor image quality, poor reimbursement, and technical limitations, overall production declined. Several newer generation HHE devices with superior image quality and reduced costs have evolved and are increasingly used in the outpatient setting, chest pain centers, the ED, and in the critical care setting. Although encouraging, the data on the efficacy of these HHE devices when compared to SE remain ambiguous. One critical argument is that in the setting of ACS a clinician experienced in performing and interpreting echocardiography should be present for rapid and accurate study interpretation. In addition, many of these HHE devices simply are not capable of providing reliable assessment of valvular disease, chamber quantitation, or diastolic heart failure information as spectral Doppler and harmonic imaging, which is required when evaluating valvular function or mechanical complications following ACS, is missing or limited. Albeit, literature has shown encouraging results for these devices. For example, Vourvourvi et al.[1,2] examined the use of the HHE device in the outpatient setting and discovered that it was quite reliable in excluding cardiac disease. In fact among 78% of the patients referred for SE, the findings from the HHE device obviated the need for a SE, which was initially ordered by the referring cardiologist. Furthermore, the positive and negative predictive values for the detection of cardiac disease with the HHE device were 100 and 96%, respectively. Among 17% of these patients, an unsuspected major cardiac abnormality, which was not suspected of being present, was discovered. The study concluded that although the devices had certain inherent limitations such as poor harmonic imaging and limited spectral Doppler, the overall benefits outweighed the limitations. An interesting point that was made in this analysis involved the training requirements for interpreting these studies. As set forth by the American Society of Echocardiography (ASE), advanced training (level II) requires the clinician to have interpreted and performed a certain number of SE studies. Many cardiologists have sufficient training for level II ASE certification. This is due to heavy emphasis on imaging during cardiology training. The echocardiographic signs of ACS require a highly experienced and trained interpreter. The difficulties arise when a clinician or noncardiologist with minimal experience interprets the study. Is it feasible or ethical to have an inexperienced or improperly trained interpreter at the controls when diagnosing ACS? Although data have shown that training individuals for the purpose of using these devices remains successful, careful thought has to be placed in this setting. The time required for this rigorous training as set by the ASE simply is not feasible for many intensivists and ED physicians. In addition, it is not possible for a unit setting or ED to have a trained cardiologist available for rapid echocardiographic interpretation present on a 24-h basis. Thus, the use of these HHE devices is often relegated to a "limited" or "focused" exam, often a screener for the more accurate SE. HHE devices can provide sufficient information regarding the presence of WMA; however, they cannot differentiate WMA from a prior myocardial infarction (MI) or ongoing ischemia. Similarly, Tsutui et al.[3] examined the role of these miniature devices among 44 patients who underwent bedside echocardiography with both a HHE device and a SE. The HHE examination was performed by an interpreter with level II training as set forth by the ASE utilizing two-dimensional imaging, color Doppler, and simple caliper measurements as opposed to the SE, which was performed by an interpreter with level III training. Their data showed that there were significant differences in cardiac chamber dimensions and LV ejection fraction between the two types of echocardiographic studies.

There was concordance between the two modalities in detecting segmental WMA, mitral valve regurgitation, and aortic regurgitation. A major limitation of the HHE device was a lack of thorough examination of pulmonary hypertension, prosthetic valves, and valvular stenosis due to its inherent lack of ability to measure these hemodynamic parameters. A recurring limitation faced daily is the fact that in contrast to this study whereby an experienced cardiologist with adequate training in echocardiography interpreted the study, many clinicians with limited training and experience are interpreting these studies. This can have detrimental consequences if a WMA is overlooked or a post-MI complication is missed. Conversely, if a WMA is absent yet interpreted as if present so by a nonexperienced clinician, then this too can lead to significant ramifications, often leading to unnecessary and invasive procedures. Atar et al.[4] examined the role of these HHE devices among patients with chest pain and an otherwise normal or nondiagnostic ECG. Seventy patients who presented to the ED for chest pain with a nondiagnostic ECG underwent a limited echocardiographic study focusing on WMA and LV function, via a portable HHE device, interpreted by an experienced cardiologist. Patients were followed for 30 days following the initial study. The HHE device was shown to have 100% sensitivity and 93% specificity for the detection of ACS. Also, the positive and negative predictive values were 71 and 100%, respectively. At 30-day follow-up, one patient with an ischemic cardiomyopathy returned to the ED and eventually suffered from a subendocardial MI. Furthermore, three additional patients with normal echocardiographic studies returned to the ED the next day with the same chest pain and were subsequently discharged home that same day. Longer duration of analysis was not analyzed. The authors concluded that HHE devices are useful in the fact that they provide important incremental information regarding chest pain, expedite chest pain triage, reduce unnecessary hospitalizations and associated costs, and also improve the sensitivity of chest pain algorithms. Moreover, the low cost when compared with SE makes these smaller devices an attractive alternative for the diagnosis of ACS. Perhaps these devices could complement the physical exam and real-time imaging techniques. Weston et al.[5] examined the hypothesis that among patients with signs suggestive of ACS in the presence of a nondiagnostic ECG and normal biochemical markers that HHE devices documented normal LV function is not associated with a poor 30-day outcome in terms of ischemia or ischemic events. LV function was analyzed in 150 patients presenting to the ED with chest pain with an ambiguous ECG and serum biomarkers using an HHE device. The incidences for the end points of death or myocardial ischemia and/or infarction were calculated. The investigators underwent a 4-h training course in an effort to learn how to perform and interpret a limited echocardiogram, in particular, for determining the presence or absence of a WMA or pericardial effusion. The miniature HHE device was capable of determining two-dimensional echo images and color Doppler, yet there were no spectral Doppler capabilities. The results showed that among patients with normal studies, 2/78 went to develop an acute MI, thereby the incidence of acute MI was 2.5%, whereas the incidence of acute MI among patients with abnormal studies was 20%, 6/30 patients. The incidence of acute MI and/or myocardial ischemia in the normal HHE group was 7.6% (6/78) vs. 14.6% (6/30) among those with abnormal studies.

The negative predictive value of these devices was 91%. The investigators concluded that there may be a role for the HHE device when the clinician is faced with a non-diagnostic ECG and serum biochemical markers for the detection of myocardial ischemia and/or ACS. They also suggested that in the ED, the use of a HHE device may serve to complement the results of the ECG for the triage of chest pain patients. Similarly, Sabia et al.[6] examined the role of two-dimensional echocardiography in the detection of acute MI in the ED setting. A low incidence of acute MI in patients who had a normal echocardiogram, with no WMA associated, was reported. A total of 2/82 patients with a normal echocardiogram subsequently suffered a subendocardial infarction, similar to the results reported by Weston et al. The highlights of the study clearly delineate the value of the HHE device and its potential ability to effectively rule out ACS in those patients with a normal or nondiagnostic ECG and its ability to determine the 30-day outcome in patients with normal HHE results. The integration of information from the ECG and HHE can provide the clinician with incremental information by both directly visualizing the LV function and assessing the electrical system. It should be emphasized though that the information yielded by the HHE device may be limited, such as the inability to differentiate if the WMA is caused by acute/ongoing vs. prior ischemia. Another major problem lies in the sensitivity of the HHE device, which correlates with the size of the ischemic zone. This area must be large enough to progress to a WMA in order for the HHE device to detect it. In other words, a non-ST-segment or nontransmural MI may not be detected as perfusion to the affected zone is preserved. In fact data suggest that >20% of the myocardium must be affected in order for LV function to be adversely affected. Moreover, myocardial ischemia can result in a very subtle WMA, less than an acute MI, leading to falsely negative studies. Thus, many patients that actually subsequently suffer from an acute coronary event are missed with an HHE device. The literature above also highlights the fact that individuals with minimal training in echocardiography can be trained to adequately detect major WMA. This has been examined by Alexander et al.[7] whereby medical students and cardiology fellows were trained via a 3-h course for the examination of LV function via a miniature HHE device. The results were encouraging in that the training was sufficient for WMA detection.

A limitation of any echocardiographic study that may arise is when the clinician is faced with a nondiagnostic study such as those experienced with an obese patient, poor echocardiographic windows, an underlying left bundle branch block, and rapid atrial fibrillation. This makes the diagnosis of WMA quite difficult and in these situations an experienced interpreter or preferably a SE is warranted.[8]

Another dilemma that is ever present today is the increasing utilization of contrast agents made of perfluorocarbon for endocardial border definition. Prior to this many WMA were underdiagnosed and missed. The use of these agents has revolutionized SE. These agents rely on tissue harmonic imaging for adequate endocardial definition. Many of these smaller HHE devices simply lack harmonic imaging capability and those that have this capacity are often underutilized as many inexperienced clinicians are unfamiliar with the safety and bioeffects and hence the proper usage and application of myocardial tissue contrast. This represents a significant problem that the nonexperienced clinician faces. The use of these agents does carry inherent risks and adverse effects such as respiratory depression and/or myocardial infarction,[9] and its mandated that patients be monitored following the dose. This takes vital time away from the possibility of looming reperfusion therapy. The patient must also be aware of the potential adverse risks and benefits regarding myocardial contrast agent, which also takes time away from viable myocardial reperfusion. Finally, the healthcare provider has to be proficient with the concept of contrast imaging including the nature of the agent, mechanism of action, and the physical properties of tissue harmonics. Hence, a course in ultrasound physics is mandated to be able to identify the true nature and effects of these contrast agents. Many ED physicians and intensivists simply do not have the time to take this course of action, often rendering them and more importantly the patient helpless.

The true value of the HHE device lies not in its ability to detect WMA in those patients with a markedly abnormal ECG and elevated cardiac enzymes but in those patients with a low likelihood of ACS in the setting of chest pain and a nondiagnostic ECG and serum cardiac markers. This ability to rule out ACS in this patient cohort along with its small size, portability, low cost, and immediate availability make it a suitable tool in the ED setting.[10] This is in stark contrast to other imaging modalities such as magnetic resonance imaging, computed tomography (CT), myocardial perfusion studies, stress echocardiography or cardiac CT, or CT angiography, which all require extensive training and certainly are not portable and are not readily available on a 24-h basis and involve substantial cost. Also as the risk of ACS is quite low in those presenting with chest pain with a nondiagnostic ECG and indeterminate cardiac markers, HHE devices may provide additional information about cardiac function, such as pericardial disease and/or effusions.[11,12] Based on the studies above the clear absence of a WMA from an adequate echocardiographic study can support grounds for patient discharge from the ED setting, reducing unnecessary costs and hospitalizations.

In conclusion, miniature HHE devices are being increasingly used effectively in the ED setting throughout the world. Although promising, they do have significant limitations. Operator and interpreter experience, poor image quality, a nondiagnostic study, and false-negative studies in the setting of a nontransmural MI can lead to fatal consequences. Therefore, its ideal use is to serve as a "screener" or first-line test to rule out ACS in a patient with a low likelihood of ACS in the setting of a nondiagnostic ECG and indeterminate serum cardiac markers. Among those higher risk patients or those patients with clear evidence of acute myocardial disease, nothing can replace or surpass a SE, the designated gold standard. At this juncture, more trials are needed to follow patients for extended periods of time to detect the presence of WMA with a normal study as determined by the HHE device. Perhaps training requirements as set by the ASE should be implemented for those set on performing and interpreting these studies from the HHE devices. This training should also include a course in ultrasound physics as the increasing use of contrast agents to enhance endocardial border definition mandates training. Also, the performance of echocardiographic studies is simply not just observing for the detection of WMA. The clinician should be familiar with valvular anomalies, pericardial disease, and right ventricular disease and the use of tissue Doppler. Finally, it is safe to assume that there simply is not a diagnostic test that will ever replace the patient history and physical examination and clinical judgment of a physician. There ceases to exist a diagnostic test with a 100% sensitivity and specificity. Until then, these tests can complement the history and physical examination. Perhaps the role of the HHE device will evolve further in the years to come; however, significant strides must be met in both the training requirements and experience of the healthcare provider in order for this to surpass SE for the detection of ACS.

# References

1. Vourvouri EC, Poldermans D, Deckers JW, et al. Evaluation of a hand carried cardiac ultrasound device in an outpatient cardiology clinic. *Heart*. 2005;91(2):171–176.
2. de Groot-de Laat LE, ten Cate FJ, Vourvouri EC, van Domburg RT, Roelandt JRTC. Impact of hand-carried cardiac ultrasound on diagnosis and management during cardiac consultation rounds. *Eur J Echocardiogr*. 2005;6(3):196–201.
3. Tsutsui JM, Maciel RR, Costa JM, et al. Hand-carried ultrasound performed at bedside in cardiology inpatient setting – a comparative study with comprehensive echocardiography. *Cardiovasc Ultrasound*. 2004;2:24.
4. Atar S, Feldman A, Darawshe A, et al. Utility and diagnostic accuracy of hand-carried ultrasound for emergency room evaluation of chest pain. *Am J Cardiol*. 2004;94(3):408–409.
5. Weston P, Alexander JH, Patel MR, et al. Hand-held echocardiographic examination of patients with symptoms of acute coronary syndromes in the emergency department: the 30-day outcome associated with normal left ventricular wall motion. *Am Heart J*. 2004;148(6):1096–1101.
6. Sabia P, Abbott RD, Afrookteh A, et al. Importance of two-dimensional echocardiographic assessment of left ventricular systolic function in patients presenting to the emergency room with cardiac-related symptoms. *Circulation*. 1991;84(4):1615–1624.
7. Alexander JH, Peterson ED, Chen AY, et al. Feasibility of point-of-care echocardiography by internal medicine house staff. *Am Heart J*. 2004;147(3):476–481.
8. Martin LD, Howell EE, Ziegelstein RC, et al. Hospitalist performance of cardiac hand-carried ultrasound after focused training. *Am J Med*. 2007;120(11):1000–1004.
9. Bhatia VK, Senior R. Contrast echocardiography: evidence for clinical use. *J Am Soc Echocardiogr*. 2008;21(5):409–416.
10. Rugolotto M, Chang CP, Hu B, et al. Clinical use of cardiac ultrasound performed with a hand-carried device in patients admitted for acute cardiac care. *Am J Cardiol*. 2002;90(9):1040–1042.
11. Spurney CF, Sable CA, Berger JT, et al. Use of a hand-carried ultrasound device by critical care physicians for the diagnosis of pericardial effusions, decreased cardiac function, and left ventricular enlargement in pediatric patients. *J Am Soc Echocardiogr*. 2005;18(4):313–319.
12. Greaves K, Jeetley P, Hickman M, et al. The use of hand-carried ultrasound in the hospital setting – a cost-effective analysis. *J Am Soc Echocardiogr*. 2005;18(6):620–625.

# Chapter 20
# Acute Complications of Myocardial Infarction

Gregory Janis, Sheila Khianey, Sandeep Joshi, and Eyal Herzog

## Introduction

Acute myocardial infarction (AMI) affects 1.7 million people in the United States. Acute complications of AMI may occur within seconds to minutes after the acute event or up to a few days after it. Echocardiography is the gold standard imaging modality to identify these complications.

In this chapter we will discuss the following complications:

- Left ventricular free wall rupture
- Ventricular septal rupture
- Pericardial effusion and tamponade
- Right ventricular infarction
- Acute mitral regurgitation

## Left Ventricular Free Wall Rupture

### Introduction

Left ventricular free wall rupture (LVFWR), in comparison to rupture of the ventricular septum, is almost entirely a fatal complication of myocardial infarction (MI). Despite great progress in the reduction of both mortality and morbidity from acute myocardial infarction, death related to LVFWR has been alarmingly high. This is primarily due to the rapid extravasation of blood into the pericardial space with resultant instantaneous acute pericardial tamponade. Because these events occur so quickly, patients usually deteriorate before any therapeutic intervention. There are less common cases of subacute rupture. In such instances, patients may have

G. Janis (✉)
Cardiology, St Luke's-Roosevelt Hospital Center, New York, NY, USA
e-mail: gjanis@chpnet.org

E. Herzog, F.A. Chaudhry (eds.), *Echocardiography in Acute Coronary Syndrome*,    269
DOI 10.1007/978-1-84882-027-2_20, © Springer-Verlag London Limited 2009

a longer therapeutic window and the acute rupture may be temporarily contained by pericardial adhesions or by thrombosis at the rupture site. It is in these patients that immediate cardiovascular surgery and repair can be undertaken with the help of emergent echocardiography as a diagnostic tool.[1] Approximately 50% of the time myocardial rupture occurs within the first 5 days after MI and within 2 weeks in over 90% of cases.[2,3] Regardless, acute or subacute myocardial rupture is a serious and predominantly fatal complication of acute MI.[4]

## *Incidence and Risk Factors*

LVFWR is a relatively common finding in patients who die as a consequence of acute MI. In such patients, many large studies have found a 14–26% incidence of cardiac rupture.[5] The incidence is much lower when all patients with acute MI are considered. According to the National Registry of Myocardial Infarction which reviewed data from 350,755 patients, the incidence of cardiac rupture was less than 1%.[6] This is consistent with a 0.85% incidence of tamponade in a review of over 100,000 patients treated with thrombolytic therapy.[7]

Studies have also suggested a higher mortality from free wall rupture with thrombolytics as cardiac rupture was responsible for 7.3% of all deaths and 12.1% with thrombolytic agents. Thrombolytic therapy has also been shown to accelerate the occurrence of cardiac rupture, often within the first 24 h of drug administration. Of note the Thrombolysis in Myocardial Infarction (TIMI) 9 study which analyzed 3759 patients found no association between cardiac rupture and the use of adjunctive thrombin inhibitors, including heparin and hirudin.[8]

In contrast to outcomes with thrombolytic agents, the incidence of cardiac rupture may be lower in patients treated with percutaneous coronary intervention. This was suggested in an observational study of 1375 patients who received a thrombolytic agent or underwent primary angioplasty; the incidence of rupture was 3.3 and 1.8%, respectively, with the two therapies.[9] Also, angioplasty was a significant independent protective factor in a multivariate analysis with an odds ratio of 0.46.

Aside from the effects of thrombolytic therapy, studies such as the Multicenter Investigation of Limitation of Infarct Size (MILIS) highlight other risk factors for myocardial rupture. The study found that myocardial rupture was 9.2 times more likely to occur in patients who had no prior history of angina or MI, ST-segment elevation or Q-wave development on the initial ECG, and peak MB creatine kinase above 150 IU/l.[5]

To summarize, both the absence of collateral blood flow, demonstrated by the lack of prior ischemic symptoms, and the greater infarct territory correlate with a higher risk of myocardial rupture. This hypothesis has been confirmed in other studies which have found that myocardial rupture is usually associated with patients with first-time infarcts, with large transmural infarcts (usually anterior or lateral), and is rarely seen in a hypertrophied ventricle or in an area of extensive collateral circulation.[10] Patients also frequently have persistent ST-segment elevation and persistent or recurrent chest pain with evidence of infarct expansion or extension. Other risk factors for rupture include anterior location of the infarction, age >70 years, and female sex.[8,9] On the other hand, beta blockers, which are routinely administered to patients with an acute MI, reduce the rate of death from free wall rupture compared to placebo.[11]

## Pathophysiology

Myocardial rupture more frequently involves the left ventricle than the right ventricle and rarely involves the atria.[6] The infarct commonly affects the anterior and lateral walls of the left ventricle near the junction of the infarct and normal myocardium. In the setting of acute MI, rupture and injury can also involve the interventricular septum, interatrial septum, chordae, papillary muscles, or valves but we will focus on LVFWR in this chapter.

Ventricular free wall rupture is defined as an acute, traumatic perforation of the ventricles which may include pericardial rupture.[4] Similar to ventricular septal rupture, during an acute infarction, the pathogenic process of the rupture changes over time. With unsuccessful or no reperfusion, coagulation necrosis develops within the first 3–5 days.[12] As the necrosis progresses, neutrophils infiltrate the myocardial space and release lytic enzymes which disintegrate the necrotic myocardium leading to perforation. Thus, the rupture is a result of transmural infarction and the actual perforation can range in size from millimeters to centimeters depending on infarct size.[12]

As mentioned, about half of the cases of myocardial rupture occur within the first 5 days post-MI and within 2 weeks in over 90% of cases.[2,3] As a result different pathological patterns can be appreciated depending in part upon the time of the event post-MI.[2] Early phase rupture is defined as within 72 h post-MI and late rupture is greater than 4 days. A study of 1450 patients with acute MI analyzed the 27 (1.9%) patients that developed free wall myocardial rupture.[13] Early rupture was described anatomically by an abrupt slit-like tear in the infarcted territory, with a preference for anterior infarction sites. Of note, the incidence of early free wall rupture was independent of successful reperfusion. Late rupture, which rarely occurs in patients with successful reperfusion, was characterized by the presence of infarct expansion, with no preferential infarction site.

## Effect of Reperfusion

Myocardial rupture after MI is less common in patients with successful reperfusion. This was demonstrated in a retrospective review assessing the perfusion status of the infarct-related coronary artery in 57 patients who had an initially nonfatal rupture and 28 patients with a postmortem diagnosis of myocardial rupture.[14] Rupture typically occurred in an area that had been infarcted without successful reperfusion. Inadequate reperfusion was shown in all 28 patients with a postmortem diagnosis of rupture. A total of 35 of the 57 patients with initially nonfatal rupture underwent coronary angiography where complete or insufficient reperfusion was documented in 30 of the 35 patients (89%).

A number of studies have shown that thrombolytic therapy early after MI improves survival and decreases the risk of cardiac rupture.[15-17] For instance, the TIMI investigators examined the hearts of 61 patients with fatal MI (death post-MI from 5 h to 42 days, median of 3 days).[16] In this subgroup, myocardial rupture of both the left ventricular free wall and the septum was a relatively common complication. The frequency of myocardial rupture, however, was lower in the 23 patients who received thrombolytic therapy than in the 38 patients who did not (22 versus 46%). Percutaneous coronary intervention (PCI) may also reduce the risk of cardiac rupture if successful reperfusion is achieved.

Despite these findings, other studies suggest that in patients older than 75 years of age, thrombolytic therapy may be associated with a significant increase in LVFWR. The magnitude of this effect was illustrated in a review of 706 patients 75 years of age with a first STEMI who were treated with primary PCI, thrombolytic therapy, or no reperfusion.[18] The patients who received thrombolytic therapy had a significantly greater likelihood of free wall rupture (17.1 versus 7.9 and 4.9% in those with no reperfusion and primary PCI, respectively). LVFWR accounted for 54% of deaths after thrombolytic therapy.

The potential benefits and risks of late reperfusion on free wall rupture have also been studied. The initial concern that late administration of thrombolytic therapy might increase the risk of cardiac rupture[15,16] was disproved by the Late Assessment of Thrombolytic Efficacy (LATE) trial.[17] This study evaluated 5711 patients randomly assigned to receive alteplase or placebo, 6–24 h after the onset of symptoms. Results showed that late thrombolysis did not increase the risk of cardiac rupture but did, as said earlier, accelerate the time of onset of rupture events usually within 24 h of treatment.

In contrast, late primary PCI may be associated with reductions in LVFWR. These benefits are suggested in a retrospective review of 2209 patients with acute MI treated with primary PCI with early reperfusion (within 12 h of presentation), late reperfusion (>12 h), or failed reperfusion.[19] The incidence of free wall rupture in those in the early and late reperfusion groups was significantly lower than for those with failed reperfusion (0.7 and 0.9 versus 3.8%). Of note, late primary PCI (after 24 h) of a totally occluded artery has not been shown to improve hard clinical outcomes, however.

## Clinical Presentation

The clinical course of myocardial rupture is variable and challenging to diagnose as patients may rapidly decompensate. Their clinical course parallels that of any patient suffering from pericardial tamponade. Thus rupture can present as sudden death in an undetected or silent MI or as incomplete/subacute rupture in those with known MI.[20]

Complete rupture of the left ventricular free wall usually leads to hemopericardium and death from cardiac tamponade. Patients may complain of transient chest pain or dyspnea. The presence of rupture is first suggested by the development of sudden profound right heart failure and shock, often progressing rapidly to pulseless electrical activity (electromechanical dissociation) and death. In one report, pulseless electrical activity in a patient with a first MI and without overt heart failure had a 95% predictive accuracy for the diagnosis of left ventricular free wall rupture.[20] In contrast, the predictive accuracy of rupture was low at 17% in those with heart failure. Emergent transthoracic echocardiography will confirm the diagnosis and emergent pericardiocentesis can further confirm the diagnosis and transiently relieve the tamponade.[20]

Incomplete/subacute rupture of the left ventricular free wall can occur when organized thrombus and the pericardium seal the ventricular perforation. This condition can progress to frank rupture with cardiac tamponade and hemodynamic compromise, to the formation of a false aneurysm walled off by pericardial tissue and communicating with the left ventricle through the perforation. Clinically an apical murmur may be appreciated with pseudoaneurysm. Left ventricular diverticulum may also form.[2,3] Patients may present with persistent or recurrent chest pain, particularly pericardial pain, nausea, restlessness and agitation, abrupt, transient hypotension, and/or electrocardiographic features of localized or regional pericarditis.[2,3] The diagnosis of incomplete/subacute rupture is confirmed by transthoracic echocardiography.[20]

## *Echocardiographic Features*

Echocardiography is the test of choice for the definitive diagnosis of LVFWR. Emergent transthoracic echocardiography when performed in the appropriate clinical settings invariably reveals a diffuse or localized pericardial effusion, intrapericardial echoes, and a discrete segmental wall motion abnormality (Figs. 20.1 and 20.2). Imaging may or may not reveal signs of cardiac tamponade, i.e., diastolic right ventricular collapse. On occasion the rupture site can be elucidated by color flow Doppler techniques, thus evaluating turbulence and flow velocities (Fig. 20.3). Echocardiography is considered to have a diagnostic sensitivity of 100% and a specificity of 93%.[21] As a guideline, although thrombolytics and glycoprotein IIb/IIIa inhibitor therapy may cause hemopericardium, LVFWR should always be considered the leading diagnosis in a patient with AMI who is hypotensive and has pericardial effusion. Occasionally when TTE is non-diagnostic, TEE can be used to visualize the free wall rupture (Fig. 20.4).

## *Treatment*

As mentioned, the mortality for acute and subacute free wall rupture is high due to the rapid clinical deterioration. Survival depends primarily upon the prompt

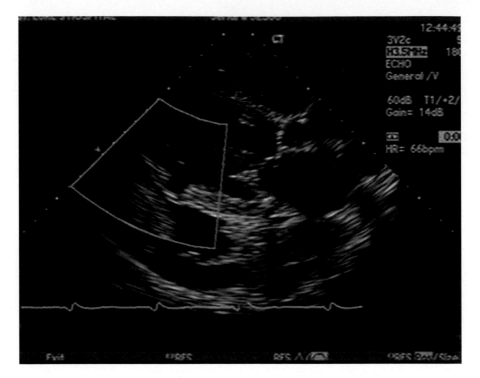

**Fig. 20.1** Transthoracic parasternal long-axis view demonstrating a posterior free wall rupture

recognition of myocardial rupture and provision of immediate therapy. Patients displaying suggestive symptoms, signs, and ECG changes require emergent bedside echocardiogram and echocardiographically guided pericardiocentesis if fluid is visualized. Immediate surgical intervention is indicated if the pericardiocentesis identifies the fluid as blood. Medical therapy aimed at hemodynamic stabilization should also be instituted. In addition to pericardiocentesis this includes fluids, inotropic support, vasopressors, and even intra-aortic balloon pump counterpulsation and percutaneous cardiopulmonary bypass when available and indicated.[2] Prompt surgical repair is also indicated for left ventricular false aneurysms because rupture of the pseudoaneurysm frequently occurs.

With rapid recognition and initiation of both medical and surgical therapy, the potential for survival particularly with subacute rupture can improve dramatically. In one study, 25 of 33 patients (76%) with subacute ventricular rupture survived the surgical procedure and 16 (48%) were long-term survivors.[21]

## Conclusion

Acute or subacute LVFWR is a serious and predominantly fatal complication of acute MI.[4] Despite great advances in mortality reduction from acute MI over the

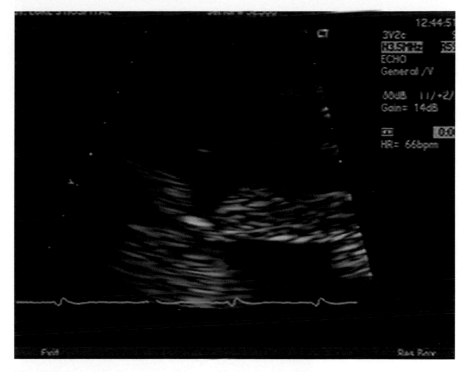

**Fig. 20.2**   Transthoracic parasternal long-axis view demonstrating a close-up view of a posterior free wall rupture

years, death related to ventricular free wall rupture has not changed. This is mostly due to the devastatingly rapid clinical deterioration of patients before the diagnosis, both clinical and echocardiographic, may be made.[22] However, in subacute ruptures the therapeutic window may be wide enough for proper diagnosis and life-saving surgical intervention. Regardless, once rupture is suspected, emergent bedside echocardiography should be performed immediately, followed by pericardiocentesis and repair of the rupture site as quickly as possible.

## Free Wall Rupture Case Presentation

A 62-year-old man presented to a local emergency room at an outside hospital for new-onset severe substernal chest pain radiating to his jaw with associated dyspnea and diaphoresis. Emergent EKG revealed 4 mm ST elevations in the anterior precordial leads with 2 mm ST depressions in the inferior leads. He was hemodynamically stable with normal ambient air oxygen saturation. A diagnosis of acute anterior wall myocardial infarction (AMI) was made; however, when cardiac catheterization was recommended to him, he refused. He was competent, agreed to medical therapy,

**Fig. 20.3** Transthoracic parasternal long-axis view using color flow Doppler demonstrating turbulent flow through a posterior free wall rupture

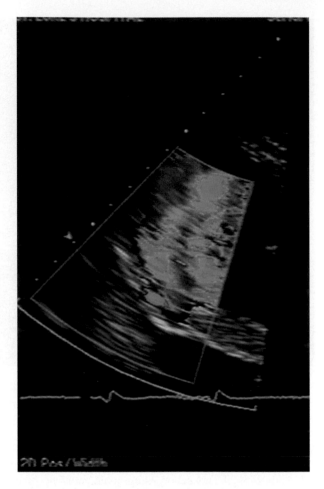

and thus thrombolytic treatment was initiated. Unfortunately, he continued to have angina without resolution of his ST-segment elevations. After further discussion of the risks of inadequate reperfusion, he agreed to undergo cardiac catheterization and was transferred to a tertiary care center for percutaneous revascularization. He was started on glycoprotein IIb/IIIa inhibitor therapy and clopidogrel. His cardiac catheterization revealed a subtotally occluded proximal left anterior descending (LAD) coronary artery, and he underwent successful revascularization with stent placement in the LAD establishing TIMI III flow. The rest of the epicardial coronary arteries were patent angiographically. The patient was admitted to the cardiac intensive care unit and his hospital course over the next 24 h was uneventful for arrhythmias or hemodynamic compromise.

On day two of his hospitalization, his blood pressure acutely fell to 64/40. His heart rate on telemetry revealed sinus tachycardia at 120 bpm. He had complained

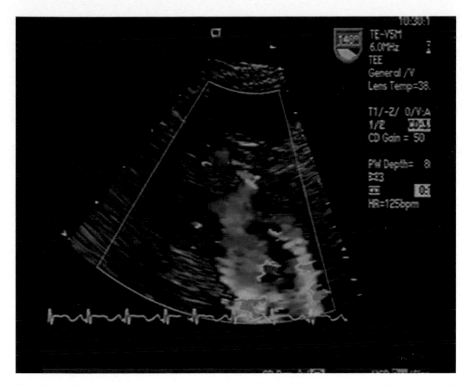

**Fig. 20.4**   Transesophageal echocardiography demonstrating color flow through posterior wall rupture post-myocardial infarction

of nausea and chest pain and then became progressively obtunded and diaphoretic. Dopamine was started. Further electrocardiography revealed sinus tachycardia, low-voltage QRS complexes with diffuse ST-segment elevations, and no electrical alternans. Auscultation revealed no audible rub or S3 gallop, no new murmurs, and clear breath sounds bilaterally. He had marked jugular venous distention and was intubated for respiratory distress. Emergent echocardiography revealed a large pericardial effusion and manifestations of cardiac tamponade but no signs of mitral regurgitation, ventricular septal defect, or free wall rupture. Intravenous fluids and dopamine were administered at the maximum rate and an emergent pericardiocentesis was performed draining 250 cc of bloody fluid. A diagnosis of free wall rupture and cardiac tamponade was made. Unfortunately before the patient was transferred for emergent surgical repair he decompensated into pulseless electrical alternans arrest. Cardiopulmonary resuscitation was attempted with placement of an intra-aortic balloon pump; however, the patient did not regain a pulse or blood pressure. He was pronounced dead after a 30-min failed resuscitation. Subsequent pathology examination confirmed myocardial wall rupture as the cause of tamponade and death.

# Ventricular Septal Rupture

## Introduction

One of the deadliest complications of acute myocardial infarction involves rupture of the interventricular septum. The need for rapid diagnosis, aggressive medical therapy, and prompt surgical intervention is essential to increase the possibility of survival. As medical therapy has advanced, the incidence and timing of ventricular septal rupture has been up for debate.

In the era before reperfusion therapy, rupture of the interventricular septum is thought to have caused complications in 1–2% of patients with acute myocardial infarction and accounts for approximately 5% of deaths in this setting.[23] It typically occurs in the first week after infarction, with a mean time from symptom onset of 3–5 days.[24] The classic risk factors for septal rupture in the pre-reperfusion era include hypertension, advanced age, female sex, and the absence of a history of myocardial infarction or angina.[25] Prognosis for ventricular septal rupture in the pre-reperfusion era was very poor, with an in-hospital mortality of about 45% in those treated surgically and about 90% in those treated medically.[24] With the advent of thrombolysis and percutaneous intervention, theories have changed.

The following will review the pathologic and clinical features of interventricular septal rupture, explain how echocardiography is the diagnostic test of choice, and present the most recent updates from the reperfusion era.

## Pathophysiology

Ventricular rupture is defined as an acute, traumatic perforation of the ventricles which may also include pericardial rupture, laceration, or rupture of the interventricular septum, interatrial septum, chordae, papillary muscles, or valves.[26] In the setting of an acute myocardial infarction, one or several of these types of rupture may occur. During an acute infarction, the pathogenic process of the rupture changes over time. Without reperfusion, coagulation necrosis develops within the first 3–5 days. The septum becomes necrotic and is infiltrated by neutrophils which release lytic enzymes, thereby disintegrating the necrotic myocardium.[25] A transmural septal infarction underlies rupture of the interventricular septum, with the tear ranging in size from millimeters to centimeters.[23]

The ventricular septum is a very vascular structure. The rarity of septal rupture and the variable infarct location relate to the fact that the interventricular septum has a dual blood supply. The anterior two-thirds is supplied by the left anterior descending coronary artery and its branches. The posterior one-third is supplied by branches of the posterior descending artery which comes from the right coronary or the left circumflex artery depending on the dominance of the circulation.[27] Studies have conflicted in determining which artery is predominantly responsible for septal rupture, but anterior myocardial infarction is most frequent followed by inferior infarction.

Edwards et al. performed a study on 53 autopsied hearts with interventricular septal rupture complicating acute myocardial infarction and classified them into two types: simple and complex.[28] A simple rupture is defined as a direct, through and through opening connecting the ventricular chambers. The left and right ventricular openings are at about the same horizontal level of the septum. A complex rupture is defined as an interventricular communication that ascribes an undulating or serpiginous course. The tract may extend into regions remote from the site of the primary infarction. Commonly, the openings into the two ventricular chambers are at different planes of the ventricular septum.[28]

The anatomical location of the septal rupture tends to predict whether it is simple or complex. As one travels from the apex to the base, interventricular septal ruptures tend to trend from simple to complex.[28] Septal ruptures complicating an anterior myocardial infarction are generally apical and simple. Conversely, septal ruptures in patients with inferior myocardial infarctions tend to involve the basal, inferoposterior septum and are often complex.[25] Edwards et al. proposed that a triad of inferior wall infarction, complete atrioventricular block, and a ventricular septal rupture can predict a complex type of rupture.[28]

## Clinical Presentation

The classic risk factors associated with ventricular septal rupture include the absence of a history of angina or infarction.[24] It is also thought that most cases occur with a total occlusion of the infarct-related artery.[29] Many hypothesize that the absence of significant pre-existing coronary disease causes less collaterals to develop. In the setting of an abrupt cessation of flow in the infarct-related artery, no collateral flow exists to support the infarcted zone, thereby making the septum prone to rupture. Autopsy series and clinical angiographic series have differed. Overall, it appears that more than 50% of these patients have at least two vessel disease, and most cases occur with a total occlusion of the infarct-related artery.[23]

Whether in the pre- or post-reperfusion era, it is generally agreed that the clinical presentation and examination of a patient with a ventricular septal rupture has remained constant. Symptoms of rupture include shortness of breath, chest pain, and signs of low cardiac output and shock.[25] In 1934, Sager proposed a set of clinical criteria for suspecting a ruptured septum.[30] The sudden onset of a systolic murmur, often accompanied by a thrill, in a patient with rapid hemodynamic decompensation is highly suggestive of a ruptured interventricular septum.[30] The rupture produces a harsh, loud holosystolic murmur along the left sternal border, radiating toward the base, apex, and right parasternal area, with a palpable thrill present in half of the patients.[25]

In the setting of cardiogenic shock, the thrill and murmur may be difficult to appreciate because turbulent flow across the defect is reduced. Pulmonary hypertension may cause the pulmonic component of the second heart sound to be accentuated. Right and left ventricular S3 gallops are often heard. Tricuspid regurgitation may be present and biventricular failure generally occurs within hours to days.[25]

Differentiating between a ventricular septal rupture and acute mitral regurgitation may be difficult.[23] Compared to acute mitral regurgitation, septal rupture has a loud murmur, a thrill, and right ventricular failure. Importantly it is less often characterized by severe pulmonary edema. Once cardiogenic shock has developed, it may be difficult to distinguish these two entities. To complicate things further, severe mitral regurgitation may be present in 20% of patients with interventricular septal rupture.[25]

## Echocardiographic Features

When a patient develops clinical findings suggestive of a possible ventricular septal rupture, the initial step is to perform an immediate bedside transthoracic echocardiogram. Bedside echocardiography has been demonstrated to be highly sensitive and specific in the diagnosis of ventricular septal defect.[1] The advantages of echocardiography include its portability, its ability to be performed at the bedside, its non-invasive nature, and its ability to provide real-time imaging of intracardiac structures.[31] Basic transthoracic two-dimensional imaging can visualize the defect in 40–70% of patients. Adding contrast increases the sensitivity to 86% while color flow Doppler imaging elevates it to 95%. When transthoracic echocardiogram is suboptimal, transesophageal echocardiogram is highly accurate and has a reported sensitivity and specificity of 100%.[1]

Both the size and the location of the defect can be estimated by a careful echocardiographic examination. All acoustic windows should be used with careful apical-to-basal and anterior-to-posterior sweeps.[27] The parasternal short-axis, the apical four-chamber, and the subcostal long-axis views can all be used to visualize the septal defect (Fig. 20.5). The highest yield will be in apical views, but frequently "off-axis" angulation to interrogate available scan planes will be necessary (Fig. 20.6).[31] In addition to visualizing the septal defect, two-dimensional echocardiography can assess and diagnose the presence of right ventricular hypokinesis and septal dysfunction.[27]

Doppler color flow mapping allows imaging of blood flow signals superimposed on "real-time" two-dimensional echocardiographic images.[32] Two-dimensional echo alone has limitations in detecting small, multiple, or serpiginous tears in the septum because of artifactual dropouts and lateral resolution limitations. A ventricular septal rupture is diagnosed when turbulent blood flow signals are observed moving from the left into the right ventricle through an area of discontinuity in the ventricular septum. This turbulent systolic blood flow across the ventricular septal rupture will result in a striking display of mosaic-colored signals and aliasing within the right ventricular cavity. This aliasing represents flow signal acceleration and convergence (Fig. 20.7).[32]

Continuous-wave Doppler across the defect can be performed to determine the right ventricular systolic pressure. The operator can align the cursor as parallel to the direction of the ventricular septal rupture jet as possible, and the maximum velocity in systole can be obtained. The pressure gradient between left and right ventricles

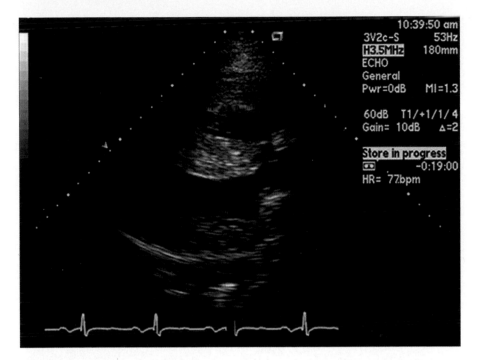

**Fig. 20.5** Transthoracic parasternal short-axis view demonstrating a ventricular septal defect

can be calculated using the simplified Bernoulli equation $(4\,V^2)$, and this value is subtracted from systemic cuff blood pressure (Fig. 20.8).[32]

Often transthoracic echocardiogram is suboptimal for identifying ventricular septal defects. Transesophageal echocardiography has been used in critically ill patients who may be technically difficult to image because of suboptimal patient positioning and increased pulmonary interference of ultrasound transmission by mechanical ventilation.[27] When TTE is suboptimal, transesophageal echocardiogram is highly accurate with a reported sensitivity and specificity of 100%.[31] TEE will improve delineation of the site of the defect, the morphology, and the presence of multiple defects. It is especially helpful with smaller defects. With echocardiography there should be no need for invasive measures to be taken to diagnose ventricular septal rupture.

## Treatment

After the diagnosis is made, medical therapy may consist of mechanical support with an intra-aortic balloon pump, afterload reduction, diuretics, and inotropic agents.[25] Prompt surgical intervention is essential as most patients have a rapid deterioration and die. It was previously believed that shortly after an acute myocardial

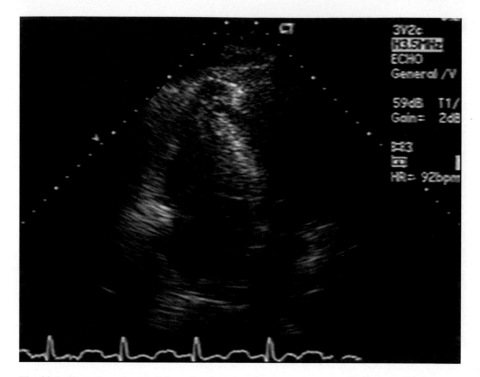

**Fig. 20.6** Transthoracic apical four-chamber view demonstrating a ventricular septal defect

infarction, the myocardium was too fragile for safe repair of the rupture. In the past, a waiting period of 3–6 weeks was standard before surgical intervention to allow the margins of the infarcted muscle to develop a firm scar to facilitate surgical repair.[33] It is now believed that immediate surgical intervention is the only option as medically managed patients generally die. This will be outlined below.

## *Update in the Reperfusion Era*

While many of the clinical characteristics and complications of acute myocardial infarction have remained the same, over the last few decades treatment strategies have advanced. Previous studies that investigated ventricular septal rupture were done in the pre-reperfusion era and contained small numbers of patients. Two pivotal studies that contained large numbers of patients are the Global Utilization of Streptokinase and TPA for Occluded Coronary Arteries (GUSTO-I) and the Should we emergently revascularize Occluded Coronaries for cardiogenic shock? (SHOCK) trials. These trials, which were performed in the thrombolysis and percutaneous intervention era, have changed the way we think about acute myocardial infarction.

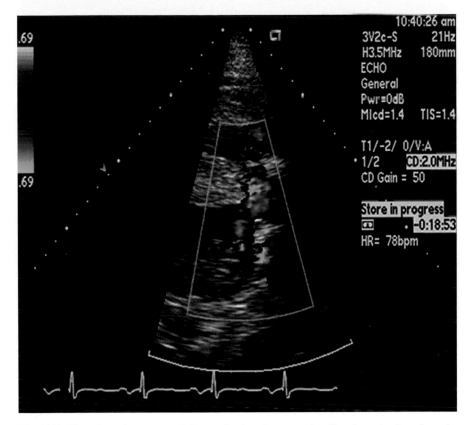

**Fig. 20.7** Transthoracic parasternal short-axis view demonstrating Doppler color flow through a ventricular septal defect

The following will review these studies as they pertain to interventricular septal rupture.

GUSTO-I enrolled 41,021 patients who presented within 6 h after the onset of symptoms, with chest pain for greater than 20 min and evidence of an ST-elevation myocardial infarction. Patients were randomized to receive streptokinase with subcutaneous heparin, streptokinase with intravenous heparin, accelerated alteplase with intravenous heparin, or the combination of alteplase and streptokinase with intravenous heparin.[34] A total of 84 patients were identified as having confirmed ventricular septal defects.[24] This represented 0.2% of the total GUSTO-I population. Echocardiography diagnosed the defect in most circumstances. The median time from MI symptom onset to septal rupture diagnosis was 1 day and 94% of cases were diagnosed within 1 week.[24]

Patients were more likely to be older, hypertensive, and female.[24] They most commonly had no history of smoking, an anterior infarction, an increased heart rate, and a worse Killip class at admission. Sixty percent of these patients underwent

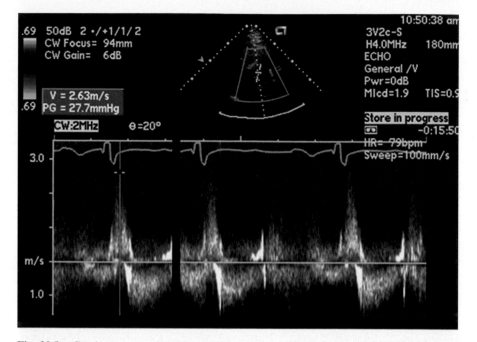

**Fig. 20.8** Continuous-wave Doppler showing a pressure gradient through a ventricular septal defect

angiography and they were more likely to have TIMI grade 0 or 1 flow at first angiography. They underwent angiography a median of 21 h after the onset of their index infarction versus 95 h in those patients without septal ruptures. Fifty-seven percent had total occlusion of the infarct-related artery which was more commonly the left anterior descending artery (64 versus 28% for the right coronary artery). Evidence of two- or three-vessel coronary disease was present in 50% and the median ejection fraction was lower in patients with ventricular septal defects (40 versus 51% in those without septal defects).[24]

In-hospital course, as well as 30-day and 1-year outcomes, varied greatly in those with interventricular septal defects versus those without. Ventricular septal defect patients were much more likely to have in-hospital procedures such as pacemakers, swan-ganz catheters, ventilators, and bypass surgery. Sixty-seven percent developed cardiogenic shock versus 5.9% of those without VSDs. A total of 34 of the 84 patients underwent surgical repair. At 30 days, patients who underwent surgical repair had 47% mortality versus 94% of those who were treated medically. At 1 year, 53% of the surgical patients died versus 97% of those medically managed. Those patients with VSDs who died at 30 days were more likely to be female and have an inferior infarction compared to those who survived. All patients with Killip class III or IV symptoms died at 30 days versus 27% of those VSD patients who were Killip class I or II.[24] Clearly, surgery was the best option, although prognosis was still poor.

GUSTO-I had a much lower incidence and an accelerated time to diagnosis inter-ventricular septal rupture than had been previously reported. About 0.2% of the population had this complication versus anywhere between 1 and 5% in the pre-thrombolytic era. Early reperfusion therapy may prevent the extensive myocardial necrosis that is associated with ventricular rupture.[24] Previously it had been reported that VSDs occur within 3–5 days of the index infarction. GUSTO-I patients had a mean time of 1 day from infarction to development of VSD. Many have postulated that this acceleration of rupture may be due to thrombolysis causing hemorrhage during the "lytic state", so that if a ventricular septal rupture occurs, its time course may be accelerated.[24]

Other differences with the previously reported data exist. Advanced age, anterior infarct location, female sex, and no current smoking were found to be the most potent predictors of VSD in GUSTO-I.[24] Previously hypertension and no history of myocardial infarction or angina had been predictors.

Mortality continues to be very high despite advances in medical and surgi-cal techniques (50% in surgical patients and 94% in medically treated patients). As Edwards et al. reported, it appeared that patients with inferior infarcts had a worse outcome than those with anterior infarcts.[24] This supports the results of their necroscopy study that reported inferior infarcts to be more complex and have right ventricular involvement versus anterior infarcts which are more likely to be sim-ple.[28] GUSTO-I patients treated medically had a very poor prognosis (30-day mor-tality of 94%) which is similar to previous reports.

The Should we emergently revascularize Occluded Coronaries in cardiogenic shock? (SHOCK) study[35] was a prospective, multicenter registry and randomized trial of cardiogenic shock complicating acute myocardial infarction. The study pri-marily looked at patients with left ventricular pump failure but patients with ventric-ular septal rupture were followed prospectively as part of the SHOCK Trial Registry. This study was performed in the interventional era. It assessed the effect of surgi-cal repair on outcomes of ventricular septal rupture and the profile and outcomes of patients with cardiogenic shock complicating acute myocardial infarction that both did and did not have septal rupture.[36]

There were 1190 patients with suspected cardiogenic shock complicating acute myocardial infarction that was prospectively registered.[37] Criteria for entry included (1) hypotension, (2) clinical evidence of end-organ hypoperfusion, and (3) confirma-tory hemodynamic or radiographic features. Only patients with cardiogenic shock due to predominant left ventricular failure with electrocardiographic evidence of recent total coronary occlusion were eligible for the original study.[37] Etiologies of cardiogenic shock due to anything other than pure left ventricular pump failure were placed in the SHOCK Trial Registry. This included patients with ventricular septal rupture.

Of the 1190 patients, 884 patients had predominant left ventricular failure and 55 were due to ventricular septal rupture. Rupture occurred within a median of 16 h after infarction which is again shorter than previously reported.[36] Patients tended to be older, more often female, and less often had previous infarction, dia-betes, or smoking history. They more often underwent invasive procedures including right heart catheterization, intra-aortic balloon pumping, and coronary artery bypass surgery. Interestingly, left ventricular ejection fraction was higher for the ventricular septal rupture group versus those with left ventricular failure without VSR (40 versus 30%). Forty-six percent of the patients with VSR involved the right coronary artery and 42% involved the left anterior descending artery. The majority had single- or double-vessel disease (26 and 43%, respectively). All culprit vessels had >90% stenosis and almost all had TIMI grade 0 or 1 flow.[36]

The overall in-hospital survival rate was only 13% for patients with ventricular septal rupture compared to 39% for patients with predominant left ventricular failure. Although patients with rupture had less severe coronary disease, their in-hospital mortality was higher (87 versus 61%). Surgery was performed in 31 patients with rupture (21 had concomitant bypass surgery) and only 6 (19%) survived. Of the 24 patients managed medically, only 1 survived.[36]

This study again had a much shorter time to rupture (16 h) than the 1 week that had been previously reported. It showed that women and the elderly with less multivessel coronary artery disease are most susceptible to ventricular septal rupture when compared to patients whose shock was due to predominant pump failure. The study highlights the dismal outcomes of those with ventricular septal defects and cardiogenic shock complicating acute myocardial infarction. Medial therapy carried a close to 100% mortality. Surgical therapy results were poor as well, but it was still considered the primary therapy.[36]

## Conclusion

Interventricular septal rupture is a rare complication of acute myocardial infarction. It appears to be more unusual in the reperfusion era. Nevertheless, its prompt diagnosis can be made by echocardiography in the appropriate clinical setting. This diagnostic tool can be used at the bedside to accelerate surgical intervention and thereby decrease the mortality rates of this deadly complication.

## Ventricular Septal Rupture Case Presentation

A 79-year-old male presented to the emergency room with severe chest pain for 5 days. He has a past medical history significant for coronary artery disease, hypertension, hypercholesterolemia, and diabetes. He is status post two myocardial infarction in 1994 and again in 1998. He formerly smoked two packs of cigarettes a day for 25 years and denies alcohol or drug use. He presented with complaints of intermittent, left-sided chest tightness for 5 days. The patient originally felt this chest pressure on exertion with associated shortness of breath. During the 3 days before presentation, his symptoms progressed in character and intensity until they were persistent at rest. The pain was very similar to his previous myocardial infarctions. The patient was supposed to be on a host of cardiac medications but he admitted to being noncompliant with all of them.

Upon arrival to the emergency room his physical exam proved to be markedly abnormal. His blood pressure was 91/52 mmHg, despite having a history of hypertension. His heart rate measured 102 bpm and respiratory rate was 24 rpm. The patient was afebrile and his oxygen saturation was 98% on 4 l of oxygen via nasal cannula. He was in obvious distress with markedly elevated jugular venous pressure. Rales were present half way up both lung fields and his lower extremities were extremely edematous. His heart sounds were rapid in rate. Both S1 and S2 were audible, and a 3/6 holosystolic ejection murmur was heard at the apex which extended into his axilla.

An electrocardiogram was done within 10 min of his arrival to the emergency room. It showed normal sinus rhythm at 100 bpm with 3 mm ST elevations in leads II, III, aVF, Q waves in leads II, III, aVF, and 2 mm ST depressions in leads I and aVL. The myocardial infarction team was activated and the patient was immediately transferred to the cardiac catheterization lab for emergent revascularization. His laboratory values showed a blood urea nitrogen of 36 mg/dl and a creatinine of 1.3 mg/dl. Glucose was 213 mg/dl. White blood cell count was 18 cells/μl. Troponin was 17 ng/ml. Creatine phosphokinase was 446 units/l, MB isozyme was 26.6 ng/ml, and MB index was 6.0. The leading diagnosis at the time was acute inferior ST-elevation myocardial infarction.

After obtaining informed consent the patient underwent coronary catheterization. He was found to have a right dominant system. His left main artery showed no angiographic stenosis. His left anterior descending artery showed a focal 90% proximal stenosis. His left circumflex artery showed an 80% proximal stenosis. His right coronary artery showed a hazy appearing total occlusion in mid-segment, no distal collaterals were present. The patient was in Killip class III decompensated congestive heart failure with an acute ST-elevation myocardial infarction. An intra-aortic balloon pump was placed and the right coronary artery was successfully stented. The patient was sent to the cardiac care unit for further monitoring.

Upon arrival he continued to be hemodynamically unstable with worsening congestive heart failure symptoms. His blood pressure fell to 80/50 mmHg and he was in severe respiratory distress with an oxygen saturation of 85% on 100% oxygen. At that time the patient was intubated and an emergent transthoracic echocardiography was performed due to his progressive hemodynamic decompensation despite adequate revascularization of the infarct-related artery.

The inferior wall was akinetic. The posterior wall was severely hypokinetic. The base and mid-septum were akinetic. Visually estimated left ventricular ejection fraction was 40%. There was a very large ventricular septal defect with left-to-right shunt. The left atrium was normal size. The right ventricle was dilated. The right ventricle was severely hypokinetic. The Doppler (spectral/color) study showed mild to moderate tricuspid regurgitation.

Due to his severe hemodynamic instability and presence of a large ventricular septal defect, detected by the bedside transthoracic echocardiogram, an emergent cardiothoracic surgery consult was called. Based on these results the patient was immediately taken to the operating room where he had triple coronary bypass graft surgery and a ventricular septal defect repair. The patient tolerated the procedure well. He was extubated on postoperative day number three. Ten days after his admission he was discharged to a rehabilitation center and has been following up in clinic without complications.

## Pericardial Effusion and Tamponade

### *Introduction*

Pericardial heart disease comprises a wide array of pathology that can eventually lead to the catastrophic complication of pericardial tamponade. Of all the diseases that affect the pericardium, tamponade can be the most acutely life threatening, thereby requiring prompt diagnosis and treatment. Echocardiography has proven to be the modality of choice to easily and accurately aid in the diagnosis of tamponade. In contrast to heart failure, coronary artery disease, valvular disease, and other topics in cardiology, there are scant data from randomized trials to guide physicians in the management of pericardial diseases.[38] There are no AHA/ACC guidelines on the topic, but the European Society of Cardiology published guidelines in 2004.[39] The following will review the pathophysiology, clinical manifestations, echocardiographic diagnostic criteria, and treatment of pericardial tamponade.

### *Pathophysiology*

An understanding of the physiology of the normal pericardium is necessary in order to comprehend the pathophysiology of tamponade. The pericardium is not essential for life, as no adverse consequences follow surgical removal or its congenital absence.[40] The pericardium is a predominantly avascular, fibrous sac that surrounds the heart. It is composed of the visceral and parietal pericardium. The visceral layer is a single layer of mesothelial cells that is adherent to the epicardium of the heart. The parietal pericardium is a fibrous structure that is less than 2 mm thick and is composed primarily of collagen and to a lesser degree elastin. The pericardial space separates the two layers and creates a potential space that normally contains 15–35 ml of serous fluid that is distributed mostly over the atrial–ventricular and interventricular grooves.[38]

The pericardium encases the heart and attaches to the sternum, the diaphragm, and the anterior mediastinum. It is invested around the great vessels and the vena cava, thereby serving to anchor the heart in the central thorax.[38] It limits distention of the four cardiac chambers and facilitates coupling of the ventricles and atria so that changes in volume and pressure on one side of the heart influence volume and pressure on the other side.[41]

The pericardium serves several other important functions. It is well innervated, giving rise to severe pain caused by pericarditis, as well as triggering vagally mediated reflexes.[38] It prevents torsion and displacement of the heart and minimizes friction with surrounding structures. It can also serve as an anatomical barrier to the spread of infection from contiguous structures.[40] The pericardium is also thought to secrete prostaglandins that modulate cardiac reflexes and coronary tone.[42]

The etiology of cardiac tamponade mirrors the various conditions that cause pericarditis. Idiopathic pericarditis and any infection, neoplasm, inflammatory or autoimmune process (including post-radiation and drug induced) can cause pericardial effusion.[43] Uremia, tuberculosis, SLE, Lyme disease, HIV, and lymphoma are just a few examples. Non-inflammatory diseases such as hypothyroidism and amyloidosis can cause effusions. Bleeding into the pericardial space after blunt and penetrating trauma as well as after a post-MI rupture of the ventricular free wall can cause disastrous tamponade. Retrograde bleeding related to an aortic dissection is also an important cause of tamponade.[43]

Pericardial effusions are reported to be associated with heart failure in 14%, valvular disease in 21%, and myocardial infarction in 15%.[44] Of all conditions, bacterial (including mycobacterial), fungal, and HIV-associated infections all have a high incidence of progression to tamponade.[43]

Post-cardiac surgery effusions are very common. However, large effusions or effusions leading to pericardial tamponade in this situation are rare.[40] Kuvin et al. did a retrospective study on over 4500 postoperative patients and only 48 were found to have moderate or large effusions on echo; and only 36 met the diagnostic criteria for tamponade. The use of preoperative anticoagulation, female sex, and valvular surgery were associated with a higher prevalence of tamponade.[45]

Cardiac tamponade occurs when fluid accumulation in the intrapericardial space is sufficient to raise the pressure surrounding the heart to the point where cardiac filling is affected.[38] The primary abnormality is compression of all cardiac chambers as a result of increasing intrapericardial pressure.[46] The key concept is that once the total intrapericardial volume has caused the pericardium to reach the noncompliant region of its pressure–volume relation, cardiac tamponade develops rapidly.[38] Clinical significance depends on how fast and how much fluid fills the pericardial space.

With slow accumulation, the parietal pericardium compliance increases. The more fluid in the pericardial space, the more intrapericardial pressure increases. In response, the central venous pressure increases via venoconstriction and fluid retention to maintain a gradient that allows cardiac filling. There comes a point where pericardial compliance can increase no more, and the intrapericardial pressure equalizes.[47] As the chambers become progressively smaller and myocardial diastolic compliance is reduced, cardiac inflow is limited, ultimately equalizing mean diastolic pericardial and chamber pressures.[46]

Since the right heart has lower pressures, it is most vulnerable to compression by a pericardial effusion. As a result, abnormal right heart filling is the earliest sign of a hemodynamically significant effusion. Because the total intrapericardial volume is fixed by the pressurized effusion, inspiratory increase in right ventricular filling crowds the left ventricle and impairs its filling. Therefore, in tamponade left heart filling takes place mainly during expiration when there is less right heart filling.[38]

When the effusion reaches its critical point, the cardiac output drops and blood pressure is maintained only through an increase in heart rate, contractility, and peripheral arteriolar vasoconstriction. When fluid accumulates slowly, the pericardium can increase compliance sufficiently before overt hemodynamic compromise can occur.[47] Inflammatory causes of pericardial effusion result in slow accumulation of fluid. Two liters or more may accumulate before life-threatening tamponade can occur.[46]

When pericardial fluid accumulates rapidly, the pericardium may not have sufficient time to stretch. With rapid filling of the pericardial space, intrapericardial pressure increases quickly, and cardiac filling is impaired often leading to a dramatic drop in cardiac output. Intrapericardial hemorrhage from wounds or cardiac rupture occurs in the context of a relatively stiff pericardium which quickly overwhelms the capacity of the pericardium to stretch before most compensatory mechanisms can be activated.[46] Life-threatening, acute cardiac tamponade can result leading to cardiogenic shock and death. Recognizing the clinical presentation can be difficult but is paramount in preventing the disastrous consequences of this clinical entity.

## Clinical Presentation

Cardiac tamponade is potentially a fatal form of cardiogenic shock, which must be recognized early and treated immediately. Symptoms are generally nonspecific, so suspicion must be high. Effusions by themselves do not cause symptoms unless tamponade is present.[43] Tachypnea and dyspnea on exertion are the typical symptoms as well as a vague chest discomfort or fullness. Patients can report nausea or abdominal pain from hepatic or visceral congestion or dysphagia from compression of the esophagus.[47] Very nonspecific symptoms can occur as well, such as lethargy, fever, cough, weakness, fatigue, anorexia, and palpitations. It is important to note that it can be impossible to obtain a history as the patient may be unconscious or obtunded. Therefore, tamponade must be suspected in many contexts, such as hypotension in patients with wounds of the chest or after cardiac surgery.[46]

Physical examination can be very nonspecific in chronic effusions but can also be very helpful when suspecting tamponade. Patients usually appear uncomfortable, with signs reflecting various degrees of reduced cardiac output and shock. These include tachypnea, diaphoresis, cool extremities, peripheral cyanosis, and depressed sensorium.[43] Tachycardia, defined as a heart rate greater than 90 bpm, is the rule. In rare cases such as hypothyroidism and uremia, the patient can be bradycardic. Heart sounds may be muffled due to the insulating effects of the pericardial fluid and to reduced cardiac output.[46]

Hypotension and elevated jugular venous distention are almost always seen. Rapid tamponade may produce exaggerated jugular pulsations without the finding of distention, due to insufficient time for the blood volume to increase.[46] The X descent seen during ventricular systole is typically the dominant jugular venous wave with a blunted or no Y descent. In 1935, Claude Schaeffer Beck[48] described the Beck triad consisting of decreasing arterial blood pressure, increasing jugular venous pressure, and a small, quiet heart. This triad was seen in surgical patients with acute tamponade due to intrapericardial hemorrhage. These findings are frequently but not always seen in tamponade caused by other conditions.

The examiner must check for pulsus paradoxus if tamponade is suspected. Described by Adolf Kussmaul in 1873, this finding is demonstrated by a fall of the radial pulse on inspiration in patients with tamponade.[49] Negative intrapleural pressures that occur during inspiration cause increased venous return and filling of the right heart, which results in bowing of the interventricular septum to the left, decreasing filling of the left heart, thereby decreasing cardiac output and peripheral blood pressure. Whether done with a sphygmomanometer or by palpating the peripheral pulse, pulsus paradoxus is considered positive when there is a greater than 10 mmHg drop in blood pressure throughout the respiratory cycle.[47] One study looked at 65 patients with known pericardial effusions and found that the likelihood ratio for tamponade was 5.9 with a pulsus paradoxus greater than 12 mmHg and 3.3 for a measurement greater than 10 mmHg.[50] Care must be taken as other conditions can cause pulsus paradoxus such as pulmonary embolism, obstructive lung disease, or various forms of severe hypotension.[46]

Findings on an electrocardiogram include reduced voltage and electrical alternans of the QRS complex. Reduced voltage is a very nonspecific finding that can be found in many other conditions. Electrical alternans is virtually specific but relatively insensitive for cardiac tamponade. It is caused by anterior–posterior movement of the heart with each heart beat. If pericarditis is present, diffuse ST elevation with PR segment depression can be present.[43]

Chest radiograph will not change until a pericardial effusion is at least moderate in size. With larger pericardial effusions, the anteroposterior cardiac silhouette assumes a rounded, flask-like appearance. In the lateral views, a linear lucency between the chest wall and the anterior surface of the heart may be seen. Lung fields are typically free of congestion.[43]

## Echocardiographic Diagnosis

When cardiac tamponade is suspected a two-dimensional Doppler echocardiography should be performed without delay. Although tamponade is a clinical diagnosis, echocardiography enhances the ability to accurately make the diagnosis. Echocardiography visualizes pericardial fluid as an echo-free space surrounding the heart. Acute hemorrhagic effusions may have an element of thrombus involved which appears as an echo-dense mass.[51] Small pericardial effusions are usually only seen posteriorly. Those that are large enough to produce cardiac tamponade are almost always circumferential (seen both anteriorly and posteriorly).[38] Occasionally effusions can be loculated or localized which most commonly happens after cardiac surgery.

There are several echocardiographic features described in patients with hemodynamic compromise and frank cardiac tamponade. The technician must use all
views to visualize the effusion. On M-mode echocardiography, pericardial effusion
appears as an echo-free space both anterior and posterior to the heart. The size of
the space is directly proportional to the amount of fluid. Care must be taken because
an anterior echo-free space may be due to mediastinal fat, fibrosis, thymus, or other
tissues.[52] Therefore, an effusion must be seen both anterior and posterior to the heart
(Fig. 20.9).

Most often two-dimensional echo is used to screen and quantify pericardial effusion. Effusions tend to be most prominent in the more depended (i.e., posterior in a
supine patient) area and appears maximal in the posterior atrioventricular groove.
Using additional views such as the parasternal short-axis, apical, and subcostal
views, the circumferential extent of an effusion can be determined.[52] In the parasternal long-axis view pericardial fluid reflects at the posterior atrioventricular groove,
while pleural fluid continues under the left atrium, posterior to the descending aorta
(Figs. 20.10 and 20.11).[39]

Once a pericardial effusion is visualized, it must be graded as small, moderate,
large, or very large. The European Society of Cardiology published guidelines in
2004 (ESU) that proposes the following grading scale. A small effusion is defined
as an echo-free space in diastole of <10 mm. Moderate is 10–20 mm, large is ≥
20 mm, and very large is ≥ 20 mm with compression of the heart.[39]

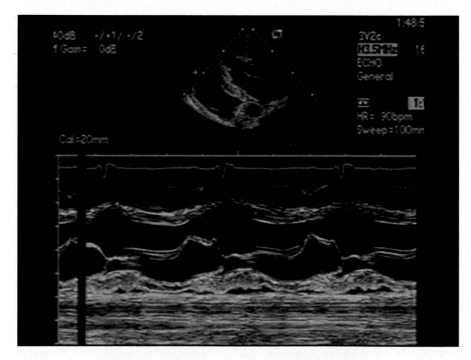

**Fig. 20.9** M-mode echocardiography demonstrating a pericardial effusion

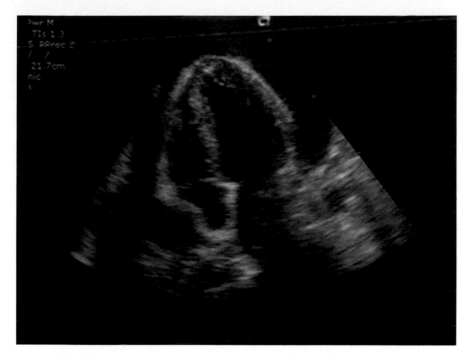

**Fig. 20.10**   Apical four-chamber view showing a large pericardial effusion

One of the earliest signs of cardiac tamponade is evidence of a swinging heart that can be detected on either two-dimensional or M-mode echo. Evidence of a swinging heart is simply a marker of a large effusion and is an indirect indicator of elevated intrapericardial pressure. The movement of the heart within the pericardial sac is the mechanism of electrical alternans seen on electrocardiography with large pericardial effusions (Fig. 20.12).[52]

More specific signs of hemodynamic compromise exist that are directly related to actual elevation of intrapericardial pressures. Diastolic right ventricular outflow collapse and exaggerated right atrial collapse during atrial systole are important indicators of tamponade. M-mode echocardiography shows a characteristic posterior motion of the anterior right ventricular wall in diastole.[52]

In patients with tamponade, intracavitary cardiac pressure may transiently fall below intrapericardial pressure in early diastole leading to hydrodynamic compression of these more distensible structures. The right ventricular outflow tract is the most compressible structure of the right ventricle and tends to collapse with significantly elevated intrapericardial pressure. Immediately after closure of the pulmonic valve in early diastole, the right ventricular outflow tract will paradoxically collapse inward. This is often best appreciated in the parasternal long- and short-axis views and occasionally in the apical four-chamber view.[52] When seen, this is indicative of a hemodynamically significant effusion.

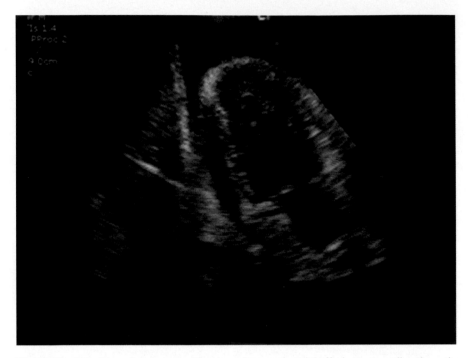

**Fig. 20.11** Apical two-chamber view showing a large pericardial effusion surrounding the entire heart

Along with right ventricular compression, exaggerated right atrial collapse is seen and indicates impeded right atrial filling. It can typically be viewed from the subcostal or apical four-chamber view. The right atrium normally contracts during atrial systole, so the degree of right atrial collapse must be quantified with respect to either the magnitude of collapse or the duration for which it remains collapsed. Right atrial collapse occurs immediately after normal atrial systole. In pericardial tamponade the right atrial wall will remain collapsed throughout atrial diastole and buckle inward.[52] Right atrial collapse is more sensitive for tamponade, but right ventricular collapse lasting more than one-third of diastole is more specific for cardiac tamponade.[38]

Doppler echocardiography also plays a crucial role when evaluating the significance of a pericardial effusion. Doppler evaluation of the mitral or tricuspid valve inflow or aortic or pulmonary outflow can be used to demonstrate exaggerated phasic variation in flow during respiration. With inspiration, the right ventricular early diastolic filling velocity is augmented, while left ventricular diastolic filling diminishes. Normally peak velocity of mitral inflow varies by 15% or more with respiration and tricuspid inflow by 25% or more.[52] These findings correlate with the pathophysiology of cardiac tamponade described earlier. For the tricuspid valve there is augmented inflow during inspiration with diminished flow during expiration. The opposite is true for the mitral valve.

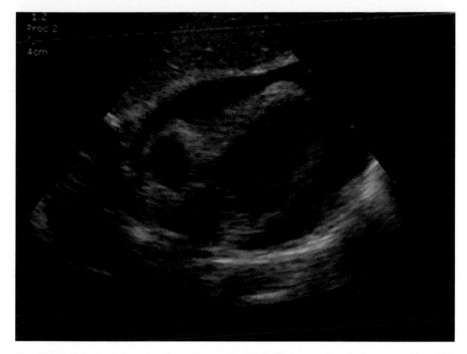

**Fig. 20.12** Subcostal view showing a large pericardial effusion causing the heart to swing within the pericardial sac

Variation in peak velocity and time velocity integral of aortic and pulmonary flow is typically less than 10%. With hemodynamically significant pericardial effusions all of these thresholds are exaggerated with respiration. There is augmented pulmonary flow with inspiration and a reciprocal decrease in left ventricular outflow at the same time in the respiratory cycle. This represents physiologic evidence of exaggerated intraventricular interdependence. These findings are the echocardiographic correlates of pulsus paradoxus described previously.[52]

Investigation of the inferior vena cava can be helpful as well. Distention of the inferior vena cavae with a less than 50% inspiratory reduction is a result of elevated venous pressure seen in tamponade. Also, because of limited cardiac volume seen in tamponade, Doppler can be used to demonstrate that venous flow predominantly occurs in systole and not in diastole as it normally does.[38]

Overall, echocardiography demonstrates the presence and size of a pericardial effusion and can reflect its hemodynamic consequence. All of the parameters described above must be evaluated to determine the significance of a pericardial effusion. Right atrial and right ventricular collapse indicates cardiac compression, while enhanced respiratory variation of ventricular filling is a manifestation of ventricular interdependence. When combined with clinical evidence of pericardial tamponade, immediate echocardiography can lead to prompt diagnosis and treatment.

## Treatment

The treatment of cardiac tamponade involves drainage of the pericardial effusion. Echocardiography-guided needle pericardiocentesis can be performed in the cardiac catheterization lab or even at the bedside in emergent situations.[38] In the paraxiphoid approach the needle is aimed toward the left shoulder, and in the apical approach, the needle is aimed internally. The needle is inserted at a 15° angle to bypass the costal margin.[46] Two-dimensional echo-guided pericardiocentesis carries about a 1.2% complication rate.[53]

Removal of small amounts of pericardial fluid can produce considerable symptomatic and hemodynamic improvement. Removal of all the pericardial fluid normalized pericardial, atrial, ventricular diastolic and arterial pressures and cardiac output. A drainage catheter can be advanced over a guide wire into the pericardial space and remain there for several days.[40] Patients should then be followed with the use of Doppler echocardiography to ensure that the pericardial space has been adequately drained to avoid recurrence. When drainage is less than 50 ml/day, the catheter may be withdrawn.[46] Malignant pericardial effusions generally recur. If the effusion recurs, sclerosing agents can be inserted into the pericardial space through the catheter to prevent further accumulation.[40]

If pericardial tissue is required for diagnosis, if the pericarditis is purulent, or if the effusion recurs, surgical drainage may be the preferred treatment.[38] Surgery is also the treatment of choice for traumatic hemopericardium.[39] Surgical drainage is usually performed through a limited subxiphoid incision. This approach allows for direct visualization and biopsy of the pericardium. Creation of a pericardial window creates a communication with the pleural space and eliminates future episodes of cardiac tamponade.[43]

Medical management of cardiac tamponade is usually ineffective and should only be used as a bridge to pericardiocentesis. Fluid resuscitation may be of transient benefit if the patient is hypovolemic. The use of inotropic agents is also largely ineffective as there is already an intense endogenous adrenergic stimulation.[38] The initiation of mechanical ventilation in a patient with cardiac tamponade may produce further drop in blood pressure because positive intrathoracic pressure will further impair cardiac filling and cardiac output.[54] Uremic tamponade often responds to intense dialysis, but if this is ineffective, drainage is required.[46] When signs of shock are evident and tamponade is diagnosed, pericardiocentesis is a life-saving procedure.

## Conclusion

Pericardial tamponade is a life-threatening entity that must be in the forefront of every physicians mind as it must be treated immediately. The clinical features of hypotension, elevated jugular venous pressure, muffled heart sounds, and pulsus paradoxus should immediately cue the physician to order an emergent two-dimensional echocardiography. When a pericardial effusion is present and right atrial and ventricular collapse is seen, emergent pericardiocentesis should be performed. In this setting, echocardiography can help diagnosis and aid in treatment, thereby leading to life-saving maneuvers.

# Right Ventricular Infarction

## *Introduction*

Right ventricular infarction had been described over 60 years ago, but for decades it was not considered to be important because it showed no hemodynamic consequence in animal models.[55] Over time, it has become important to diagnose as it defines a specific clinical entity that is associated with considerable immediate morbidity and mortality.[56] Right ventricular infarction complicates up to half of inferior left ventricular infarctions.[55] Prompt recognition of this mechanical complication of acute myocardial infarction is crucial as its initial management differs from that of other types of infarction. The following will review the pathophysiology, clinical features, diagnosis, and treatment of right ventricular infarction.

## *Pathophysiology*

The right side of the heart varies considerably from the left side. It is a low pressure system that has one-sixth of the muscle mass of the left ventricle and performs one-fourth of the stroke work. Despite this, both ventricles have the same cardiac output.[55] This is due to the fact that the pulmonary vascular resistance is one-tenth that of the peripheral systemic resistance.[57] These factors are important in the hemodynamic consequences of right ventricular infarction.

Coronary blood flow to the right ventricle is unique in that it occurs in both systole and diastole.[55] The right coronary artery supplies the lateral wall through the acute marginal branches in the majority of patients, as well as the posterior wall and posterior interventricular septum through the posterior descending artery in right dominant systems. Typically, right ventricular infarction occurs when there is occlusion of the right coronary artery proximal to the acute marginal branches. It can also occur with an occlusion of the left circumflex in those who have a left dominant system. Although quite rare, occlusion of the left anterior descending artery may result in infarction of the anterior right ventricle.[55]

The incidence of right ventricular infarction in association with left ventricular infarction ranges from 14 to 84%, depending on the study performed. Incidence of isolated right ventricular infarction accounts for less than 3% of all cases of infarction.[55] When isolated to the right ventricle, the occlusion is usually in the acute marginal vessels or of a non-dominant right coronary artery.[58] Many right coronary artery occlusions do not result in right ventricular necrosis.[56] Up to half of inferior myocardial infarctions involve the right ventricle. This may be due to the lesser right ventricular myocardial oxygen demand as a result of its smaller muscle mass or from its improved oxygen delivery from the biphasic nature of the coronary blood flow during both systole and diastole. A rich left-to-right collateral system is also thought to play a part.[55]

The hemodynamic consequences of right ventricular infarction are interesting. Acute underperfusion of the right ventricular free wall and adjacent interventricular septum leads to a stunned and noncompliant right ventricle. Loss of right ventricular contractility results in a serious deficit in left ventricular preload with a resultant drop in cardiac output, thereby causing systemic hypotension.[59] Augmented atrial contractility is necessary to overcome the increased myocardial stiffness associated with right ventricular infarction.[60] Factors that impair filling of the noncompliant right ventricle and cause decreased preload are likely to have profound adverse effects on hemodynamics in patients with large right ventricular infarctions. These factors include intravascular volume depletion due to the use of diuretics and nitrates or any diminution in atrial function caused by concomitant atrial infarction or the loss of atrioventricular synchrony.[55]

To complicate matters, acute right ventricular dilatation causes a leftward shift of the interventricular septum, increasing left ventricular end-diastolic pressure with a resultant decrease in left ventricular compliance and cardiac output. Left ventricular compliance is further aggravated by increased intrapericardial pressure as a result of right ventricular dilatation. As a consequence, even if the patient shows signs of increased right-sided pressure, the left ventricular filling and systolic function may be below normal.[56] If significant left ventricular dysfunction complicates right ventricular infarction, the results can be disastrous.

## Clinical Presentation

Given that management of right ventricular infarction is quite different from left ventricular infarction, recognizing its clinical presentation is important. When a patient presents with an inferior myocardial infarction the triad of hypotension, clear lung fields, and elevated jugular venous pressure is virtually pathognomonic for right ventricular infarction.[55] This triad is very specific, but has a sensitivity of less than 25%.[61] Auscultation may reveal a right-sided S3 and S4.[62] Tricuspid regurgitation may also be noted if the right ventricle is sufficiently dilated.

Pulsus paradoxus (decreased systolic blood pressure with inspiration) and Kussmaul's sign (elevated jugular venous distention with inspiration) have also been reported in RV infarction.[62] The presence of Kussmaul's sign and elevated jugular venous distention in the presence of an acute inferior myocardial infarction indicate a hemodynamically significant right ventricular infarction with a sensitivity of 88% and a specificity of 100%.[61] Careful examination of neck veins in the setting of an inferior myocardial infarction should alert the physician to the drastic consequences that the use of nitrates and morphine can have. These agents should be avoided as they reduce preload and can promote or exacerbate hypotension.

The electrocardiogram is crucial for the diagnosis of right ventricular infarction. The most frequent finding is any degree of ST elevation in leads II, III, and aVF with or without Q waves. Occlusion sufficiently proximal in the right coronary artery to cause right ventricular free wall injury also frequently compromises the blood supply to the sinoatrial node, atrium, and atrioventricular node, producing such effects as sinus bradycardia, atrial infarction, atrial fibrillation, and AV block.[59] Involvement of the right ventricular free wall may be suspected with the presence of ST depression in precordial leads V2 and V3 when compared to V1. Confirmation of RV ischemia can be quickly obtained when right-sided leads V4R through V6R show ST-segment elevations greater than 1 mm.[59] A 1-mm ST elevation in V4R is 70% sensitive and 100% specific for right ventricular infarction.[55]

ST-segment elevation in V4R has been shown to be a strong independent predictor of major complications and in-hospital mortality.[56] A prospective study of 200 consecutive patients with ST elevation in V4R strongly identified a group of patients prone to cardiogenic shock, ventricular fibrillation, and third-degree heart block. The patients with ST elevation in lead V4R had a higher in-hospital mortality rate (31 versus 6%) and a higher incidence of major in-hospital complications (64 versus 28%) compared to patients without these electrocardiographic changes.[63] This ST elevation can be rather transient in nature. One study showed that 48% of patients had resolution of these changes within 10 h of symptom onset. For this reason, prompt recognition of the diagnostic electrocardiographic changes is imperative. Right bundle branch block and complete atrioventricular block are the most common conduction disturbances seen although atrial fibrillation and sinus bradycardia can be seen as well.[55]

## Echocardiographic Features

Electrocardiographic signs of right ventricular infarction are both sensitive and specific for the presence of right ventricular infarction, but they do not provide information as to the extent of myocardial involvement. Two-dimensional echocardiography is a quick and easy way to quantify the amount of dysfunction. The subcostal view provides an excellent view of the right ventricular wall. When this view is inadequate, apical and parasternal views can be used (Figs. 20.13 and 20.14). The right ventricular wall is divided into three segments: the apical, middle, and basal segments.[64] From M-mode recordings in the parasternal long-axis view, right ventricular end-diastolic diameter can be measured and it can be assessed according to body surface area (normal end-diastolic diameter is greater than or equal to 20 mm/m$^2$).[65] M-mode studies demonstrate right ventricular dilatation and an increased ratio of right ventricular to left ventricular end-diastolic dimensions in patients with right ventricular infarction.

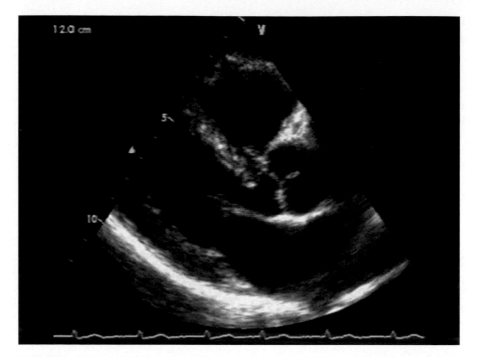

**Fig. 20.13** Transthoracic parasternal long-axis view demonstrating a dilated right ventricular outflow tract

The echocardiographic signs of right ventricular infarction include right ventricular dilatation, decreased right ventricular function, segmental wall motion abnormalities, and paradoxical septal wall motion. Decreased descent of the right ventricular base is commonly used to describe decreased function.[1] In many instances, the wall motion abnormality of the inferior wall of the left ventricle may be relatively small and overall left ventricular systolic function may appear preserved.[52] Right ventricular failure with high right atrial pressures results in bowing of the interatrial septum into the left atrium and dilatation of the inferior vena cava with lack of inspiratory collapse.[1] The elevation of right heart pressure may result in substantial amounts of right-to-left shunting through a patent foramen ovale.[52] The presence of interatrial septal bowing, indicating a concomitant right atrial infarction, is an important prognostic marker and is predictive of more hypotension, atrioventricular blocks and higher mortality in right ventricular infarction (Figs. 20.15 and 20.16).[56]

Some other important features that can be seen on two-dimensional echo are the presence of tricuspid regurgitation, tricuspid papillary muscle rupture, and a dilated inferior vena cava. The pressure half-time of the pulmonary regurgitant jet reflects the compliance of the right ventricular chamber.[1] In one study, a short pressure half-time of the pulmonary regurgitant jet of less than 150 ms was a predictor of in-hospital events.[66] Increased right ventricular and right atrial pressures can cause

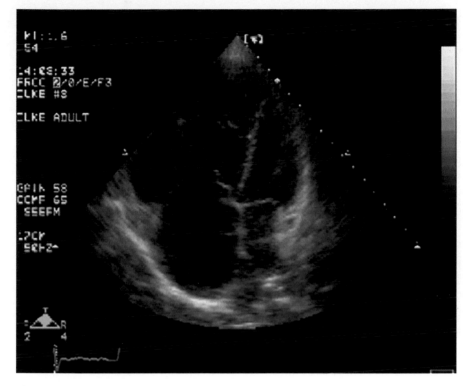

**Fig. 20.14** Transthoracic apical four-chamber view demonstrating a dilated and severely hypokinetic right ventricle

right-to-left flow across a patent foramen ovale. Doppler echocardiography can also determine premature opening of the pulmonic valve, indicating a noncompliant right ventricle.[56]

## *Treatment*

The treatment strategy of right ventricular infarction includes early maintenance of right ventricular preload, reduction of right ventricular afterload, inotropic support of the dysfunctional right ventricle, and early reperfusion.[55] When the right ventricle is ischemic, use of drugs such as nitrates and diuretics will reduce preload and may reduce cardiac output and cause severe hypotension. Volume loading alone with normal saline will often increase filling of the right ventricle and in turn increase filling of the underfilled left ventricle and increase cardiac output.[56] This treatment strategy is different from therapy for pump failure that accompanies left ventricular infarct where nitrates and diuresis are often critical. When bilateral pump failure is

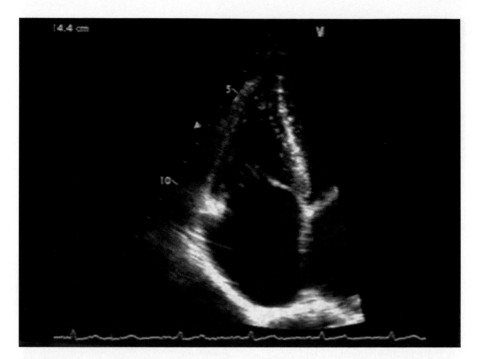

**Fig. 20.15** Transthoracic apical four-chamber view demonstrating a dilated right atrium and a hypokinetic right ventricle

present, use of afterload reducing agents like sodium nitroprusside or an intra-aortic balloon pump is often necessary to unload the left ventricle and the right ventricle.[55]

Fluid administration can further elevate right-sided filling pressures without improvement in cardiac output. In some cases, volume loading will cause further dilatation of the right ventricle, which in turn further compromises left ventricular output through pericardial restraining effects.[55] Inotropic support with dobutamine should be initiated if the cardiac output fails to improve with up to 1 l of fluid administration.[56]

Often inferior myocardial infarction can result in bradyarrhythmias and atrioventricular dyssynchrony. When stroke volume is impaired cardiac output depends on heart rate and bradycardia can be deleterious. The development of high-degree atrioventricular block has been reported in as many as 48% of patients with right ventricular infarction.[67] Atrioventricular dyssynchrony causes loss of right atrial contribution to preload and can lead to further hemodynamic compromise. Several investigators have shown that atrioventricular sequential pacing in patients with complete heart block leads to significant increase in cardiac output and reversal of shock when ventricular pacing alone has no benefit.[68] Prompt cardioversion for atrial fibrillation should be considered in order to restore atrioventricular synchrony at the earliest signs of hemodynamic compromise.[55]

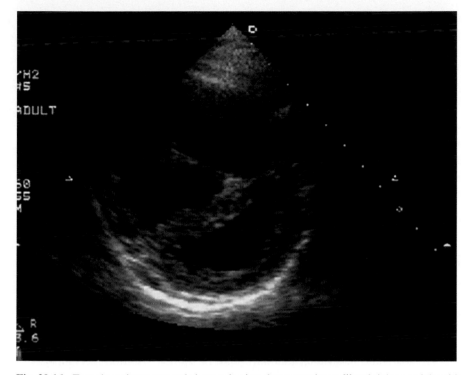

**Fig. 20.16** Transthoracic parasternal short-axis view demonstrating a dilated right ventricle with pressure and volume overload on the left ventricle with septal flattening

Reperfusion should be considered in the initial management of right ventricular infarction. Some studies suggest that right ventricular function improves only after successful reperfusion, while others report improvement even in the absence of a patent infarct-related vessel.[56] In the second Thrombolysis in Myocardial Infarction trial, there was a reduction in the incidence of right ventricular infarction among patients with inferior myocardial infarctions who had patent infarct-related arteries as compared with the rate in those whose arteries remained occluded.[69] Moreyra et al. showed rapid hemodynamic improvement when primary angioplasty has been used to treat RV infarction.[70] In a study of 53 patients, Bowers et al. showed that mortality in those with incomplete reperfusion was 58% at 1 month versus 2% in those who were completely revascularized.[71]

The Should we emergently revascularize Occluded Coronaries in cardiogenic shock? (SHOCK) study[72] was a prospective, multicenter registry and randomized trial of cardiogenic shock complicating acute myocardial infarction. The study primarily looked at patients with left ventricular pump failure but patients with right ventricular infarction were followed prospectively as part of the SHOCK Trial Registry.[73] Of the 933 patients with cardiogenic shock entered into the registry, 49 had predominantly right ventricular failure and 884 had predominantly left ventricular failure. They were followed prospectively. A total of 31 of the 49 patients underwent coronary angiography. The investigators were surprised to find that the in-hospital mortality for those with right ventricular failure was similar to those with left ventricular failure complicating acute myocardial infarction (53 versus 61%). The rates of recurrent ischemia and reinfarction were very similar as well.[73]

Those patients with predominant right ventricular failure who underwent revascularization with either percutaneous angioplasty or coronary artery bypass grafting had much better outcomes. Mortality was 42% for those revascularized versus 65% for those not revascularized. These numbers were similar for those with predominant left ventricular failure (40 and 73%). The conclusion was made that right ventricular failure complicating acute myocardial infarction carries a very high mortality risk similar to that for left ventricular failure. Revascularization helps improve these numbers and should be considered immediately.[73]

## Conclusion

Long-term prognostic data for those suffering from right ventricular infarction are conflicting. It is generally thought that when patients survive to discharge, prognosis is favorable but large-scale studies are needed to confirm this theory.[55] Zehender et al. showed that when inferior myocardial infarction is complicated by right ventricular infarction, in-hospital mortality may be as high as 31% as compared to 6% in those without RV involvement, but no long-term data were given.[63] Some have shown that right ventricular dysfunction after acute myocardial infarction is an independent risk factor for higher long-term mortality, while others have shown no difference.[55]

Even without long-term prognostic data, prompt diagnosis of right ventricular infarction, by electrocardiographic and echocardiographic means, must be made to direct the appropriate therapy and prevent the potential disastrous consequences of this complication of acute myocardial infarction.

## Right Ventricular Infarction Case Presentation

A 53-year-old woman presented to the emergency room with complaints of left-sided chest pain for 2 h. Her past medical history was significant only for hyperlipidemia for which she was recently started on medication. She formerly smoked one pack of cigarettes a day for 20 years but quit 5 years ago. She admitted to drinking occasional alcohol but denied drug use. She presented with complaints of a constant left-sided chest tightness that began while watching television 2 h earlier. The patient felt this chest pressure at rest with associated shortness of breath and diaphoresis. During the 3 days before presentation, she noticed these symptoms while she walked up the stairs but they were not as severe. In the emergency room she was nauseous and vomited twice.

Upon arrival to the emergency room her blood pressure was 125/75 mmHg and her heart rate measured 110 bpm with a respiratory rate of 20 rpm. The patient was afebrile and her oxygen saturation was 98% on 4 l of oxygen via nasal cannula. She was in obvious distress with diaphoresis and bilious vomiting. Her jugular venous pressure was markedly elevated to 15 mmHg. Her lungs were completely clear to auscultation and her heart sounds were rapid in rate. Both S1 and S2 were audible, and a 2/6 holosystolic ejection murmur was heard at the left sternal border in the fifth intercostal space.

An electrocardiogram was done within 10 min of her arrival to the emergency room. It showed normal sinus rhythm at 110 bpm with 3 mm ST elevations in leads II, III, aVF and 2 mm ST depressions in leads I and aVL. The myocardial infarction team was activated and the patient was prepared for immediate cardiac catheterization. The leading diagnosis was acute inferior myocardial infarction.

She was given aspirin, heparin, and sublingual nitroglycerin for her chest pressure and her blood pressure fell to 70/50 mmHg. At that time she became obtunded. She was immediately intubated for airway protection and placed on dopamine. All laboratory values were normal including a troponin of 0.0 ng/ml and a creatine phosphokinase level of 78 units/l. While waiting for the cath lab team to arrive an emergent bedside echocardiogram was performed by the cardiology fellow due to her hemodynamic instability.

The left atrium was normal. The left ventricular chamber size was normal. No left ventricular wall motion abnormalities were noted. Visually estimated left ventricular ejection fraction was 55%. The right atrium was dilated. The right ventricle was severely dilated. The right ventricle was severely hypokinetic. The Doppler (spectral/color) study showed mild to moderate tricuspid regurgitation. There was evidence of bowing of the interatrial septum. She was also noted to have a patent foramen ovale with right-to-left shunting of blood.

At that time a right-sided electrocardiogram was performed which showed Q waves in leads RV3 through RV5 with 2 mm ST elevations in RV3 through RV5. The patient was diagnosed with an isolated right ventricular infarction. The dopamine was discontinued and she was given two consecutive 1 l boluses of normal saline and started on a dobutamine infusion. Her blood pressure increased to 110/80 mmHg and cardiac catheterization was performed.

Catheterization revealed a proximal total occlusion of her right coronary artery, proximal to the acute marginal coronary arteries. Her system was left dominant. The left main coronary artery showed no stenosis. The left anterior descending artery and left circumflex artery also showed no angiographic disease. There was presence of grade 3 collaterals filling the distal right coronary artery, coming from the left anterior descending artery. Her right coronary artery was successfully opened with a drug-eluting stent. The patient tolerated the procedure well and she was transferred to the cardiac care unit for further monitoring.

After receiving sublingual nitroglycerin, the patient became obtunded and required intubation. The stat bedside echo revealed a severely hypokinetic right ventricle, thereby diagnosing right ventricular infarction in the setting of an inferior wall myocardial infarction. The left ventricular function was normal, likely due to adequate collaterals supplying the right coronary artery and because her system was left dominant. This echo changed management drastically. Instead of withholding intravenous fluids, as one would do with left ventricular failure, the patient was judiciously given fluids and put on the appropriate inotropes. She became hemodynamically stable and underwent successful percutaneous intervention without difficulty.

In the cardiac care unit intravenous fluids were discontinued. The dobutamine was tapered off as she became hemodynamically stable. She was successfully extubated about 3 h later. Follow-up echocardiogram showed normalization of her right ventricular function. She was discharged home after day three of her hospitalization and has returned to her normal daily activities without consequence.

# Acute Mitral Regurgitation

## Introduction

Acute mitral regurgitation (MR) is one of the major fatal mechanical complications of acute myocardial infarction (MI). The three main causes of MR in the setting of acute MI include ischemic papillary muscle dysfunction, papillary muscle or chordal rupture, and left ventricular dilatation or true aneurysm.[74] In the setting of an inferior MI, a high index of suspicion for this complication should be entertained. It usually occurs 2–7 days post-infarct and is associated with both ST-elevation and non-ST-elevation infarcts.[75] In such predisposed patients, the various risk factors for any post-myocardial infarction rupture include delayed hospitalization (over 24 h), undue in-hospital physical activity, and post-infarction angina. These complications are all clinically significant as if undiagnosed and untreated they invariably result in cardiogenic shock and an estimated 5% patient mortality.

## Pathophysiology

The mitral valve is located retrosternally at the fourth costal space, consisting of an anterior and posterior leaflet. In addition to both leaflets the mitral valve apparatus consists of chordae tendinae, papillary muscles, ventricular wall, and annulus connected to the atria. Each leaflet is supported by chordae tendinae that are attached to both anterolateral and posteromedial papillary muscles which become taut with each ventricular contraction ensuring valvular competence.

Any portion of the mitral apparatus can become anatomically disrupted and result in a portion of the mitral valve becoming flail and dysfunctional. The degree of resultant regurgitation is directly related to the extent of anatomic disruption. Most of the time in the setting of acute MI, the rupture of an entire papillary muscle or muscle head typically results in acute severe mitral regurgitation.[52] Depending on whether the infarct expansion includes one of the heads or both the rupture may be termed complete or partial. In most patients, the anterolateral papillary muscle receives dual blood supply from the left anterior descending and circumflex coronary arteries and is less likely to be involved by the ischemic process than is the posteromedial papillary muscle which is supplied solely by the posterior descending artery. Because of its single-vessel blood supply the posteromedial papillary muscle is 6–12 times more vulnerable to vascular compromise and rupture than the anterolateral papillary muscle. Often, the infarct expansion is relatively small with poor collaterals, and up to 50% of patients have single-vessel disease, with many of them being a consequence of a first-time MI.[76,77] Several studies support that acute MR is not only a common complication post-acute MI but that the degree of MR is predictive of patient survival. In the "Should we emergently revascularize Occluded Coronaries in cardiogenic shock?" (SHOCK) trial of early revascularization in cardiogenic shock after acute MI, 169 patients had echocardiograms.[78,79] Those with noted moderate or severe MR (39%) had a significantly lower 1-year survival than patients with mild or no MR (31 versus 58%). Larger studies calculate the mortality of patients with moderately severe to severe MR during an acute MI to be 24% at 30 days and 52% at 1 year.[75] Mild MR in the setting of acute MI, however, is not associated with clinically adverse events as it is likely reversible and secondary to the acute ischemic insult.

Of note select patients with moderate to severe MR, but without papillary muscle rupture, are hemodynamically stable. In this setting patients respond well to medical therapy and revascularization with or without eventual surgical intervention (mitral valve repair or replacement or coronary artery bypass grafting).[80] Thus papillary muscle rupture is a poor prognostic factor.

## Clinical Presentation

The clinical signs of papillary muscle rupture or severe dysfunction are consistent with those of cardiogenic shock and are invariably seen in all mechanical complications of acute MI. The most common and alarming signs include hemodynamic collapse and a new systolic murmur. Patients will present with acute onset, hypotension, pulmonary edema, a hyperactive precordium, and many times a new systolic murmur but usually no thrill.

One must be careful in clinically assessing the murmur of acute MR as it can vary significantly from the murmur of classic chronic MR in terms of timing in systole, harshness, and radiation. The reason for this is the different etiologies and hemodynamics behind acute or chronic mitral regurgitation. The murmur of acute MR may be a mid-, late-, or holosystolic murmur that may or may not have widespread radiation. The intensity of the murmur of acute MR does not always correlate with the severity of the murmur. As many as 50% of patients with severe MR secondary to papillary muscle rupture have early equalization of left ventricular and left atrial pressures resulting in silent MR or a relatively soft, short, and nonspecific murmur.[75]

## *Echocardiographic Features*

Despite the advent of higher resolution cardiac imaging modalities such as computed tomography and magnetic resonance imaging, emergent transthoracic echocardiography has remained the imaging modality of choice to identify acute mitral regurgitation in the setting of acute myocardial infarction. Transthoracic echocardiography is extremely helpful in evaluating the presence and severity of acute mitral regurgitation and can assess papillary muscle rupture with a diagnostic sensitivity of 65–85%. Due to the close proximity of the ultrasound transducer to the mitral apparatus, transesophageal echocardiography is often used to better elucidate the cause of MR and improves the diagnostic yield to between 95 and 100% (Figs. 20.17 and 20.18).[81–83]

Color flow imaging and continuous-wave Doppler ultrasound are crucial in assessing the various etiologies of acute mitral regurgitation. Color Doppler imaging is performed in several tomographic planes in order to construct a three-dimensional impression of the extent, shape, and direction of the regurgitant jet. An eccentric jet suggests pathologic regurgitation and provides clues about the mechanism of regurgitation. Abnormalities of the posterior leaflet tend to result in an anteriorly directed jet, while anterior leaflet or papillary muscle dysfunction tends to result in posteriorly directed jet. Both the anterior and posterior leaflets of the mitral valve

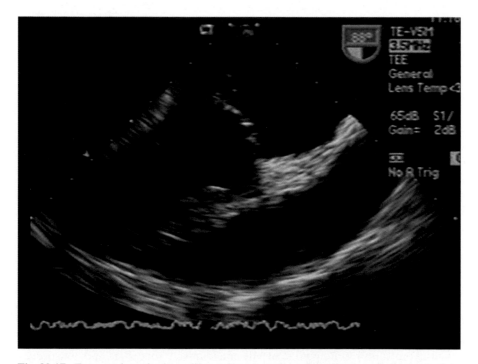

**Fig. 20.17** Transesophageal echocardiogram demonstrating a flail posterior mitral valve leaflet

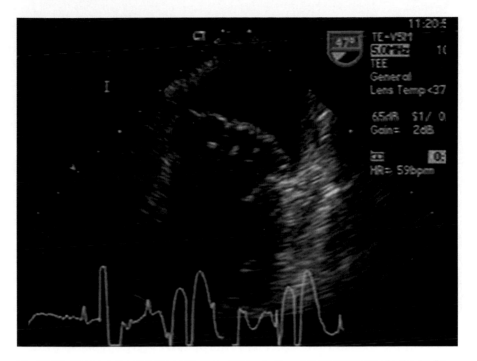

**Fig. 20.18** Transesophageal echocardiogram demonstrating a bilateral flail mitral valve leaflet

are attached to both papillary muscle heads. Thus, the direction and eccentricity of the mitral regurgitant jet on echocardiography helps to locate the leaflet involved, but not necessarily the coexisting papillary muscle pathology (Figs. 20.19 and 20.20),[52]

Often from a transthoracic window, the actual ruptured papillary muscle head cannot be directly visualized. However, detection of an eccentric mitral regurgitation jet with a relatively normal-sized left atrium is indirect evidence that a mechanical disruption has occurred. Partial rupture of a papillary muscle, defined as rupture of one of several "heads" or as partial disconnection of the base of the papillary muscle, is seen more often than complete rupture as these patients are more likely to survive long enough to undergo diagnostic evaluation. Classically, in this situation transthoracic echocardiography shows a thin, attenuated, excessively mobile papillary muscle.[1] If one head has ruptured, about 60–70% of the time a mass may be seen attached to the flail segment of the leaflet prolapsing into the left atrium in systole and the left ventricle in diastole.[84] Left ventricular function is usually hyperdynamic as a result of ventricular contraction against the low-impedance left atrium.[75] Again, if the entire papillary muscle is disconnected from the underlying left ventricular wall, few patients survive due to acute severe mitral regurgitation.

Dilatation of the left ventricle or mitral annulus may also result in significant mitral regurgitation usually as a central, symmetric jet. Thus in addition to anatomic

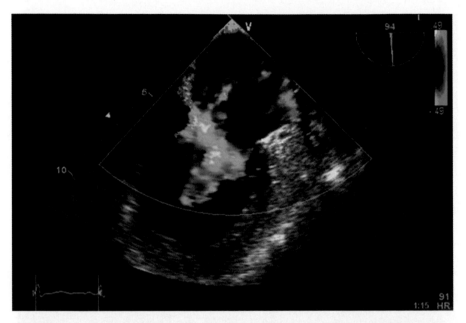

**Fig. 20.19** Transesophageal echocardiogram demonstrating severe mitral regurgitation represented by a posteriorly directed color flow Doppler jet due to a flail mitral valve leaflet

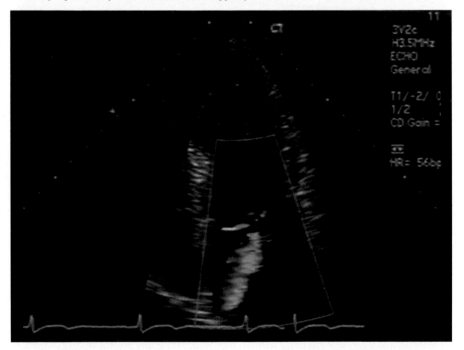

**Fig. 20.20** Transthoracic echocardiogram demonstrating severe mitral regurgitation due to a flail mitral valve

disruption of the mitral valve apparatus, mitral regurgitation can be the result of functional disturbances in mitral valve coaptation. Ischemic mitral regurgitation may be due to regional left ventricular dysfunction with abnormal contraction of the papillary muscle or underlying ventricular wall. In patients with a myocardial infarction, myocardial scarring results in mitral regurgitation at rest. In patients with normal resting myocardial function but inducible ischemia with stress, mitral regurgitation may be intermittent. Ischemic mitral regurgitation is characterized by restricted leaflet motion, with tethering of valve closure and interfering with normal valvular coaptation and giving an appearance of "tenting" of the mitral valve in systole.[1] Depending on the degree of displacement and which leaflet is involved, the mitral regurgitant jet is often central and symmetric or eccentric and ranges from mild to severe. In some cases it is difficult to determine if mitral regurgitation is the cause or consequence of ventricular dilatation and systolic dysfunction.

As mentioned, although transthoracic echocardiography may suffice to establish the diagnosis, transesophageal echocardiography is often necessary to confirm the precise anatomic defect. It is often necessary to fully exclude ventricular septal defect (VSD), especially in patients who may have had pre-existing mitral regurgitation. This distinction is important as both complications have similar clinical presentations and separate emergent surgical treatments. On occasion, one may image a patient with papillary muscle necrosis but without frank rupture. In these instances, one may note an abnormal shape of the papillary muscle. Three-dimensional echocardiography has shown tremendous promise for localization of the specific area of anatomic description.[52]

There are several pitfalls in echocardiography that can lead to over or underestimating MR. We would like to discuss some key confounding variables that should be considered to ensure the correct assessment of acute MR. It is important to adjust Doppler gains appropriately to avoid inappropriately low Nyquist limits. Incorrect settings of both these parameters can artifactually overstate the mitral regurgitant jet size. Of note, the jet size varies throughout systole and thus it is inaccurate to calculate MR in any one still frame. In general, the severity of mitral regurgitation is directly proportional to the area of the regurgitation jet in the left atrium. The assessment of severity can be further assessed by indexing the regurgitant jet area to left atrial size. Additionally, the width of the regurgitant jet at its origin, the vena contracta, can be measured from the color Doppler image and has been correlated with regurgitation severity as well.[52] It is important to note that color flow Doppler imaging of an eccentric layer along the left atrial wall will underestimate the regurgitation volume by approximately 40% when compared with an identical regurgitant volume that is centrally located.[76] However, Colombo et al. demonstrated that the sensitivity of assessing acute eccentric mitral regurgitation in the setting of acute myocardial infarction with TTE and TEE can improve by using color Doppler and calculating the angle of the proximal MR jet and the plane of the mitral annulus with an angle of $\leq 47°$ on TEE and $\leq 45°$ on TTE. The calculated sensitivity and specificity was 88% for flail mitral leaflet.[85]

An additional parameter called spectral density is directly proportional to the severity of the regurgitation.[76] In the presence of a flail leaflet, the mitral regurgitation spectral signal may have an atypical appearance. Depending on where the interrogation beam intersects the jet it can alter the density and velocity of the signal, resulting in a less than holosystolic jet. Also flail portions of the mitral apparatus that oscillate in the regurgitation flow stream can result in bright structures embedded in the regurgitant jet termed "tiger stripe". This atypical appearance of the spectral signal results from the oscillating tissue densities in the regurgitant jet. It is also associated with a "whistling" sound on the audible signal.[76]

With acute MR an increase in left atrial pressure during late systole may be present due to a steep pressure–volume relationship of the nondilated, noncompliant left atrium. In this situation, the pressure gradient between the left ventricle and the left atrium is high initially but then it equalizes in late systole as left atrial pressure rises. The corresponding Doppler velocity curve indicates a high initial velocity with a subsequent rapid fall in velocity in mid- to late systole. This pattern of Doppler velocities is termed a $v$ wave. Signal intensity of the mitral regurgitant signal in comparison with antegrade flow is related to mitral regurgitation severity. In addition, significant regurgitation is associated with an increase in the antegrade velocity due to increased transmitral volume flow. Pulmonary artery pressures also increase in the setting of acute mitral regurgitation. Thus it is prudent to derive pulmonary artery pressures from the tricuspid regurgitant jet velocity, estimated by right atrial pressure.

## Treatment

According to the 2004 American College of Cardiology/American Heart Association guidelines on ST-elevation MI and on coronary artery bypass surgery (CABG), treatment for any mechanical complication of acute MI including acute MR is emergent surgical correction of the mitral valve and CABG when indicated. Prompt diagnosis and initiation of medical therapy in the interval to emergent surgery are all important for a favorable outcome. Prompt diagnosis and aggressive medical therapy prior to surgery markedly improve patient outcomes. When considering hemodynamic compromise secondary to significant acute mitral regurgitation, aggressive medical resuscitation involves improving forward flow by afterload reduction and thus improving the regurgitant fraction. Afterload reduction is accomplished with the use of nitrates, sodium nitroprusside, diuretics, and intra-aortic balloon pump counterpulsation.

The operative mortality for these patients is an estimated 20–25% and heavily dependent on the timing of diagnosis and treatment. Despite such a high mortality, survival in patients restricted to medical therapy alone is significantly lower. Thus, emergent surgical intervention remains the treatment of choice for papillary muscle rupture.[86] Of note, mitral valve repair rather than replacement should be attempted in centers experienced in performing this procedure[75,80] and patients must meet the strict criteria for mitral valve repair which includes the preserved integrity of the mitral apparatus (i.e., intact papillary muscles and chordae). Interestingly, long-term results in one small study of 22 patients revealed a perioperative mortality of 27% and a 7-year survival for the survivors of surgery of 64% (the overall 7-year survival was 47%).[86] The only factor which improved both immediate and long-term survival was the concomitant performance of coronary artery bypass grafting.

## Conclusion

Acute mitral regurgitation is a serious and frequently fatal complication of acute myocardial infarction. It is important to recognize symptoms of cardiogenic shock in these patients and to have a high clinical suspicion for mechanical complications. The diagnosis should then be quickly confirmed with emergent echocardiography. This diagnostic tool can be used at the bedside to accelerate surgical intervention and thereby improve patient outcomes and survival from this deadly complication.

## Acute Mitral Regurgitation Case Presentation

A 68-year-old female with no significant past medical history presented to the hospital with a 2-day history of progressive substernal chest pressure, shortness of breath, and diaphoresis. She had never experienced such symptoms before. She did not take any regular medications other than a multivitamin and denied any past or present substance use.

Upon arrival to the emergency room the patient appeared in acute distress and was only able to respond in brief sentences. Her breathing was labored with a respiratory rate of 28 rpm and her ambient air oxygen saturation was 83% which normalized only with supplemental oxygen. She was tachycardic with a heart rate of 116 bpm and was hypotensive with a blood pressure of 82/50. Her jugular venous pressure was elevated to the angle of the jaw with a prominent v wave. Her initial cardiorespiratory examination was remarkable for an S3 with bilateral crackles.

A bedside electrocardiogram showed normal sinus rhythm at 110 bpm with 2 mm ST elevations in leads II, III, aVF, Q waves in leads II, III, aVF, and 2 mm ST depressions in leads I and aVL. The myocardial infarction team was activated and the patient was immediately transferred to the cardiac catheterization lab for emergent revascularization. Her chest X-ray demonstrated pulmonary vascular redistribution. The complete blood count, electrolytes, and liver function tests were within normal limits. The cardiac enzymes including troponin I and creatine kinase were elevated consistent with myocardial injury. The leading diagnosis at the time was acute inferior ST-elevation myocardial infarction.

After obtaining informed consent the patient underwent cardiac catheterization. The catheterization revealed a totally occluded mid-right coronary artery stenosis with no distal collaterals. A right coronary artery stent was successfully placed with resultant TIMI III flow. However, toward the end of the case, the patient decompensated further. She grew increasingly obtunded, hypoxic, and her systolic blood pressure fell to the mid-70s. At this point she was emergently intubated, an intra-aortic balloon pump was placed, and she was started on dopamine for pressure support. Due to her continued hemodynamic collapse despite revascularization, a stat transthoracic echo (TTE) was performed emergently. The TTE revealed an eccentric, anteriorly directed jet of severe mitral regurgitation with a presumed diagnosis of a ruptured posteromedial papillary muscle attached to the flail posterior mitral valve leaflet. The cardiothoracic surgery team was alerted of the patient's clinical status and she was taken to the OR. Intraoperative transesophageal echocardiography (TEE) confirmed the TTE diagnosis of posteromedial papillary muscle rupture with resultant acute and severe eccentric mitral regurgitation.

During cardiopulmonary bypass, one head of the posterior papillary muscle was ruptured and attached via chordae to the flail posterior mitral leaflet. A mechanical mitral valve was implanted without complication. The patient postoperatively did well and was discharged from the hospital on the fifth postoperative day.

# References

1. Otto C. The practice of clinical echocardiography. *Chapter 12: Echocardiography in the Coronary Care Unit*. Philadelphia, PA: WB Saunders Co.; 2002.
2. Purcaro A, Costantini C, Ciampani N, et al. Diagnostic criteria and management of subacute ventricular free wall rupture complicating acute myocardial infarction. *Am J Cardiol*. 1997;80:397.
3. Batts KP, Ackerman DM, Edwards WD. Postinfarction rupture of the left ventricular free wall: clinicopathologic correlates in 100 consecutive autopsy cases. *Hum Pathol*. 1990;21:530.
4. Reeder GS. Identification and treatment of complications of myocardial infarction. *Mayo Clin Proc*. 1995;70:880.
5. Pohjola-Sintonen S, Muller JE, Stone PH, et al. Ventricular septal and free wall rupture complicating acute myocardial infarction: experience in the Multicenter Investigation of Limitation of Infarct Size. *Am Heart J*. 1989;117:809.
6. Becker RC, Gore JM, Lambrew C, et al. for the National Registry of Myocardial Infarction Participants. A composite view of cardiac rupture in the United States National Registry of Myocardial Infarction. *J Am Coll Cardiol*. 1996;27:1321.
7. Patel MR, Meine TJ, Lindblad L, et al. Cardiac tamponade in the fibrinolytic era: analysis of >100,000 patients with ST-segment elevation myocardial infarction. *Am Heart J*. 2006;151:316.
8. Becker RC, Hochman JS, Cannon CP, et al., for the TIMI 9 Investigators. Fatal cardiac rupture among patients treated with thrombolytic agents and adjunctive thrombin antagonists. Observations from the Thrombolysis and Thrombin Inhibition in Myocardial Infarction 9 study. *J Am Coll Cardiol*. 1999;33:479.
9. Moreno R, Lopez-Sendon J, Garcia E, et al. Primary angioplasty reduces the risk of left ventricular free wall rupture compared with thrombolysis in patients with acute myocardial infarction. *J Am Coll Cardiol*. 2002;39:598.
10. Pasternak RC, Braunwald E, Sobel BE. Acute myocardial infarction. In: Braunwald EB, ed. *Heart Disease*. 4th ed. Philadelphia, PA: Saunders; 1992:200.
11. Mechanisms for the early mortality reduction produced by beta-blockade started early in acute myocardial infarction: ISIS-1. ISIS-1 (First International Study of Infarct Survival) Collaborative Group. *Lancet*. 1988;1:921.
12. Batts KP, Ackerman DM, Edwards WD. Postinfarction rupture of the left ventricular free wall: clinicopathologic correlates in 100 consecutive autopsy cases. *Hum Pathol*. 1990;21:530.

13. Nakatsuchi Y, Minamino T, Fujii K, Negoro S. Clinicopathologic characterization of cardiac free wall rupture in patients with acute myocardial infarction: difference between early and late phase rupture. Int J Cardiol. 1994;47:S33.

14. Cheriex EC, de Swart H, Dijkman LW, et al. Myocardial rupture after myocardial infarction is related to the perfusion status of the infarct-related coronary artery. Am Heart J. 1995;129:644.

15. Honan MB, Harrell FE Jr, Reimer KA, et al. Cardiac rupture, mortality and the timing of thrombolytic therapy: a meta-analysis. J Am Coll Cardiol. 1990;16:359.

16. Gertz SD, Kragel AH, Kalan JM, et al. Comparison of coronary and myocardial morphologic findings in patients with and without thrombolytic therapy during fatal first acute myocardial infarction. The TIMI Investigators. Am J Cardiol. 1990;66:904.

17. Becker RC, Charlesworth A, Wilcox RG, et al. Cardiac rupture associated with thrombolytic therapy: impact of time to treatment in the late assessment of thrombolytic efficacy (LATE) study. J Am Coll Cardiol. 1995;25:1063.

18. Bueno H, Martinez-Selles M, Perez-David E, Lopez-Palop R. Effect of thrombolytic therapy on the risk of cardiac rupture and mortality in older patients with first acute myocardial infarction. Eur Heart J. 2005;26:1705.

19. Nakatani D, Sato H, Kinjo K, et al. Effect of successful late reperfusion by primary coronary angioplasty on mechanical complications of acute myocardial infarction. Am J Cardiol. 2003;92:785.

20. McMullan MH, Maples MD, Kilgore TL Jr, Hindman SH. Surgical experience with left ventricular free wall rupture. Ann Thorac Surg. 2001;71:1894.

21. Lopez-Sendon J, Gonzalez A, Lopez de Sa E, et al. Diagnosis of subacute ventricular wall rupture after acute myocardial infarction: sensitivity and specificity of clinical, hemodynamic and echocardiographic criteria. J Am Coll Cardiol. 1992;19:1145–1153.

22. Feigenbaum H, Armstrong W, Ryan T. Feigenbaum's Echocardiography. Chapter 15: Coronary Artery Disease. 6th ed. Philadelphia, PA: Lippincott Williams and Wilkins; 2005.

23. Topaz O, Taylor AL. Interventricular septal rupture complicating acute myocardial infarction: from pathophysiologic features to the role of invasive and noninvasive diagnostic modalities in current management. Am J Med. 1992;93:683–688.

24. Crenshaw BS, Granger CB, Birnbaum Y, et al. Risk factors, angiographic patterns, and outcomes in patients with ventricular septal defect complicating acute myocardial infarction. Circulation. 2000;101:27–32.

25. Birnbaum Y, Fishbein MC, Blanche C, Siegel RJ. Ventricular septal rupture after acute myocardial infarction. N Engl J Med. 2002;347(18):1426–1432.

26. Davis N, Sistino JJ. Review of ventricular rupture: key concepts and diagnostic tools for success. Perfusion. 2002;17:63–67.

27. Buda AJ. The role of echocardiography in the evaluation of mechanical complications of acute myocardial infarction. Circulation. 1991;84(3 suppl):109–121.

28. Edwards BS, Edwards WD, Edwards JE. Ventricular septal rupture complicating acute myocardial infarction: identification of simple and complex types in 53 autopsied hearts. Am J Cardiol. 1984;54:1201–1205.

29. Cheriex EC, de Swart H, Dijkman LW, et al. Myocardial rupture after myocardial infarction is related to the perfusion status of the infarct-related artery. Am Heart J. 1995;129:644–650.

30. Sager RV. Coronary thrombosis; perforation of the infracted interventricular septum. Arch Intern Med. 1934;53:140–148.

31. Fortin DF, Sheikh KH, Kisslo J. The utility of echocardiography in the diagnostic strategy of postinfarction ventricular septal rupture: a comparison of two-dimensional echocardiography versus Doppler color flow imaging. Am Heart J. 1991;121:25–32.

32. Helmcke F, Mahan EF, Nanda NC, et al. Two-dimensional echocardiographic and Doppler color flow mapping in the diagnosis and prognosis of ventricular septal rupture. Circulation. 1990;81(6):1775–1783.

33. Giuliani ER, Danielson GK, Pluth JR, Odyniec NA, Wallace RB. Postinfarction ventricular septal rupture: surgical considerations and results. Circulation. 1974;49:455–459.

34. GUSTO Investigators. An international randomized trial comparing four thrombolytic strategies for acute myocardial infarction. *N Engl J Med.* 1993;329:1615–1622.
35. Hochman JS, Sleeper LA, Webb JG, et al. Early revascularization in acute myocardial infarction complicated by cardiogenic shock. *N Engl J Med.* 1999;341:625–634.
36. Menon V, Webb JG, Hillis LD, et al. Outcome and profile of ventricular septal rupture with cardiogenic shock after myocardial infarction: a report from the SHOCK Trial Registry. *J Am Coll Cardiol.* 2000;36(suppl A):1110–1116.
37. Hochman JS, Jacobs ML, Sleeper LA, et al. Cardiogenic shock complicating acute myocardial infarction – etiologies, management and outcome: a report from the SHOCK Trial Registry. *J Am Coll Cardiol.* 2000;36(suppl A):1063–1070.
38. Little WC, Freeman GL. Pericardial disease. *Circulation.* 2006;113:1622–1632.
39. Maisch E, Seferovic PM, Ristic AD, et al. for the Task Force on the Diagnosis and Management of Pericardial Diseases of the European Society of Cardiology. Guidelines on the diagnosis and management of pericardial diseases: executive summary. *Eur Heart J.* 2004;25:587–610.
40. Hoit BD. Pericardial disease and pericardial tamponade. *Crit Care Med.* 2007;35(8 suppl):S355–S364.
41. Shabetai R. The pericardium: an essay on some recent developments. *Am J Cardiol.* 1978;263:H1657–H1681.
42. Miyazaki T, Pride HP, Zipes DP. Prostaglandins in the pericardial fluid modulate neural regulation of cardiac electrophysiological properties. *Circulation Res.* 1990;66:163–175.
43. LeWinter MM, Kabbani S. Pericardial diseases. In: Zipes DP, Libby P, Monow RO, Braunwald E, eds. *Braunwald's Heart Disease.* 7th ed. Philadelphia, PA: Elsevier Saunders; 2005:1757–1780.
44. Maisch B. Pericardial diseases, with a focus on etiology, pathogenesis, pathophysiology, new diagnostic imaging methods, and treatment. *Curr Opin Cardiol.* 1994;9:379–388.
45. Weitzman LB, Tinker WP, Kronzon I, et al. The incidence and natural history of pericardial effusion after cardiac surgery: an echocardiographic study. *Circulation.* 1984;69:506–511.
46. Spodick DH. Acute cardiac tamponade. *N Engl J Med.* 2003;349(7):684–690.
47. Roy LR, Minor MA, Brookhart MA, Choudhry NK. Does this patient with a pericardial effusion have cardiac tamponade? *J Am Med Assoc.* 2007;297(16):1810–1818.
48. Beck C. Two cardiac compression triads. *J Am Med Assoc.* 1935;104:714–716.
49. Kussmaul A. Uber schwielige Mediastinoperikarditis und den paradoxen. *Puls Berl Klin Wochenschr.* 1873;10:433–435.
50. Curtiss El, Reddy PS, Uretsky BF, Cecchetti AA. Pulsus paradoxus: definition and relation to the severity of cardiac tamponade. *Am Heart J.* 1988;115:391–398.
51. Knopf WD, Talley JD, Murphy DA. An echo-dense mass in the pericardial space as a sign of left ventricular free wall rupture during acute myocardial infarction. *Am J Cardiol.* 1987;59:1202.
52. Faigenbaum H, Armsrtong WF, Ryan T. *Pericardial Diseases in Faigenbaum's Echocardiography.* 6th ed. Philadelphia, PA: Lippincott Willams and Wilkins; 2005:247–270.
53. Tsang TS, Enriquez-Sarano M, Freeman WK, et al. Consecutive 1127 therapeutic echocardiographically guided pericardiocenteses: clinical profile, practice patterns, and outcomes spanning 21 years. *Mayo Clin Proc.* 2002;77:429–436.
54. Tsang TS, Barnes ME, Hayes SN, et al. Clinical and echocardiographic characteristics of significant pericardial effusions following cardiothoracic surgery and outcomes of echo-guided pericardiocentesis for management. *Mayo Clin Exp.* 1979–1988. *Chest.* 1999;116:322–331.
55. Kinch JW, Ryan TJ. Right ventricular infarction. *N Engl J Med.* 1994;330:1211–1219.
56. Haji SA, Movahed A. Right ventricular infarction – diagnosis and treatment. *Clin Cardiol.* 2000;23:473–482.
57. Lee FA. Hemodynamics of the right ventricle in normal and disease states. *Clin Cardiol.* 1992;10:59–67.

58. Anderson HR, Falk E, Nielsen D. Right ventricular infarction: frequency, size and topography in coronary heart disease: a prospective study comprising 107 consecutive autopsies from a coronary care unit. *J Am Coll Cardiol*. 1987;10:1223–1232.

59. Horan LG, Flowers NC. Right ventricular infarction: specific requirements of management. *Am Fam Physician*. 1999;60(6):1727–1734.

60. Goldstein JA, Barzilai B, Rosamond TL, Eisenberg PR, Jaffe AS. Determinants of hemodynamic compromise with severe right ventricular infarction. *Circulation*. 1990;82:359–368.

61. Dell'Italia LJ, Starling MR, O'Rourke RA. Physical examination for exclusion of hemodynamically important right ventricular infarction. *Ann Intern Med*. 1983;99:608–611.

62. Cintron GB, Hernandez E, Linares E, Aranda JM. Bedside recognition, incidence and clinical course of right ventricular infarction. *Am J Cardiol*. 1981;47:224–227.

63. Zehender M, Kasper W, Kauder E, et al. Right ventricular infarction as an independent predictor of prognosis after acute inferior myocardial infarction. *N Engl J Med*. 1993;328: 981–988.

64. Bellamy GR, Rasmussen HH, Nasser FN, Wiseman JC, Cooper RA. Value of two-dimensional echocardiography, electrocardiography, and clinical signs in detecting right ventricular infarction. *Am Heart J*. 1986;112:304–309.

65. Moller JE, Sondergaard E, Poulsen SH, et al. Serial Doppler echocardiographic assessment of left and right ventricular performance after a first myocardial infarction. *J Am Soc Echocardiogr*. 2001;14:249–255.

66. Cohen A, Logeart D, Costagliola D, et al. Usefulness of pulmonary regurgitation Doppler tracings in predicting in-hospital and long term outcome in patients with inferior wall acute myocardial infarction. *Am J Cardiol*. 1998;81:276–281.

67. Braat SH, deZwann C, Brugada P, Coenegracht JM, Wellens HJJ. Right ventricular involvement with acute inferior wall myocardial infarction identifies high risk of developing atrioventricular nodal conduction disturbances. *Am Heart J*. 1984;107:1183–1187.

68. Love JC, Haffajee CI, Gore JM, Alpert JS. Reversibility of hypotension and shock by atrial or atrioventricular sequential pacing in patients with right ventricular infarction. *Am Heart J*. 1984;108:5–13.

69. Berger PB, Ruocco NA Jr, Ryan TJ, et al. Frequency and significance of right ventricular dysfunction during inferior wall left ventricular myocardial infarction treated with thrombolytic therapy (results from the Thrombolysis in Myocardial Infarction. [TIMI] II trial. *Am J Cardiol*. 1993;71:1148–1152.

70. Moreyra AE, Suh C, Porway MN, Costis JB. Rapid hemodynamic improvement in right ventricular infarction after coronary angioplasty. *Chest*. 1988;94:197–199.

71. Bowers TR, O'Neil WW, Grines C, Pica MC, Safian RD, Goldstein JA. Effect of reperfusion on biventricular function and survival after right ventricular infarction. *N Engl J Med*. 1998;338:933–942.

72. Hochman JS, Sleeper LA, Webb JG, et al. Early revascularization in acute myocardial infarction complicated by cardiogenic shock. *N Engl J Med*. 1999;341:625–634.

73. Jacobs AK, Leopold JA, Bates E, et al. Cardiogenic shock caused by right ventricular infarction: a report from the SHOCK registry. *J Am Coll Cardiol*. 2003;41:1273–1279.

74. Tcheng JE, Jackman JD, Nelson CL, et al. Outcome of patients sustaining acute ischemic mitral regurgitation during myocardial infarction. *Ann Intern Med*. 1992;117:18.

75. Lavie CJ, Gersh BJ. Mechanical and electrical complications of acute myocardial infarction. *Mayo Clin Proc*. 1990;65:709.

76. Feigenbaum H, Armstrong W, Ryan T. *Feigenbaum's Echocardiography*. Chapter 11: Mitral Valve Disease. 6th ed. Philadelphia, PA: Lippincott Williams and Wilkins; 2005.

77. Reeder GS. Identification and treatment of complications of myocardial infarction. *Mayo Clin Proc*. 1995;70:880.

78. Hochman JS, Jacobs ML, Sleeper LA, et al. Cardiogenic shock complicating acute myocardial infarction – etiologies, management and outcome: a report from the SHOCK Trial Registry. *J Am Coll Cardiol*. 2000;36(suppl A):1063–1070.

79. Picard MH, Davidoff R, Sleeper LA, et al. Echocardiographic predictors of survival and response to early revascularization in cardiogenic shock. *Circulation*. 2003;107:279.
80. David TE. Techniques and results of mitral valve repair for ischemic mitral regurgitation. *J Card Surg*. 1994;9:274.
81. Himmelman RB, Kusumoto F, Oken K, et al. The flail mitral valve: echocardiographic findings by precordial and trans-esophageal imaging and Doppler color flow mapping. *J Am Coll Cardiol*. 1991;17:272–279.
82. Enriquez-Sarano M, Freeman WK, Tribouilloy CM, et al. Functional anatomy of mitral regurgitation: accuracy and outcome implication of transesophageal echocardiography. *J Am Coll Cardiol*. 1999;34:129–1136.
83. Sochowski RA, Chan KL, Ascah KJ, Bedard P. Comparison of accuracy of transesophageal versus transthoracic echocardiography for the detection of mitral valve prolapse with ruptured chordae tendinae (flail mitral leaflet). *Am J Cardiol*. 1991;67:1251–1255.
84. Moursi MH, Bhatnagar SK, Vilacosta I, et al. Transesophageal echocardiographic assessment of papillary muscle rupture. *Circulation*. 1996;94:1003.
85. Colombo PC, Wu RH, Weiner S, et al. Value of quantitative analysis of mitral regurgitation jet eccentricity by color flow Doppler for identification of flail leaflet. *Am J Cardiol*. 2001;88:534–540.
86. Kishon Y, Oh JK, Schaff HV, et al. Mitral valve operation in postinfarction rupture of a papillary muscle: immediate results and long-term follow-up of 22 patients. *Mayo Clin Proc*. 1992;67:1023.

# Chapter 21
# Chronic Complications of Acute Myocardial Infarction

Sandeep Joshi, Gregory Janis, and Eyal Herzog

Acute myocardial infarction (AMI) affects 1.7 million individuals within the United States annually and is an inevitable fatal in 25% of these patients and thus is one of the leading causes of sudden cardiac death (SCD). Among those who survive the immediate effects of an AMI, long-term complications can occur following the event, which may manifest within the acute-phase period or weeks following the infarction. These entities can be readily diagnosed via echocardiography, the gold standard, for imaging cardiac structures. Acute complications have been discussed in a previous chapter. This chapter will discuss the chronic complications of an AMI, which include ventricular aneurysm, ventricular pseudoaneurysm, left ventricular thrombus formation, and infarct expansion/cardiac remodeling.

## Ventricular Aneurysm

Left ventricular aneurysm (LVA) is a common mechanical complication follow ing an AMI, occurring between 10 and 15% of patients. Prior to the era of current management strategies such as thrombolytic therapy, percutaneous coronary intervention, and the administration of afterload-reducing agents, the incidence was approaching 40%.[1,2] An analysis of 350 patients has shown that the incidence of LVA among 350 consecutive patients with ST segment AMI, treated with thrombolytic therapy, was significantly lower in those with a patent infarct-related artery (7.2% vs. 18.8%).[3]

It has been described as a well delineated and distinct break ("hinge point") in the LV geometry and contour present in both systole and diastole. The walls consist of thin, scarred, or fibrotic myocardium, completely devoid of muscle, a resultant of a healed transmural AMI. The pathogmonic features include a wide mouth that enables communication with the aneurysmal cavity. Often this is evident

S. Joshi (✉)

Cardiology, St Luke's Roosevelt Hospital Center, 1111 Amsterdam Ave, New York, NY, USA

e-mail: sjoshi@chpnet.org

E. Herzog, F.A. Chaudhry (eds.), *Echocardiography in Acute Coronary Syndrome*, 319
DOI 10.1007/978-1-84882-027-2_21, © Springer-Verlag London Limited 2009

at 4–6 weeks following an AMI. The involved wall segment is either akinetic or dyskinetic during systole and collapses inward when the ventricle is fully vented during surgery. LVA of the apex and the anterior wall are approximately four times more common than those of the inferior or the inferoposterior walls (Figs. 21.1 and 21.2).

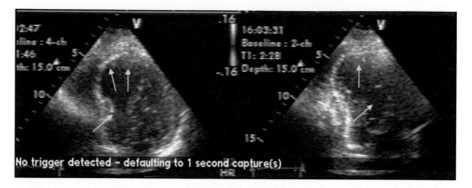

**Fig. 21.1** Apical four-chamber view (*left*) and two-chamber (*right*) views obtained during stress echocardiography depicting a large apical AMI with a large aneurysm (*arrows*). Notice the distinct break in wall thickness and function (*arrows*)

Approximately 70–85% of LVAs are located in the anterior or apical walls due, in most cases, to complete occlusion of the left anterior descending (LAD) coronary artery and the absence of collateralization. However, 10–15% of cases involve the inferior-basal walls due to right coronary artery occlusion. A rare finding is a lateral LVA, which is the result of an occluded left circumflex coronary artery. Among patients with multivessel disease, LVA is uncommon if there is extensive collateralization or a nonoccluded left anterior descending artery.

Although the size of an aneurysm varies widely, most are within 1–8 cm in diameter. The wall of the aneurysm typically consists of a hybrid of necrotic myocardium and white fibrous scar tissue. This wall is extremely thin and delicate and may calcify over an extended period of time. Of note, it is imperative to distinguish between an LVA and a pseudoaneurysm, which is characterized by a narrow neck and a distinct "shelf-like" opening.

The endocardial surface is smooth and nontrabeculated. The aneurysm is filled with organized thrombus in more than 50% of cases, which has the tendency to calcify over time.[4] Dense adhesions between the aneurysm and the overlying pericardium are common phenomena. On a molecular level, initially, the ventricular wall is characterized by myocardial muscle necrosis and a concomitant intense inflammatory reaction, which eventually is replaced with scar tissue formation, and a mature aneurysm consists mostly of hyalinized fibrous tissue. The "border zone", i.e., the layer between the aneurysm and the healthy myocardium, is characterized by patchy fibrosis and abnormal alignment of the muscle fibers.

**Fig. 21.2** ( *Top*) Apical three-chamber view obtained from transthoracic echocardiogram revealing a large left ventricular aneurysm enhanced with color flow Doppler (*bottom*) establishing an area of communication between the normal left ventricle and the aneurysmal portion

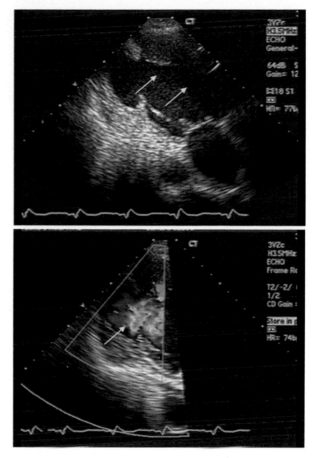

## *Diagnosis*

A prior history of AMI is almost universally present in patients with an LVA that is not associated with other etiologies such as hypertrophic cardiomyopathy or Chagas disease. The physical examination may reveal one or more of the following findings:

- Cardiac enlargement with a diffuse apical impulse located to the left of the midclavicular line.
- An area of dyskinesis can occasionally be appreciated with palpation of the apex or the left lateral chest wall, in the area of the anterior wall of the LV.
- A third and/or fourth heart sound (S3 or S4) is often heard, which heralds the onset of coronary blood flow into a dilated and stiffened LV chamber.

- A mitral regurgitation like systolic murmur may be appreciated due to the distortion of LV geometry that results in the absence of leaflet apposition, papillary muscle dysfunction, and/or annular dilatation.

The electrocardiogram (ECG) usually reveals evidence of a large AMI and there may be persistent ST segment elevation; however, this finding is usually the result of a large area of scar and does not necessarily imply an aneurysm.

Although limited and rarely used today, chest radiography may aid in the diagnosis of an LVA; however, given the extreme limitations of chest radiography, the diagnosis is definitively made via two-dimensional echocardiography. A simple definition of an LVA on echocardiography imaging is the presence of a dyskinetic wall motion abnormality with the feature of diastolic deformity.[5,6] Transthoracic echocardiography (TTE) is most often used and has globally emerged as the diagnostic tool of choice. The benefits of echocardiography over other imaging modalities include its relatively noninvasiveness, simplicity, the ability to perform at the bedside, and the ability to yield immediate results when interpreted by an experienced physician.

Radionuclide ventriculography or contrast ventriculography at the time of cardiac catheterization are alternatives; however, they are rarely used. Three-dimensional echocardiography and cardiac magnetic resonance imaging (MRI) are newer modalities that are increasingly used for diagnosis, measurement of left ventricular volume, and for postoperative follow-up. These modalities are also useful to distinguish between a true and pseudoaneurysm.[7] MRI can be useful to assess myocardial viability particularly in patients with akinetic segments; however, data are more limited on the use of cardiovascular MRI. Given the limitations of MRI imaging, such as excluding patients with pacemakers, intracardiac defibrillators, or prosthetic joints, echocardiography remains the test of choice for diagnosis.

## Complications

There are a number of serious complications that can result from an LVA.

A. *Heart Failure and Angina:* During ventricular systole, the paradoxical bulging of the aneurysmal segment results in "stealing" part of the LV stroke volume, resulting in decreasing cardiac output and predisposing to LV volume overload. As the LV dilates, the wall stiffens and LV end-diastolic pressure rises. As per Laplace's law, a consequential increase in wall tension and LV cavity enlargement occurs. This increase yields a greater degree of circumferential wall stress and therefore increased oxygen demand. In the setting of underlying coronary artery disease, the increase in oxygen demand may lead to relative or absolute myocardial ischemia with subsequent angina. The end-result of long-standing volume overload and prolonged ischemia is a globally dilated, failing left ventricle.

B. *Ventricular Arrhythmias:* Ventricular arrhythmias, a substrate for SCD, are common in patients with an LVA. Two principal mechanisms appear to be contributing the following:

1. Myocardial ischemia and increased myocardial stretch can lead to enhanced cardiac automaticity.
2. The myocardium located at the border zone is made up of a mix of fibrotic tissue, inflammatory cells, and damaged muscle fibers, which is a suitable substrate for a reentrant tachycardia as it may develop when two or more electrically heterogeneous pathways having different conduction velocities and refractoriness are connected proximally and distally.

C. *Systemic Embolization:* As previously mentioned, a mural thrombus is identified in autopsy or surgery in >50% of patients with LVA. Furthermore, two factors play a pivotal role in clot formation in this setting. The first is stasis of flow in the aneurysm cavity and the second is direct contact of blood with potentially procoagulant fibrous tissue in an LVA rather than normal endocardium. A possible fatal consequence of thrombus formation is systemic embolization.

D. *Ventricular Rupture:* LVAs may enlarge over time. However, unlike false aneurysms, a true LVA rarely ruptures because of the dense fibrosis that comprises the walls.[8,9]

## *Natural History*

The natural history of patients with LVA continues to remain ambiguous. Very early data suggest that among patients with pathologically proven LVA, the 3- and 5-year survival rates were 27% and 12%.[9]

In contrast, the 5-year survival in the subset of patients with LVA from the Coronary Artery Surgery Study (CASS) was much better at 71%.[10] These differing views are emblematic of differences in several major variables such as the size and magnitude of the aneurysm, whether the aneurysmal segment is dyskinetic or akinetic, the extent of coronary disease (single vs. multivessel), and the function of the nonaneurysmal part of the LV. An important caveat that lies herein is that much of the data presented are based on treatment strategies prior to the institution of current medical therapies with the widespread use of primary percutaneous coronary intervention or thrombolytic therapy. Therefore, the use of these as absolute markers against which surgical results should be compared is limited.

## *Treatment*

### Medical Therapy

Mild-to-moderate size asymptomatic aneurysms can be safely treated medically with an anticipated 5-year survival of up to 90%. Therapy is aimed at reduction of afterload of the LV enlargement via angiotensin-converting enzyme inhibitors, nitrates, and anticoagulation in the setting of significant LV dysfunction or evidence of thrombus within the aneurysm or LV. The optimal approach to the patient with a large, asymptomatic LVA remains a clinical dilemma. Concomitant repair of the aneurysm has been advocated when coronary artery bypass surgery (CABG) or valve surgery is performed. In the absence of such indications for surgery, these patients should otherwise be treated with the same regimen as those with a small LVA; they should also be followed closely for progressive left ventricular dilation. Similar to other settings of chronic volume overload, a progressive increase in LV diameter and/or decrease in LV ejection fraction are a clear indication for surgery even prior to the presence of advanced heart failure or other symptoms.

## Indications for Surgical Repair

As per the 2004 American College of Cardiology/American Heart Association (ACC/AHA) guidelines on ST elevation MI, aneurysmectomy, accompanied by CABG, in patients with an LVA who have repetitive ventricular arrhythmias and/or heart failure unresponsive to medical and catheter-based therapy[11] is a Class Ia recommendation and is therefore reasonable. Surgical repair should be considered for symptomatic patients with either akinetic or dyskinetic segments, as they represent variants in the spectrum of the same disease. Surgical repair of an LVA is very effective and results in a significant improvement in patient survival, symptoms, and functional class compared to medical treatment.[12,13,14]Furthermore, a marked decrease in surgical mortality has been achieved in the past 25 years, resulting in an expansion of indications for surgery.

Endocardial mapping with subsequent endocardial resection and possible cryoablation are performed in patients with malignant ventricular arrhythmias. Nonguided endocardectomy also may be an effective approach. In a review of 106 patients with LVA and spontaneous or inducible ventricular tachycardia (VT) who underwent this procedure, no patient had spontaneous VT at late follow-up and only 11% had inducible VT.[15]

## Ventricular Pseudoaneurysm

A left ventricular pseudoaneurysm (LVPA) or false aneurysm forms when cardiac rupture is more or less contained by adherent pericardium or scar tissue. Unlike a true aneurysm, an LVPA is devoid of endocardium or myocardium and since these aneurysms are prone to rupture, a quick and accurate diagnosis is of extreme importance. Unlike a true LVA whereby the walls consist of dense fibrous tissue with excellent tensile strength, the wall of an LVPA is comprised of thrombus, varying portions of the epicardium, and parietal pericardium. It is the result of an AMI with myocardial rupture and hemorrhage into the pericardial space, becoming progressively compressive. Cardiac tamponade occurs, thereby preventing further hemorrhage into the pericardium. Over time, thrombus organizes, with overall poor structural integrity, and is thus prone to inevitable rupture, a fatal and catastrophic event.[16]

## Etiology

Majority of cases of an LVPA are products of an AMI, particularly of the inferior wall, which was twice as common as the anterior wall. There are some cases that are the complications from surgery, such as mitral valve replacement and aneurysmectomy itself. Trauma accounted for a small percentage as well.

The site of an LVPA varies with the underlying etiology. Data suggest that LVPAs are primarily noted in the inferior or the posterolateral wall following an AMI, which is consistent with inferior infarction, in the right ventricular outflow tract after congenital heart surgery, in the posterior subannular region of the mitral valve after mitral valve replacement, and in the subaortic region after aortic valve replacement.[17]

## Clinical Presentation

It has been suggested that the most frequent symptoms associated with LVPA include chest pain and dyspnea. However, often symptoms can be somewhat vague and nonspecific. The other symptomatology includes that of tamponade, heart failure, syncope, arrhythmia, or systemic embolism. Cardiac murmurs are present in about two-thirds of patients. The murmur is often indistinguishable from that of mitral regurgitation. Almost all patients have some degree of underlying ECG changes, which include ST segment elevation and nonspecific T wave changes. Evidence of a mass on chest x-ray is seen in more than one-half of patients; however, as previously mentioned, this is not specific or sensitive for the diagnosis of an LVPA.[17]

## Diagnosis

The most reliable method for diagnosis of an LVPA is via echocardiography. A transthoracic echocardiogram (TTE) is a reasonable first step, but a definitive diagnosis is made in only a fraction of patients. Echocardiography can usually distinguish a pseudoaneurysm from a true aneurysm by the appearance of the connection between the aneurysm and the ventricular cavity. Small discrete ruptures of the ventricular wall are compatible with survival. Thus, as a result, LVPA have a narrow neck, typically less than 40% of the maximal aneurysm diameter, which causes an abrupt interruption in the ventricular wall contour (Figs. 21.3 and 21.4). In contrast, true aneurysms are nearly as wide at the neck as they are at the apex.

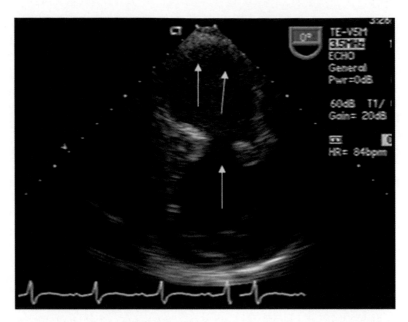

**Fig. 21.3** Short-axis view of the left ventricle (*lower cavity*) during transesophogeal echocardiography. Large pseudoaneurysm (*top cavity*) noted in a 65-year-old female 2 months following an AMI. Notice the narrow "bottleneck" opening (*arrows*)

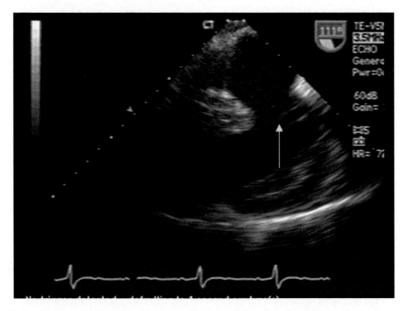

**Fig. 21.4** Short-axis view from transesophogeal echocardiogram depicting a large pseudoaneurysm. Notice the narrow "shelf-like" opening into the aneurysmal cavity

Interestingly, the LVPA is comprised of aneurysmal cavity and organizing hematoma; the true sized is often underrepresented on echocardiography since a hematoma has a similar appearance to many soft tissue densities like surrounding structures. Therefore, it is not uncommon to notice a large pericardial mass on computed tomography or on a chest x-ray. This makes it difficult to ascertain the ratio of the size of the opening to the LV cavity to the actual aneurysmal size since the blood-filled aspect can be visualized. Cardiovascular MRI is an alternative to angiography or echocardiography that may be useful in order to distinguish a pseudoaneurysm from a true aneurysm. However given the extreme limitations of MRI, it is rarely used, as in the case with LVA which was discussed earlier in this chapter.

## Treatment

Untreated LVPA has a 30–45% risk of rupture and, with medical therapy, a mortality of almost 50%. Thus, surgery is the preferred therapeutic option. With current techniques, the perioperative mortality is less than 10%, although the risk is greater among patients with severe mitral regurgitation requiring concomitant mitral valve replacement.[18]

## Left Ventricular Thrombus

A mural LV thrombus is a frequent sequelae of an AMI and most commonly develops in the presence of a large infarction. Its formation is prone to originate in regions of stasis. It is most commonly noted to occur in the apex of the left ventricle but may also occur in the lateral and inferior aneurysms. Prior to conventional medical therapy such as thrombolytics, the incidence was between 25 and 40%[19] and has since decreased substantially. The major risk of a thrombus is subsequent embolization, which is highest during the first 2 weeks following an AMI with eventual reduction of risk by 6–8 weeks. This is attributed to a relative endothelialization of the thrombus with reduction in its embolic potential. Echocardiography has high sensitivity (95%) and high specificity (85%) for identification of a left ventricular thrombus and has emerged as the diagnostic modality of choice. Certain echocardiographic features are important for diagnosis. These include size, the character of the thrombus, i.e., whether it is a laminar type, which has the formation of a layer against the akinetic wall, or whether it is pedunculated or protruding, an entity that is prone to embolize. Fresh thrombi have a cystic appearance secondary to a combination of thrombus maturity and display acoustic boundaries between fresh and organized regions. These may also often have a distinct echolucency within the center. Furthermore, when using new generation high-frequency transducers, spontaneous contrast is noted in the LV cavity, which is seen in the area of a wall motion abnormality. This is most likely a product of stagnant blood in the region of aneursymal dila-

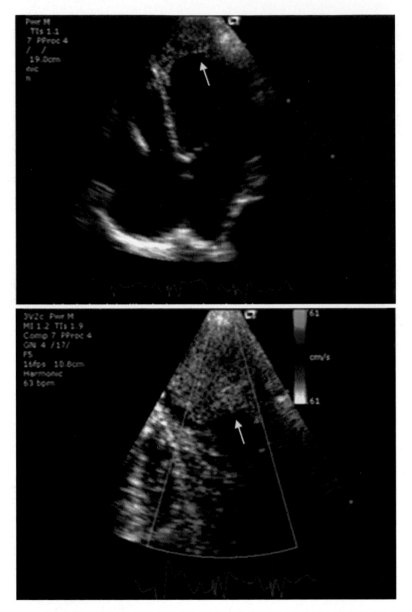

**Fig. 21.5** Apical four-chamber transthoracic view and two-chamber view (*bottom*) from a 74-year-old patient 3 months following AMI. Notice the large protruding apical thrombus (*arrow*). Color flow imaging may be used to demonstrate abnormal swirling patterns of blood

tion. Also, abnormal swirling patterns of blood may be observed via color flow imaging at low velocities. In addition, the use of intravenous contrast agents that are perfluorocarbon-based, passing into the LV cavity, completely opacifies the LV apex and by doing so a filling defect can be noted which can confirm the presence of a thrombus. Characteristically, a thrombus has a nonhomogeneous echo density with a margin distinct from the underlying wall, which is akinetic to dyskinetic (Fig. 21.5). A thrombus is more likely to occur following an AMI in the LAD artery distribution (up to 33%) vs. the right coronary or circumflex (<1%) coronary arteries. False positives may occur. For instance, false chordae or false tendon spanning the LV apex as well as coarse trabeculations associated with LV hypertrophy and near-field artifacts (commonly present in low-frequency transducers) may mimic the echocardiographic findings. High-frequency transducers can differentiate true thrombus from these artifacts and color Doppler flow or intravenous contrast agents may outline the contours of the thrombus, creating a filling defect and improving the detection of the thrombus. TEE may not visualize the apex as well as transthoracic echocardiography.[18,19]

## Cardiac Remodeling After Myocardial Infarction

Observations in patients with AMI depict the frequency and significance of cardiac remodeling in patients with LV dysfunction. The GISSI-3-Echo Substudy[20] examined the frequency with which remodeling occurs in this setting via serial echocardiograms, which were performed in 614 patients with an average infarct size that was relatively small (26%). Using the end-diastolic volume index (EDVI) as a marker of remodeling, the following observations were noted:

- Between 24 and 48 h after symptom onset to hospital discharge, the EDVI diminished to 26%, and then subsequently increased modestly in 32%, and increased more than 20% in 19%, representing severe early remodeling.
- Between hospital discharge and 6 months after infarction, the EDVI fell in 31%, was stable in 25%, increased modestly in 28%, and increased more than 20% in 16%, indicative of severe late remodeling.

In-hospital LV enlargement was not predictive of subsequent remodeling, but late remodeling, which most often occurred in the absence of in-hospital LV enlargement, was associated with a progressive deterioration of global LV function and more extensive wall motion abnormalities. Determinants of infarct expansion and LV remodeling include large infarct size, ST segment AMI, anterior location, lack of patency of the infarct vessel, elevated intraventricular pressure, and the use of thrombolysis. Data from the GISSI-3 trial suggest that serial ECG changes can predict postinfarction remodeling.[20] Lack of negative T wave resolution or the late appearance of new negative T waves was associated with less recovery of wall motion abnormalities, more pronounced LV enlargement, and progressive deterioration of LV function; in contrast, normalization of negative T waves was related to functional recovery of viable myocardium and was more useful than QRS changes.

## *Use of Imaging Techniques*

Both radionuclide imaging and echocardiography provide a simple assessment of LV systolic function and chamber size. Although echocardiography is reliable in clinical trials, repeat measurements of LV mass and volume or LVEF may vary considerably and methods are poorly standardized between centers. Further limiting its use is the inability to obtain good images in some patients, such as those who are obese or have airway disease. Thus, one must be cautious in using standard echocardiographic monitoring to guide management. Echocardiography using harmonic imaging and contrast injection improves the accuracy and reproducibility of standard echocardiography and therefore, echocardiography has emerged globally as the diagnostic tool of choice, even further expanded with the advent of three-dimensional echocardiography.

Cardiac MRI provides better accuracy and reliability than echocardiography. However, it is both difficult to access and expensive, which limits routine use.

## *Use of LVEF to Guide Management*

The LVEF, regardless of how it is measured, is an important predictor of outcome. For instance, the Val-HeFT[21] trial identified LVEF as a powerful predictor of all-cause mortality in patients with HF. The mortality increased in a nonlinear fashion as LVEF diminished, with the mortality rate increasing steeply in patients with an LVEF <0.25. However, using LVEF to estimate survival in an individual patient is of limited value. Another dilemma is that the LVEF is of limited utility in some situations, as in the immediate postinfarction period where LV dysfunction may be caused by large areas of hibernating or stunned myocardium. Despite these limitations, information about the LVEF, generated from echocardiography, often results in management decisions. Increases in LVEF have been linked to improved prognosis. Although the degree of improvement is important, it must be considered in the context of other responses that may affect mortality. An analysis of the combined data from a Val-HeFT substudy[22] showed that, although enalapril failed to increase LVEF as much as hydralazine/isosorbide dinitrate, it was associated with a greater reduction in mortality; these observation suggest that inhibition of the renin–angiotensin system conferred additional survival benefit. The V-HeFT data also found that serial measurements of LVEF provided additional prognostic information, suggesting that there is some merit to monitoring LVEF or chamber size to assess response to therapy and altering it accordingly. However, randomized clinical trials have yet to prospectively test this hypothesis.

## References

1. Friedman BM, Dunn MI. Postinfarction ventricular aneurysms. *Clin Cardiol.* 1995;18(9):505–511.

2. Glower DG, Lowe EL. Left ventricular aneurysm. In: Edmunds LH, ed. *Cardiac Surgery in the Adult.* New York, NY: McGraw Hill; 1997.677.
3. Tikiz H, Balbay Y, Atak R, Terzi T, Genç Y, Kütük E. The effect of thrombolytic therapy on left ventricular aneurysm formation in acute myocardial infarction: relationship to successful reperfusion and vessel patency. *Clin Cardiol.* 2001;24:656.
4. Feigenbaum H, Armstrong WF, Ryan T. *Feigenbaum's Echocardiography.* Philadelphia, PA: Lipincott Williams and Wilkins; 2005:469–473.
5. Nicolosi AC, Spotnitz HM. Quantitative analysis of regional systolic function with left ventricular aneurysm. *Circulation.* 1988;78:856.
6. Matsumoto M, Watanabe F, Goto A, et al. Left ventricular aneurysm and the prediction of left ventricular enlargement studied by two-dimensional echocardiography: quantitative assessment of aneurysm size in relation to clinical course. *Circulation.* 1985;72:280.
7. Konen E, Merchant N, Gutierrez C, et al. True versus false left ventricular aneurysm: differentiation with MR imaging – initial experience. *Radiology.* 2005;236:65.
8. Vlodaver Z, Coe JL, Edwards JE. True and false left ventricular aneurysms: propensity for the latter to rupture. *Circulation.* 1975;51:567.
9. Dubnow MH, Burchell HB, Titus JL. Postinfarction ventricular aneurysm. a clinicomorphologic and electrocardiographic study of 80 cases. *Am Heart J.* 1965;70:753.
10. Faxon DP, Ryan TJ, Davis KB, et al. Prognostic significance of angiographically documented left ventricular aneurysm from the Coronary Artery Surgery Study (CASS). *Am J Cardiol.* 1982;50:157.
11. Antman EM, Anbe DT, Armstrong PW, et al. ACC/AHA guidelines for the management of patients with ST-elevation myocardial infarction. Available at: www.acc.org/ qualityand-science/clinical/statements.htm
12. Rao G, Zikria EA, Miller WH, et al. Experience with sixty consecutive ventricular aneurysm resections. *Circulation,* 1974;50:II149.
13. Antunes PE, Silva R, Ferrão de Oliveira J, et al. Left ventricular aneurysms: early and long-term results of two types of repair. *Eur J Cardiothorac Surg.* 2005;27(2):210–215.
14. Shapira OM, Davidoff R, Hilkert RJ, et al. Repair of left ventricular aneurysm: long-term results of linear repair versus endoaneurysmorrhaphy. *Ann Thorac Surg.* 1997;63:701.
15. Waldo AL, Arciniegas JG, Klein H. Surgical treatment of life-threatening ventricular arrhythmias: the role of intraoperative mapping and consideration of the presently available surgical techniques. *Prog Cardiovasc Dis.* 1981;23:247.
16. Frances C, Romero A, Grady D. Left ventricular pseudoaneurysm. *J Am Coll Cardiol.* 1998;32:557.
17. Dachman AH, Spindola-Franco H, Solomon N. Left ventricular pseudoaneurysm: its recognition and significance. *JAMA.* 1981;246:1951.
18. Yeo TC, Malouf JF, Oh JK, Seward JB. Clinical profile and outcome in 52 patients with cardiac pseudoaneurysm. *Ann Intern Med.* 1998;128:299.
19. Reeder GS, Lengyel M, Tajik AJ, et al. Mural thrombus in left ventricular aneurysm: incidence, role of angiography, and relation between anticoagulation and embolization. *Mayo Clin Proc.* 1981;56:77.
20. Popes BA, Antonini-Canterin F, Temporelli PL and the GISSI-3 Echo Substudy Investigators, Right ventricular functional recovery after acute myocardial infarction: relation with left ventricular function and interventricular septum motion. GISSI-3 echo substudy. *Heart.* 2005;91(4):484–488.
21. Cohn JN, Tognoni G, and the Valsartan Heart Failure Trial Investigators. A randomized trial of the angiotensin-receptor blocker valsartan in chronic heart failure. *N. Engl. J. Med.* 2001;345(23):1667–1675.
22. Wong M, Staszewsky L, Latini R, and the Val-HeFT Heart Failure Trial Investigators. Valsartan benefits left ventricular structure and function in heart failure: Val-HeFT echocardiographic study. *J Am Coll Cardiol.* 2002;40(5):970–975.

# Chapter 22
# Echocardiographic-guided Pericardial Drainage in Acute Coronary Syndrome

Mark V. Sherrid, Gregory S. Sherrid, and Seth Uretsky

When patients with acute chest pain present to the hospital, 2D echocardiography is often one of the first tests performed. This is because of the unique ability of echocardiography to visualize not only myocardial motion but also myocardial thickening, valvular pathology and function, proximal aortic root, and the pericardium. Moreover, since echocardiography can be performed at the bedside, such evaluation can be done quickly on the very sickest patients.

Not infrequently, a patient thought initially to have an acute coronary syndrome will be found to have a large pericardial effusion and normal left ventricular wall motion. With this information, there is an abrupt shift, and new diagnostic and therapeutic possibilities arise. In this chapter, we discuss how echocardiography cannot only help diagnosis but also treat large pericardial effusions. On occasion in selected patients, the decision will be made after consideration of risks and benefits to drain the pericardial fluid and examine its contents for diagnostic purposes. Also, a pigtail catheter may be left in the pericardial space to drain the fluid.

Echocardiographic-guided pericardial drainage has been introduced as a less invasive technique than subxiphoid surgical window pericardiostomy.[1-5] It is indicated for drainage of symptomatic large pericardial effusions.

## Technique

The patient is placed in a shallow right anterior decubitus position by placing a pillow or a wedge underneath the right shoulder. Two-dimensional echocardiography is performed, specifically searching for the area of the chest wall where the pericardial fluid is closest to the skin.[1,2] Our preferred location is at the apex of the left ventricle. As pericardial fluid accumulates, the lung is pushed out of the way and the apex becomes completely occupied by the pericardial effusion (Fig. 22.1). An excellent ultrasound window offers assurance that one is not over the lung. This window often extends as far as the left anterior axillary line in very large effusions. The pericardial

M.V. Sherrid (✉)
Cardiology, St Luke's-Roosevelt Hospital Center, 1000 10th Ave, New York, NY 10019, USA
e-mail: msherrid@chpnet.org

E. Herzog, F.A. Chaudhry (eds.), *Echocardiography in Acute Coronary Syndrome*,
DOI 10.1007/978-1-84882-027-2_22, © Springer Verlag London Limited 2009

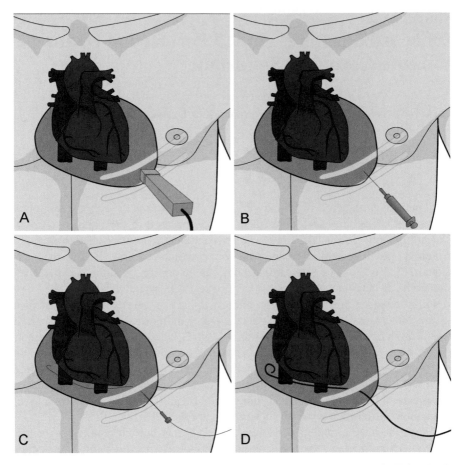

**Fig. 22.1** The technique of echocardiographic guided pericardial drainage. (**A**) Using the 2D echocardiographic transducer the physician searches for the interspace location on the chest wall with the closest access to the large pericardial effusion. Generally the fluid will be 2−3 cm from the transducer. The transducer angle, cranio-caudad, and medial-lateral from the center of the chest is noted. The interspace location is marked with a marker. The patient is prepped and draped. (**B**) Local anesthesia and low dose sedation is administered. Using the same position and angle noted above, the pericardial needle is gently advanced over the top of the rib into the pericardial space. (**C**) A J wire is advanced though the needle and into the pericardial space. If fluoroscopy is available the J wire is noted to course from the left side into the right without any intervening boundaries. This is a good confirmer that the wire is in the pericardial space and not in the heart. A sheath is placed over the wire, using standard Seldinger technique. Agitated saline may be injected at this point. (**D**) The pigtail catheter is then advanced into the pericardial space and evacuation of the fluid is begun

fluid is generally 2−3 cm below the skin in this location. Other sites of entry are possible, including the parasternal spaces and the traditional subxiphoid entry. The subxiphoid route always requires a longer needle track with associated discomfort and demands a more precise direction of needle angle. The parasternal spaces, while completely accessible, require one to avoid the internal thoracic artery.[6] We have generally required an effusion >1 cm in AP direction; attempting to place the needle in a smaller effusion risks hitting the heart.

The ideal interspace is chosen and a mark is made there with an indelible marker (Fig. 22.1A). With the transducer showing a "straight shot" into pericardial fluid, one observes the transducer angle relative to the center of the chest: both medial-lateral and cranio-caudad. Note also how far from the skin the fluid would be expected, and also the distance to the heart. Next, the ultrasound gel is cleaned off and the patient is prepped and draped.

The site of entry is just over the top of the rib. Local anesthesia is instilled, including both the skin and the intercostal muscle. The patient is lightly sedated. A 0.5 cm incision is made with a #14 scalpel blade.

The pericardiocentesis needle is gently inserted through the incision with the precise angle that had been indicated by the echo probe (Fig. 22.1B). The trocar is left in place until the needle is almost at the depth where fluid might be expected. It is then removed and gentle aspiration is applied using a 3 cc syringe. The pericardium is usually entered with a small pop. Once pericardial fluid is found, it is important to keep the needle still to avoid lacerating the heart. One advantage of the apical route is that the coronary arteries are small at the apex and there is less danger of lacerating a major coronary artery. Such a complication is possible from the parasternal entry.

Bloody fluid is often aspirated in patients who have malignant effusions or post-surgical cases. However, on close inspection, the fluid is serosanguineous not frank blood. Throughout the insertion of the needle and the sheath, a nurse observer watches the electrocardiogram; the occurrence of ventricular tachycardia indicates that the heart has been hit and the needle should be withdrawn.

A guide wire with a small J is placed through the needle into the pericardial space (Fig. 22.1C). If the procedure has been done in the cardiac catheterization laboratory, typically the wire is seen to pass from the left chest into the right chest on fluoroscopy, as there are no intracardiac borders to confine it. This is a good marker of entry into the pericardial space. The needle is removed and then, using standard Seldinger technique, a sheath and introducer are inserted into the pericardial space and the guide wire and introducer are removed, leaving just the sheath.

At this point, agitated saline may be injected into the sheath to confirm location during echocardiography recording. This may also be done earlier when just the needle is in place. It is not necessary to record the echocardiographic transit of the needle and the sheath because the needle and the sheath are rarely clearly seen. A pigtail catheter 6−8 F is inserted through the sheath and the sheath is withdrawn (Fig. 22.1D).

## Removal of the Fluid

The first aliquot should go for bacterial and fungal culture, Gram stain, AFB smear, and AFB culture. The next aliquot should go for cells, protein and sugar, and LDH.

The last aliquot, the largest, should be sent in its entirety to the cytology laboratory. If tamponade had been present, after removal of 200 cc, the patient's vital signs will often improve. The catheter is then sewn to the chest wall with three restraining sutures and taped thoroughly. The fluid is collected by gravity drainage or attachment to a hemovac collector.

The catheter is left for at least 4 days until fluid drainage is <40 cc per shift. This allows for apposition of the two layers of the pericardium with each other. This apposition fosters fibrous adhesions to form between the two layers of the pericardium and prevents new fluid accumulation. Adhesions are also the mechanism whereby surgical window pericardiostomy works, as well. Surgical windows close after several days. To avoid clotting of the catheter, 3 cc of heparinized saline should be injected, using sterile technique, and left in the pericardial tube every 8 h.

There may be oozing of pericardial fluid around the catheter through the insertion site. This is not of concern, and we have not seen infection. It is managed by sterile dressing changes. If there is suspicion of malignancy, we generally wait until the cytology returns. If cytology is positive, in many cases, after consultation with the oncology service, we will inject intrapericardial bleomycin 30 units diluted in 50 cc normal saline. This is done to foster adhesions between the visceral and the parietal pericardium. However, others indicate that bleomycin is not necessary to prevent recurrence.[3]

When the catheter is removed, the sutures are cut and the catheter is simply pulled back, gentle pressure is placed on the entry site for a minute, and then a small dressing is placed; chest X-ray is checked.

Echocardiographic guidance of pericardial drainage was pioneered at the Mayo Clinic. A first report came from Callahan and coworkers[1] which demonstrated the value of 2D echo-guided pericardiocentesis in 117 patients. This was followed by the report of Kopecky and colleagues[2] which detailed pericardial catheter drainage in 42 patients; of note, only 6 patients (14%) required subsequent surgical pericardiectomy. More recent review described 1127 patients from a 21-year experience.[3,4] The most common etiologies for the effusion were malignant 25%, postoperative 28%, and cardiac perforation from invasive procedure 14%. Virtually all of the patients had either tamponade clinically or echocardiographic tamponade (84%). The recurrence rate was only 14% for the patients who had extended drainage. The major complication rate was 1.2%. Echo-guided drainage has been extended to the pediatric population.[5]

Others have detailed their experience with percutaneous echo-guided pericardial drainage.[7–22] Comparison of surgical subxiphoid pericardiostomy and percutaneous drainage has been described.[21,22] In these series, pericardial drainage has generally acquitted itself well with little advantage shown by the surgical technique. Allen and colleagues found higher complication rates with the percutaneous technique, but pericardial drainage was not echocardiographically guided.[22] A similar comparison was reported by McDonald and coworkers.[21] This series was retrospective and not randomized; moreover, echocardiographic guidance was not universal. Hospital mortality and effusion recurrence was higher in the percutaneous group, but this could be due to selection of patients.[20] Regardless, if symptomatic pericardial effusion recurs, a repeat drainage procedure can be performed or surgical pericardiostomy may be selected at this time.

Surgery requires anesthesia and intubation. In patients with hypotension or hemodynamic instability, induction of anesthesia may be complicated by cardiac arrest. Surgical subxiphoid pericadiostomy often requires prolonged hospitalization. It is more painful. Risks of pneumonia and infection are increased. Also, in patients with pericardial malignancy chemotherapy may be started sooner with the percutaneous technique.

## Diagnostic Yield for Malignancy

In the study of McDonald and coworkers, in patients with previously known malignancy, there was no difference in the frequency that malignancy was confirmed in the percutaneous group vs. the open pericardiostomy group, 59% vs. 62%. The lack of incremental yield occurred despite pathological examination of the pericardial specimens. Of 52 patients with open drainage, only 4 (7%) had negative cytology and positive pathology. A conclusion was that this makes "selection of the open procedure for enhanced diagnostic purposes a questionable strategy".[21]

A high frequency of finding malignant cells in patients with malignant effusions has also been reported by others.[9,14] In patients suspected of having malignant effusions, Lindenberger and colleagues found malignant cells in 82% of cases and suspicious cells in 7%.[9] These investigators recommend percutaneous drainage for the wider spectrum of large effusions, including late postoperative effusions (median 12 days post-op), uremia, inflammatory disease, idiopathic as well as malignant disease. Indeed, they would only exclude immediate postoperative hemorrhagic effusions. In the late postoperative effusions valve surgery had been performed in 2/3; the high frequency of late postoperative pericardial effusion was thought due to anticoagulation. The average INR in patients on anticoagulation was 2.28 at the time of percutaneous drainage; ongoing anticoagulation is not a contraindication to percutaneous drainage. In contrast, systemic anticoagulation would generally be reversed before open pericardiostomy.

The most feared complication of 2D echo-guided catheter drainage is chamber perforation, which occurs infrequently, 16 patients (1.4%) in the largest experience of 1127 patients. Of these, five (0.4%) had lacerations that required surgery and one patient died postoperatively.[3] This complication may be avoided by careful selection of patients: Avoid patients without a clear target – a >1 cm anterior effusion under the needle. The >1 cm clearance should be maintained throughout the cardiac cycle. Avoid patients with just posterior effusions. Monitor the ECG and if ventricular arrhythmias occur, withdraw the needle. If perforation does occur and the catheter is placed in the right ventricle, the best course of action is to insert another catheter correctly into the pericardial space. Once its correct position is assured, withdraw the first catheter. Generally the right ventricular puncture will seal. If hemopericardium ensues at any time surgery should be done. Pneumothorax is also a possible complication of echo-guided pericardial drainage occurring in 1.1% of patients. Of these, five (0.4%) of the patients required chest tube for lung re-expansion. This may be avoided by selecting an interspace that is directly over a large, clearly visualized, pericardial effusion, with minimal distance for the needle to traverse.

# References

1. Callahan JA, Seward JB, Nishimura RA, et al. Two-dimensional echocardiographically guided pericardiocentesis: experience in 117 consecutive patients. *Am J Cardiol*. 1985;55:476–479.
2. Kopecky SL, Callahan JA, Tajik AJ, Seward JB. Percutaneous pericardial catheter drainage: report of 42 consecutive cases. *Am J Cardiol*. 1986;58:633–635.
3. Tsang TS, Enriquez-Sarano M, Freeman WK, et al. Consecutive 1127 therapeutic echocardiographically guided pericardiocenteses: clinical profile, practice patterns, and outcomes spanning 21 years. *Mayo Clin Proc*. 2002;77:429–436.
4. Tsang TS, Freeman WK, Sinak LJ, Seward JB. Echocardiographically guided pericardiocentesis: evolution and state-of-the-art technique. *Mayo Clin Proc*. 1998;73:647–652.
5. Tsang TS, El-Najdawi EK, Seward JB, Hagler DJ, Freeman WK, O'Leary PW. Percutaneous echocardiographically guided pericardiocentesis in pediatric patients: evaluation of safety and efficacy. *J Am Soc Echocardiogr*. 1998;11:1072–1077.
6. Kronzon I, Glassman LR, Tunick PA. Avoiding the left internal mammary artery during anterior pericardiocentesis. *Echocardiography*. 2003;20:533–534.
7. Vaitkus PT, Herrmann HC, LeWinter MM. Treatment of malignant pericardial effusion. *JAMA*. 1994;272:59–64.
8. Wei JY, Taylor GJ, Achuff SC. Recurrent cardiac tamponade and large pericardial effusions: management with an indwelling pericardial catheter. *Am J Cardiol*. 1978;42:281–282.
9. Lindenberger M, Kjellberg M, Karlsson E, Wranne B. Pericardiocentesis guided by 2-D echocardiography: the method of choice for treatment of pericardial effusion. *J Intern Med*. 2003;253:411–7.
10. Kabukcu M, Demircioglu F, Yanik E, Basarici I, Ersel F. Pericardial tamponade and large pericardial effusions: causal factors and efficacy of percutaneous catheter drainage in 50 patients. *Tex Heart Inst J*. 2004;31:398–403.
11. Selig MB. Percutaneous transcatheter pericardial interventions: aspiration, biopsy, and pericardioplasty. *Am Heart J*. 1993;125:269–271.
12. Maisch B, Ristic AD. Practical aspects of the management of pericardial disease. *Heart*. 2003;89:1096–1103.
13. Gibbs CR, Watson RD, Singh SP, Lip GY. Management of pericardial effusion by drainage: a survey of 10 years' experience in a city centre general hospital serving a multiracial population. *Postgrad Med J*. 2000;76:809–813.
14. Meyers DG, Meyers RE, Prendergast TW. The usefulness of diagnostic tests on pericardial fluid. *Chest*. 1997;111:1213–1221.
15. Wang PC, Yang KY, Chao JY, Liu JM, Perng RP, Yen SH. Prognostic role of pericardial fluid cytology in cardiac tamponade associated with non-small cell lung cancer. *Chest*. 2000;118:744–749.
16. de la Gandara I, Espinosa E, Gomez Cerezo J, Feliu J, Garcia Giron C. Pericardial tamponade as the first manifestation of adenocarcinoma. *Acta Oncol*. 1997;36:429–431.
17. Girardi LN, Ginsberg RJ, Burt ME. Pericardiocentesis and intrapericardial sclerosis: effective therapy for malignant pericardial effusions. *Ann Thorac Surg*. 1997;64:1422–1427; discussion 1427–8.
18. Celermajer DS, Boyer MJ, Bailey BP, Tattersall MH. Pericardiocentesis for symptomatic malignant pericardial effusion: a study of 36 patients. *Med J Aust*. 1991;154:19–22.

19. Zipf RE Jr, Johnston WW. The role of cytology in the evaluation of pericardial effusions. Chest 1972;62:593–6.
20. Salem K, Mulji A, Lonn E. Echocardiographically guided pericardiocentesis – the gold standard for the management of pericardial effusion and cardiac tamponade. *Can J Cardiol.* 1999;15:1251–1255.
21. McDonald JM, Meyers BF, Guthrie TJ, Battafarano RJ, Cooper JD, Patterson GA. Comparison of open subxiphoid pericardial drainage with percutaneous catheter drainage for symptomatic pericardial effusion. *Ann Thorac Surg.* 2003;76:811–815; discussion 816.
22. Allen KB, Faber LP, Warren WH, Shaar CJ. Pericardial effusion: subxiphoid pericardiostomy versus percutaneous catheter drainage. *Ann Thorac Surg.* 1999;67:437–440.

# Chapter 23
# Risk Stratification Following Acute Myocardial Infarction: Role of Dobutamine Stress Echocardiography

**Raaid Museitif, Mohamed Djelmami-Hani, and Kiran B. Sagar**

## Introduction

The role of dobutamine stress echocardiography (DSE) in risk stratification post-acute myocardial infarction (AMI) has rapidly evolved. In the pre-stent era it helped identify patients who were at higher risk of developing adverse events. These patients were thought to benefit from more invasive therapy. In the post-stent era our paradigm has shifted to an early invasive strategy for patients with non-ST-segment elevation acute coronary myocardial infarction (NSTEMI). Since the majority of NSTEMI patients undergo early angiography, the role for DSE has been diminished. However, when myocardial viability is of question, DSE still is an effective tool.

## Background

The treatment of acute myocardial infarction has changed significantly over the last decade. Mortality has been significantly reduced with the widespread use of aspirin, statins, beta-blockers, clopidogrel, IIb/IIIa inhibitors, thrombolytics, and coronary stents. Risk stratification is an integral part of managing patients with acute myocardial infarction. Early risk stratification guides triage to clinical pathways of patient care, optimizes use of hospital resources, and directs high-intensity pharmacologic and technologic care to high-risk patients. In addition, risk stratification is extremely important for patient and family counseling.

Bedside clinical criteria are excellent for identifying high-risk patients after an acute myocardial infarction.[1,2,3,4]Patients presenting with cardiogenic shock and/or heart failure have a significantly high morbidity and mortality. They need urgent

R. Museitif (✉)

Cardiology, Aurora Sinai Medical Center, Milwaukee, Wisconsin, USA

e-mail: museitif@yahoo.com

E. Herzog, F.A. Chaudhry (eds.), *Echocardiography in Acute Coronary Syndrome*,
DOI 10.1007/978-1-84882-027-2_23, © Springer-Verlag London Limited 2009

primary coronary intervention without further testing to preserve large area of jeopardized myocardium. This concept is the driving force behind primary intervention and thrombolytic therapy in acute coronary syndromes. It is difficult to detect patients who may be stratified as low to intermediate risk initially but may be at risk of adverse events in the long term. Pre-discharge dobutamine stress echocardiography can assess preservation of viable myocardium and ischemia at a distance, indicator of multivessel coronary artery disease.

In the pre-stent/pre-thrombolytic era, patients presenting with acute MI were treated medically. Given the high rate of adverse outcomes, the need to identify high-risk patients was evident. In 1979, Theroux et al. studied the role of submaximal exercise stress testing in post-MI patients.[5] A total of 210 consecutive post-AMI patients underwent submaximal treadmill exercise stress testing prior to discharge. Patients had to be free from chest pain for at least 4 days and without clinical signs of congestive heart failure prior to stressing. They reported no procedural complications. They found that 63% of patients who reported chest pain during stress testing went on to report angina within the following year compared with 36% of those who reported no chest pain during testing. Mortality was 2.1% in patients without ST-segment changes during exercise compared to 27% in those with ST-segment depressions. They concluded that submaximal exercise stress testing could be performed safely in post-MI patients and predicts mortality. This was a significant step forward in post-MI risk stratification; however, the sensitivity was still too low.

Ambulatory electrocardiography (ECG) monitoring can also provide prognostic information early after acute MI. Gill et al. took 406 patients with acute myocardial infarction and performed submaximal exercise testing before discharge and 48-h ambulatory ECG.[6] The primary outcome was death, nonfatal myocardial infarction, and hospital admission for unstable angina at 1-year follow-up. ECG monitoring detected signs of ischemia in 23.4% of patients. Mortality was 11.6% among patients with ischemia and 3.9% ($p = 0.009$) for those without. Patients with a positive stress test had a 3.9% mortality compared with 3.0% for those with a negative test. Patients not tested had a 16.4% mortality ($p < 0.001$). Having signs of ischemia on ambulatory ECG carried an odds ratio of 2.3 (95% CI 1.2–4.5) for death, nonfatal myocardial infarction, or hospital readmission for unstable angina ($p < 0.001$). Figure 23.1 below shows the cumulative risk of ischemia.

Quantitative exercise thallium-201 scintigraphy was studied by Gibson et al. and was shown to predict future cardiac events when performed pre-discharge in post-MI patients treated medically without thrombolytics.[7] They evaluated 140 patients with acute myocardial infarction and compared them to both submaximal exercise treadmill testing and coronary angiography. Patients were divided into high- and low-risk categories. High-risk patients demonstrated Tl-201 defects in more than one vascular region, redistribution, increased lung uptake, ST-segment depression >1 mm, angina, or angiographic evidence of multivessel disease. Low-risk patients had single-region scintigraphic defects, no redistribution, no lung uptake, no ST-segment depression, no angina, and no more than one vessel disease on angiography. At $15 \pm 12$ months follow-up there were 50 cardiac events, 7 deaths, 9 recurrent myocardial infarctions, and 34 patients experienced Class III or IV angina.

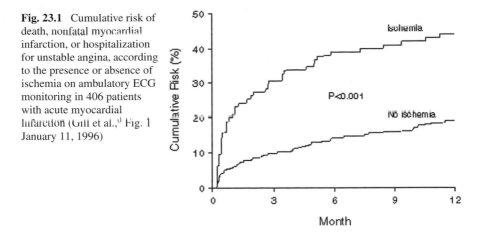

**Fig. 23.1** Cumulative risk of death, nonfatal myocardial infarction, or hospitalization for unstable angina, according to the presence or absence of ischemia on ambulatory ECG monitoring in 406 patients with acute myocardial infarction (Gill et al.,[6] Fig. 1 January 11, 1996)

Scintigraphy identified 94% of the high-risk patients compared with 56% with exercise testing ($p < 0.001$). Scintigraphy was also more sensitive than angiography (94 vs. 71%; $p < 0.01$). In addition, 12 out of 13 patients with single-vessel disease, who had an event, demonstrated redistribution on scintigraphy. This study demonstrated that submaximal exercise Tl-201 scintigraphy can enhance our ability to risk stratify patients post-myocardial infarction.

These findings are shown in Fig. 23.2. Given the enhanced sensitivity using cardiac imaging with Tl-201 scintigraphy, could echocardiography add prognostic value to exercise stress testing? Ryan et al. prospectively studied 40 patients with acute myocardial infarction.[8] Patients underwent exercise stress echocardiography 10–21 days post-infarct. They were followed for 6–10 months. Primary end points included death, recurrent myocardial infarction, unstable angina, or coronary artery bypass grafting. They found that the sensitivity and specificity of exercise stress testing was 55 and 65%, respectively. However, when echo was added, the sensitivity increased to 80% and specificity to 95%. This clearly showed that two-dimensional echocardiography could significantly add to the prognostic value of exercise stress testing in post-MI patients.

## Dobutamine Stress Echo in Thrombolytic Era

Most of the above studies were performed in the pre-thrombolytic era. With the introduction of thrombolytics, patients' profiles changed. Lysis of the offending clot left behind residual plaque with the potential to cause further injury to viable cardiac muscle. This posed a new clinical problem: should these patients be sent for cardiac catheterization or could they be treated medically? Was there a role for stress testing to risk stratify patients post-thrombolytics?

Carlos et al. attempted to answer this question.[9] They studied 214 patients with acute myocardial infarction. Patients underwent dobutamine stress echocardiograms

**Fig. 23.2** Cumulative probability of cardiac events as a function of time for different subgroups formed by the exercise test response (*top*), scintigraphic findings (*middle*), or angiographic findings (*bottom*) before hospital discharge. The *solid* and *dashed lines* represent the high-risk and low-risk cumulative probability, respectively (from Gibson et al.[7])

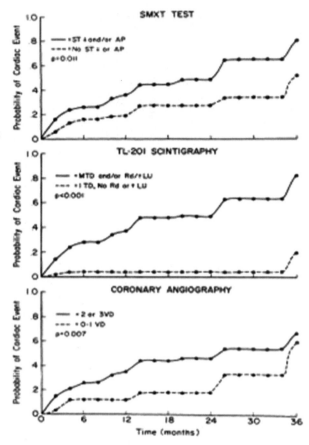

2–7 days post-infarction. Primary end point was the occurrence of a major cardiac event (cardiac death, nonfatal MI, sustained ventricular tachycardia or fibrillation, unstable angina, and congestive heart failure). Mean follow-up was 494 ± 182 days and occurred via chart review and telephone interviews. A total of 121 patients received thrombolytics. Angiography was performed at the discretion of the attending physician who was blinded to the test results. Coronary angiography was performed in 193 patients and 39% of the patients underwent revascularization prior to discharge based on coronary anatomy. There were a total of 80 events. Death occurred in 15 patients, nonfatal MI in 15, ventricular arrhythmia in 5, congestive heart failure in 14, and unstable angina in 31. They found that significant predictors of adverse outcomes were history of previous MI ($p = 0.005$), anterior infarct ($p = 0.006$), multivessel coronary artery disease ($p < 0.0001$), nonviable infarct zone ($p = 0.0001$), and ischemia/infarction at a distance ($p < 0.0001$). They also demonstrated that nonviability and the extent of the infarcted area correlated to the severity of cardiac events. Clinical, angiographic, and DSE variables were assessed via multivariate analysis. Ischemia/infarction at a distance and nonviability were the only independent predictors of adverse outcomes ($p < 0.0001$), both of which were obtained by DSE. This study provided the first evidence that DSE can be used to help predict cardiac events in patients who received thrombolytic therapy (see Figs. 23.3, 23.4, 23.5, and 23.6 for the result summary).

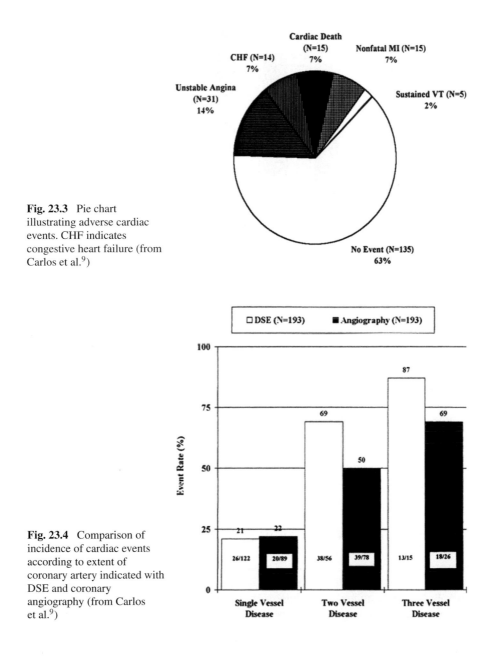

**Fig. 23.3** Pie chart illustrating adverse cardiac events. CHF indicates congestive heart failure (from Carlos et al.[9])

**Fig. 23.4** Comparison of incidence of cardiac events according to extent of coronary artery indicated with DSE and coronary angiography (from Carlos et al.[9])

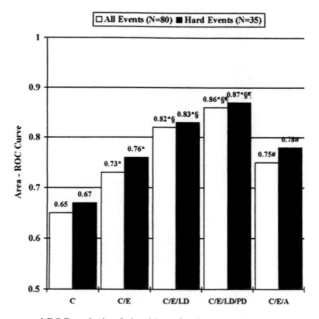

**Fig. 23.5** Incremental ROC analysis of algorithms for the prediction of all and hard events after MI. DSE provided incremental value (see text for details). C, clinical; Alg, algorithm C/E, clinical and resting echocardiography; C/E/LD, clinical, resting, and low-dose dobutamine echocardiography; C/E/LD/PD, clinical, resting, low-dose dobutamine, and peak-dose dobutamine echocardiography; C/E/A, clinical and resting echocardiography and angiography. $*p < 0.05$ vs. C Alg; $\S p < 0.05$ vs. C/E Alg; $\P p < 0.05$ vs. C/E/LD Alg; $\#p =$ NS vs. C/E Alg (from Carlos et al.[9])

In a large study by Picano et al., 925 patients underwent dipyridamole stress echocardiography (DSE) at a mean time of 10 days post-myocardial infarction and followed for a mean of 14 days.[10] Univariate analysis found that the most important predictor of angina, death, or re-infarction was inducible wall motion abnormality after dipyridamole administration ($\chi^2 = 45.8$). A Cox analysis found that the most important predictors of death were age and wall motion score index during dipyridamole administration. Both motion score index and age were found to be independent predictors of death. Mortality was 2% in patients with negative DSE, 4% in patients with positive high-dose DSE, and 7% in patients with low-dose DSE. This study proved the importance of DSE in stratifying patients post-myocardial infarction based on the absence or presence of wall motion abnormality and its severity.

## Myocardial Contrast Echocardiography

The prognostic value of myocardial contrast echocardiography (MCE) as a tool to assess myocardial viability in post-myocardial infarction patients treated with thrombolysis was studied by Swinburn et al.[11] They enrolled 99 post-AMI patients and evaluated them with MCE. During a mean follow-up time of $46 \pm 16$ months,

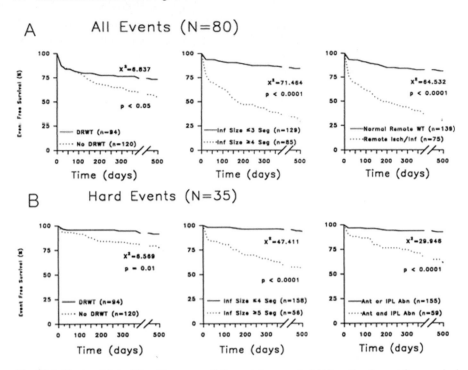

**Fig. 23.6**  Kaplan–Meier life table curves of all event-free survival (**A**) and hard event-free survival (**B**) on the basis of dobutamine-responsive wall thickening (DRWT) at low dose, infarct size (Inf size), and remote ischemia/infarction (Isch/Inf) (from Carlos et al.[9])

the extent of residual myocardial viability was found to be an independent predictor of cardiac death ($p = 0.01$) and cardiac death or MI ($p = 0.002$). They concluded that the extent of residual myocardial viability as assessed by MCE is a powerful and independent predictor of death and re-infarction in post-MI patients.

## *Dobutamine Stress Echo in Era of Primary Coronary Intervention*

With the introduction and advancement of primary coronary intervention (PCI) and angioplasty, strong evidence surged in favor of early invasive strategy using coronary angiography with angioplasty and stenting in post-AMI patients.

A meta-analysis of seven large randomized trials with 8375 patients was recently published in the *Journal of the American College of Cardiology*.[12] The authors sought in this study to answer, again, the everlasting question of the role and effect of early invasive therapy post-NSTEMI on mortality, re-infarction, and recurrent unstable angina. At a mean follow-up time of 2 years, the incidence of all-cause mortality was significantly lower in the early invasive therapy group compared to the conservative therapy group (4.9 vs. 6.5%, $p = 0.001$). During the same follow-up time, the incidence of nonfatal MI was also significantly lower in the early invasive group (7.6 vs. 9.1%, $p = 0.012$). This study proved that early invasive therapy improves long-term survival and reduces re-infarction rate and angina.

With this compelling evidence, the current practice and recommendation is to intervene early in AMI patients with coronary angiography and revascularization.[13] This approach takes away the principal role of DSE as a stratifying test post-AMI, since most, if not all, patients undergo early coronary angiography to determine their anatomy and lesions and at the same time revascularize with angioplasty and stenting of the culprit lesion.

Even though AMI patients can present with multiple coronary lesions on angiography, the current recommendation is to intervene only on the culprit vessel/lesion in early post-MI patients and stage the intervention on other lesions later on once the patient is stable.[13] The main and probably only role of DSE in post-AMI patients in this era is, in our opinion, to assess the myocardial viability and help guide any further revascularization (percutaneously or surgically).

## Dobutamine Stress Echo in Myocyte Replacement Therapy

Since the results of myocardial salvage are less than ideal, there is great interest in myocyte regeneration or replacement therapy. Early studies have documented a modest improvement in left ventricle with circulating progenitor cells, bone marrow-derived cells, and skeletal myoblasts. The mechanism of improvement is under investigation. Whether it is the result of functioning cells, of paracrine effects, or some other mechanisms is not clear. Assessment of functioning myocytes may be done with low-dose dobutamine.

## Summary and Conclusions

In the current era of early PCI and stenting, dobutamine stress echocardiography plays no major role in the treatment of post-myocardial infarction patients. It can, however, play a valuable role in assessing myocardial viability and directing further revascularization efforts in patients with multiple coronary lesions other than the stented culprit one(s).

# References

1. Abdissa A, Scott ME, Bang JY, Vankeepuram S. Tree structured risk stratificationof inhospital mortalityafter primary coronary intervention for patients with acute myocardial infarction. *Am Heart J.* 2007;154:322–329.
2. Eagle KA, Lim MJ, Dabbous OH, et al. A validated prediction model for all forms of acute coronary syndrome: estimating the risk of 6-month post discharge death in an international registry. JAMA 2004, 291:2727–2733.

3. Halkin A, Singh M, Nikolsky E et al. Predictors of mortality after primary coronary intervention for acute myocardial infarction The Cadllac Risk Score. *JAAC*. 2005;45:1391–1405.
4. Moller JE, Hillis GS, Reeder GS, Gersh BJ, Pallikka PA. Wall motion score index and ejection fraction after acute myocardial infarction. *Am Heart J*. 2006;151:419–425.
5. Theroux P, Waters DD, Halphen C, Debaisieux JC, Mizgala HF. Prognostic value of exercise testing soon after myocardial infarction. *N Engl J Med*. 1979;301:341–345.
6. Gill JB, Cairns JA, Roberts RS, et al. Prognostic importance of myocardial ischemia detected by ambulatory monitoring early after acute myocardial infarction *N Engl J Med*. 1996;334.65–71.
7. Gibson RS, Watson DD, Craddock GB, et al. Prediction of cardiac events after uncomplicated myocardial infarction: a prospective study comparing predischarge exercise thallium-201 scintigraphy and coronary angiography. *Circulation*. 1983;68:321–336.
8. Ryan T, Armstrong WF, O'Donnell J, Feigenbaum H. Risk-stratification following myocardial infarction using exercise echocardiography. *Am Heart J*. 1987;114:1305–1316.
9. Carlos ME, Smart SC, Wynsen JC, Sagar KB. Dobutamine stress echocardiography for risk stratification after myocardial infarction. *Circulation*. March 1997;95:1402–1410.
10. Picano E, Landi P, Bolognese L, et al. Prognostic value of dipyridamole echocardiography early after uncomplicated myocardial infarction: a large-scale, multicenter trial. The EPIC Study Group. *Am J Med*. December 1993;95(6):608–618.
11. Swinburn JMA, Senior R. Myocardial viability assessed by dobutamine stress echocardiography predicts reduced mortality early after acute myocardial infarction: determining the risk of events after myocardial infarction (DREAM) study. *Heart*. January 2006;92:44–48.
12. Bavry AA, Kumbhani DJ, Rassi AN, Bhatt DL, Askari AT. Benefit of early invasive therapy in acute coronary syndromes. A meta-analysis of contemporary randomized clinical trials. *J Am Coll Cardiol*. 2006;48:1319–1325.
13. Smith SC Jr, Feldman TE, Hirshfeld JW Jr, et al. ACC/AHA/SCAI 2005 guideline update for percutaneous coronary intervention: a report of the American College of Cardiology/American Heart Association Task Force on Practice Guidelines (ACC/AHA/ACAI Writing Committee to Update the 2001 Guidelines for Percutaneous Coronary Intervention). *J Am Coll Cardiol*. 2006;47:216–235.

# Chapter 24
# Echo Assessment of Myocardial Viability

Sripal Bangalore and Farooq A. Chaudhry

Heart failure is a leading cause of morbidity and mortality with a 5-year mortality rate as high as 50%, making it the leading cause of hospitalization in patients over the age of 65 years.[1] The leading cause of heart failure is coronary artery disease/acute coronary syndromes. Numerous studies have shown that left ventricular (LV) systolic function is a strong predictor of future cardiovascular events and LV dysfunction is a potentially reversible condition related to myocardial stunning, hibernation, or a combination of the two mechanisms. Segments that lose function as a result of an acute ischemic insult despite the restoration of normal perfusion are known as *stunned myocardium* (transient postischemic dysfunction). Myocardial stunning results from a mismatch between coronary flow and myocardial function and these segments are likely to recover function spontaneously over time. On the other hand, *hibernating myocardium* is the term used to refer to segments rendered dysfunctional secondary to chronic ischemia. Hibernating myocardium results from a compensatory decrease in myocardial function as a consequence of chronic ischemia. Both stunned and hibernating myocardium can potentially improve their function and are collectively referred to as "viable myocardium".[2]

In patients with ischemic cardiomyopathy, 40% of patients have improvement in ejection fraction after revascularization.[3] This would mean that there is a substantial subset of patients with ischemic cardiomyopathy undergoing revascularization that has little clinical or prognostic benefit from revascularization. The perioperative mortality rates from coronary artery bypass grafting in patients with ischemic cardiomyopathy range from 5 to >30%.[4] Furthermore, revascularization of nonviable myocardium has not proven to be beneficial for either mortality[5] or improvement in global LV function. In fact, in a meta-analysis of 24 viability studies, revascularization of patients without viable myocardium was associated with a trend toward higher annual mortality rate compared with medical management alone (7.7% vs. 6.2%, $p = 0.23$).[5] On the contrary, revascularization of viable myocardium has been shown to be associated with increased ejection fraction,[4] decreased congestive heart

S. Bangalore (✉)
Cardiology, Brigham and Women's Hospital, Harvard Medical School, Boston, MA, USA
e-mail: sbangalore@partners.org

E. Herzog, F.A. Chaudhry (eds.), *Echocardiography in Acute Coronary Syndrome*,     351
DOI 10.1007/978-1-84882-027 2_24, © Springer-Verlag London Limited 2009

failure symptoms,[4] and improved survival[5] compared to those treated medically. On the contrary, patients with viability who do not undergo revascularization are annual mortality rates five times higher than those who were revascularized.[5] The mortality benefit of revascularization of a viable myocardium increases with decreasing LV function as well as increasing number of viable segments.[5] Identifying patients with ischemic cardiomyopathy who have viable myocardium is thus important at risk stratifying patients who might benefit from revascularization.

Given the risk of revascularization, there is need for accurate identification of viability in these patients to tailor treatment. Currently, the methods used for predicting myocardial viability include assessment of contractile reserve in dysfunctional region using low-dose dobutamine stress echocardiography (DSE), assessment of cell membrane integrity using single-photon emission tomography (SPECT) with thallium-201 (stress–redistribution–reinjection, stress–reinjection–24-h imaging, or rest–redistribution imaging), and assessment of myocyte metabolic activity using F-18 fluorodeoxyglucose (FDG) positron emission tomography (PET) (Table 24.1). Other techniques which are currently being developed include myocardial contrast echocardiography (MCE) and contrast-enhanced magnetic resonance imaging; both of which hold great promise.[6,7]

**Table 24.1** Imaging techniques to detect myocardial viability

| Imaging technique | Definition of viability | Measure | Disadvantage |
| --- | --- | --- | --- |
| FDG-PET | Myocardial segments with decreased perfusion but with intact metabolic activity | Identifying myocyte metabolic activity. Measures viability in the endocardium, myocardium, and epicardium | May overestimate viability; requires radiotracer and equipment; low-resolution study; no information on wall motion or ejection fraction; long acquisition time; and higher cost |
| [201]Tl-SPECT | Myocardial segments with decreased perfusion with delayed uptake | Identifying cell membrane integrity. Measures viability in the endocardium, myocardium, and epicardium | May overestimate viability; involves radio tracer; low resolution; and higher cost |
| DSE | Wall motion abnormality at rest which improves with low-dose dobutamine infusion | Identifying inotropic contractile reserve. Measures viability in the endocardium and inner myocardium | May underestimate viability; subjective interpretation; and limited by poor acoustic window |
| MRI | Delayed enhancement (5–20 min) indicates fibrosis or scar | Identifying stunned myocardium | Cost and not portable |

DSE = dobutamine stress echocardiography; FDG-PET = fluorine-18 fluorodeoxyglucose positron emission tomography; MRI = magnetic resonance imaging; [201]Tl-SPECT = thallium single-photon emission tomography.

# Dobutamine Stress Echocardiography

## *Rationale*

Dobutamine is a synthetic catecholamine with both positive inotropic and chronotropic effects mediated predominantly through $\beta_1$-adrenergic receptor stimulation. The principle of dobutamine stress echocardiography is based on the detection of "inotropic contractile reserve" (CR) in dysfunctional but viable myocardial segments with dobutamine. At low doses (4–8 μg/kg/min), dobutamine is a positive inotrope, but at doses >10 μg/kg/min it exhibits a positive chronotropic effect in addition to the inotropic effect.[8] In order to assess myocardial viability, only low doses of dobutamine which produce inotrophy predominantly with minimal chronotropy are effective. This is because at higher doses, the increased heart rate resulting from a chronotropic effect will increase myocardial demand with consequent ischemia.[9,10] Consequently, low-dose dobutamine is the standard protocol used for the assessment of myocardial viability.

## *Protocol*

There is wide variation in the protocol used to assess viability. The commonly used protocol involves administering dobutamine intravenously beginning at a dose of 2.5–5.0 μg/kg/min and increasing by 5–10 μg/kg/min every 3–5 min up to a maximum of 50 μg/kg/min, or until a study endpoint is achieved. The endpoints for termination of the dobutamine infusion typically include development of new segmental wall motion abnormalities, attainment of 85% of age-predicted maximum heart rate, or the development of significant adverse effects related to the dobutamine infusion. Five standard echocardiographic views are obtained with each acquisition: parasternal long axis, parasternal short axis, apical four-chamber, apical three-chamber, and apical two-chamber views. Echocardiographic images are acquired at baseline, with each stage of stress and during the recovery phase. Cardiac rhythm is monitored throughout the stress echocardiography protocol, and 12-lead electrocardiograms and blood pressure measurements are obtained at baseline, at each stage of stress and during the recovery phase.

    There are four characteristic responses of dysfunctional myocardial segments with dobutamine infusion (Fig. 24.1):

(1) *Monophasic (sustained) response*: improvement at low dose that persists or further improves at high dose. This indicates *viable myocardium* with no stenosis of the coronary artery subtending the akinetic/hypokinetic myocardium;

(2) *Biphasic response*: augmentation of function at low dose followed by deterioration at high dose. This indicates the presence of *viable myocardium* but the coronary artery that supplies the myocardium has flow-limiting stenosis;

## Response to Dobutamine

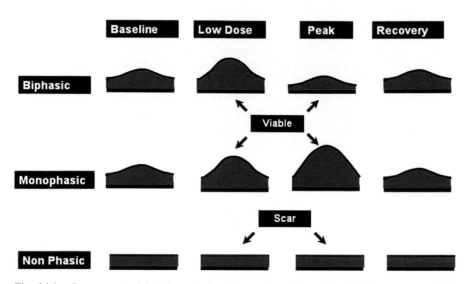

**Fig. 24.1** Response to dobutamine during stress echocardiography. Varying response of the myocardium to different doses of dobutamine in segments with and without viability

(3) *Ischemic response*: worsening of function, without contractile reserve. This indicates stress-induced ischemic myocardium due to flow-limiting stenosis (ischemia);

(4) *Nonphasic response*: no change. This indicates scarred myocardium with no viability.

A contractile response to dobutamine requires at least 50% viable myocytes in a given segment and correlates inversely with the extent of interstitial fibrosis on myocardial biopsy.[11] Atropine may be given with dobutamine to enhance the diagnostic value of the technique.[12] Other recent techniques to improve diagnostic yield of dobutamine stress echocardiography include combining with myocardial contrast echocardiography[13] and strain rate imaging with tissue Doppler.[14] Administration of nitroglycerine as an adjunct to dobutamine may enhance accuracy for detection of hibernating myocardium.[15]

## Prognostic Value

The identification of myocardial viability by low-dose dobutamine stress echocardiography is of prognostic significance in patients with ischemic cardiomyopathy. In a study by Chaudhry et al.,[16] the prognostic implications of myocardial contractile reserve were evaluated in patients with coronary artery disease and left ventricular (LV) dysfunction (ejection fraction ≤40%). In patients undergoing medical therapy alone, those with contractile reserve (identified by low-dose dobutamine stress echocardiography) had a better initial survival compared to those without contractile reserve, but this was not maintained beyond 3 years. In patients undergoing revascularization, those with contractile reserve had better survival compared to those without contractile reserve (Fig. 24.2). By multivariate analysis, the number of dysfunctional segments demonstrating contractile reserve was the strongest predictor of survival. Thus, myocardial viability as determined by low-dose dobutamine stress echocardiography is a significant predictor of survival in patients with CAD and LV dysfunction undergoing either medical therapy or revascularization, independent of symptoms, baseline LV function, or coronary anatomy (Fig. 24.2).[16]

Several other studies have evaluated the usefulness of low-dose dobutamine stress echocardiography in the prediction of improvement in regional contractile function following revascularization. Cusick et al.[17] evaluated the utility of dobutamine stress echocardiography in patients with severe left ventricular dysfunction and showed similar accuracy (Fig. 24.3). Pooled analysis of studies shows that low-dose dobutamine stress echocardiography has a good sensitivity (81%) and specificity (80%) for the prediction of improvement of regional and global LV function following revascularization.[18] It thus has a good positive predictive value (77%) and an excellent negative predictive value (85%) (Fig. 24.4).[18]

Prior studies evaluated the presence of viability in a binary fashion. However, Afridi et al.[19] evaluated the prognostic value of varying responses to dobutamine infusion (monophasic, biphasic, ischemic, and nonphasic responses). A biphasic response had the highest predictive value (72%), followed by ischemia (35%), whereas the lowest predictive value was observed in segments with either nonphasic (13%) or monophasic response (15%) during dobutamine. Combining biphasic and ischemic responses resulted in a sensitivity of 74% and specificity of 73% (Fig. 24.5).[19] Dobutamine-responsive wall motion was most often detected at doses of 5 or 7.5 μg/kg/min, and worsening was usually seen at doses >20 μg/kg/min,

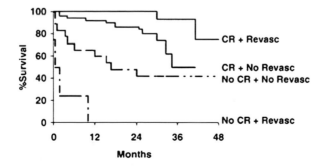

**Fig. 24.2** Myocardial viability and response to treatment. (Adapted from Chaudhry et al.[16]) CR = contractile reserve. In patients with left ventricular dysfunction and coronary artery disease, those with contractile reserve who were revascularized had the best prognosis

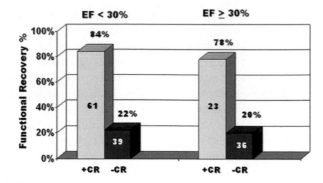

**Fig. 24.3** Assessment of myocardial viability in patients with severe left ventricular dysfunction. (Adapted from Cusick et al.[17]) CR = contractile reserve; EF = ejection fraction. The predictive accuracy of dobutamine stress echocardiography for functional recovery after revascularization was maintained in patients with or without severe left ventricular dysfunction

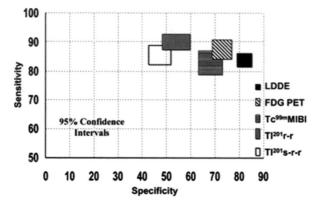

**Fig. 24.4** Sensitivity and specificity of the different imaging techniques in predicting functional recovery after revascularization (Bax[31]). FDG = fluorine-18-fluorodeoxyglucose; LDDE = low-dose dobutamine stress echocardiography; SPECT = single-photon emission computed tomography; PET = positron emission tomography. Dobutamine stress echocardiography had the best specificity

although it was seen in some patients as early as a 7.5 µg/kg/min dose. These data underscore the complex nature of dobutamine responsiveness that must be considered when interpreting clinical viability studies that use dobutamine echocardiography. Dobutamine should be started at a low dose with slow increments for optimal results.[20] However, test for viability should not be terminated after low doses of dobutamine if it is safe to continue testing at higher doses, as the demonstration of contractile reserve and inducible ischemia in the same segment (biphasic response) is a fairly definitive proof that the segment will improve with revascularization.[20,32]

Other studies have evaluated the "amount" of viable myocardium as a prognostic marker. In a study by Meluzin et al.,[21] those with large amount of viable

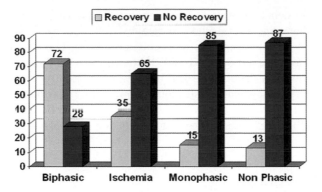

**Fig. 24.5** Response to dobutamine predicts recovery of left ventricular function following revascularization. (Adapted from Cornel et al.[32]) Patients with biphasic response (which represents both ischemia and viability) had the best recovery of function after revascularization, emphasizing the need to continue dobutamine infusion till endpoint is reached for the assessment of viability

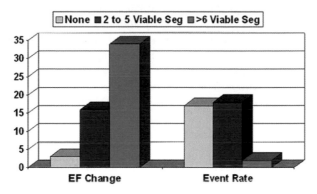

**Fig. 24.6** Importance of the amount of viable myocardium to predict improvement in ejection fraction and cardiovascular outcomes. (Adapted from Meluzin et al.[21]) The degree of improvement in ejection fraction increased with increasing number of viable segments and correlated with decrease in cardiac event rate

myocardium (≥ 6 segments) had a greater percentage increase in EF and lower cardiac event rate during a mean follow-up of 20 months compared to patients with modest amount of viable myocardium (2–5 segments) or no viable myocardium (Fig. 24.6).[21]

## Comparison with Other Modalities

Compared with other techniques for the prediction of functional recovery after revascularization, low-dose dobutamine stress echocardiography has comparable sensitivity with very good specificity (Fig. 24.4).[18] Bax et al.[18,31] in a pooled analysis of studies showed that the highest sensitivity was observed for FDG-PET, followed by the other nuclear imaging techniques, whereas the lowest sensitivity was observed for dobutamine stress echocardiography. However, the specificity was highest for dobutamine stress echocardiography, followed by FDG-PET, nuclear SPECT, whereas the lowest specificity was observed for [201]Tl reinjection. Thus, the highest NPV was observed for FDG-PET, followed by dobutamine stress echocardiography, followed by the other nuclear imaging techniques. Whereas, the highest PPV for recovery of segmental wall motion abnormality was observed for dobutamine stress echocardiography, followed by FDG-PET, [201]Tl rest–redistribution, and the lowest PPV was observed for [201]Tl reinjection (Fig. 24.4).[18,31]

## *Thallium Scintigraphy*

Arnese et al.[22] evaluated the predictive value of poststress reinjection thallium SPECT imaging and dobutamine echocardiography in 38 patients with severe LV dysfunction. Segments that had akinesis or severe hypokinesis were examined for improvement in function 3 months after coronary artery bypass surgery, as assessed by regional wall thickening on echocardiography. Thallium scintigraphy detected three times the number of viable segments as did low-dose dobutamine echocardiography (103 vs. 33 segments), with a higher sensitivity for an improvement of segmental function (89% for thallium SPECT and 74% for echocardiography). Low-dose dobutamine echocardiography, however, had a higher specificity and positive predictive value (95 and 85%, respectively) than did thallium reinjection imaging (48% vs. 33%, respectively).

Pooled analysis from various studies has shown that dobutamine stress echocardiography has a higher specificity, yielding a 14% higher positive predictive value compared to thallium SPECT.[23] However, the sensitivity of thallium SPECT is reported to be higher yielding a 9% higher negative predictive value than that for dobutamine stress echocardiography.[23] This seems to suggest that many myocardial segments with baseline systolic dysfunction will manifest thallium uptake but lack inotropic reserve during dobutamine administration resulting in "overestimation" of viability by nuclear SPECT (Table 24.1).

## *F-18 Fluorodeoxyglucose Positron Emission Tomography*

Pierard et al. evaluated 17 patients after thrombolytic therapy for acute myocardial infarction by low-dose dobutamine echocardiography and PET imaging with FDG. Repeated imaging $9 \pm 7$ months later was performed to assess the ability of these studies to predict recovery of regional function. PET and dobutamine echocardiography were concordant regarding the presence and absence of viability in 62 of the 78 myocardial segments (79%). However, among the segments with discordant results by the two modalities, 7 (16%) with viability on dobutamine stress had no viability based on PET study, and among the segments considered without viability on the dobutamine study, 9 (26%) had PET evidence of viability. At the follow-up examination, the regions with viability by both PET and dobutamine echocardiography improved in function, and the regions with concordance regarding the absence of viability by the two techniques had persistent dysfunction. However, all nine of the discordant regions thought to be viable by PET but without contractile reserve did not improve in function, and six had metabolic evidence of necrosis on the follow-up study; among the seven regions predicted to be viable by echocardiography but necrotic by PET, five had improved function and normal metabolism on the follow-up study. Thus, although PET and dobutamine echocardiography provided concordant findings in the majority of regions, these data indicate that PET might overestimate the presence and extent of viability, and that dobutamine echocardiography had at least similar negative predictive value and better positive predictive value than PET for functional recovery after thrombolytic therapy.

## Reasons for Discordant Finding Between Various Modalities to Assess Viability

Studies such as that described above indicate that a greater number of dysfunctional myocardial segments have been identified as viable by PET/nuclear than by echocardiography, indicating that some regions of viable myocardium are metabolically active and/or have intact cell membrane but lack inotropic reserve. The regions with discordant findings between the two techniques tend to be those in which blood flow is reduced at rest and those that are presumably hibernating.[20]

Discrepancies between dobutamine echocardiography and SPECT or PET imaging may reflect the underlying alternations in cellular metabolism, membrane integrity, and myocyte function. Blood flow and flow reserve may be reduced to such an extent that contractile reserve is lost but transmembrane pump activity is preserved. This could be imaged directly with thallium or sestamibi or could be assessed by investigating the metabolic processes necessary to generate the high-energy processes to maintain membrane integrity.[20] In such cases, "viability" may be detected by PET or SPECT and not by dobutamine stress echocardiography.

On the other hand, data of other investigators have shown that the magnitude of regional perfusion tracer activity reflects the mass of viable tissue, which in turn correlates with systolic function.[22,24,25] The "overestimation" of viability with techniques such as rest–redistribution thallium scintigraphy or PET imaging with FDG may be a result of the detection of small regions of viability that are of inadequate size to permit improvement in regional or global systolic function.[20] The distribution of viable cells may also be important, especially with regard to the recovery of ventricular function. A heterogeneous admixture of necrotic and viable cells may not demonstrate improved contraction, in spite of the presence of adequate metabolic function in at least some of the cells.[20] However, even without the return of cardiac function, the presence and maintenance of viability may be crucial for long-term prognosis, perhaps by the prevention of infarct expansion, ventricular remodeling, and the development of heart failure.

# Future Advances

## *Nitroglycerine Dobutamine Stress Echocardiography*

Ling et al.[15] compared nitroglycerine dobutamine stress echocardiography (NTG-DE) with intracoronary myocardial contrast echocardiography (MCE) and rest–redistribution thallium 201 single-photon emission computed tomography on the recovery of myocardial function following revascularization in patients with chronic ischemic LV dysfunction. Nitroglycerine (0.4 mg) was sprayed sublingually, followed by echocardiography 5 min later, followed by dobutamine infusion and standard dobutamine stress echocardiography protocol. Nitroglycerin alone increased regional thickening in 20% of viable akinetic segments. Among the various techniques for detecting myocardial viability, NTG-DE had the best specificity hypothesizing that nitroglycerin may be a useful adjunct to dobutamine stimulation. Nitroglycerin has been shown to increase contractility of viable asynergic segments by ventriculography,[26] enhance radionuclide uptake,[25] and augment end-systolic wall thickening by magnetic resonance.[27] Some of the mechanisms which have been postulated include direct vasodilation, recruitment of collateral circulation, or optimization of loading.[15,28,29]

## *Enoximone Stress Echocardiography*

Lu et al.[22] evaluated the role of enoximone, a phosphodiesterase inhibitor, with positive inotropic action but less hemodynamic effects compared to dobutamine, for the prediction of functional recovery following revascularization in patients with chronic ischemic LV dysfunction. Compared with dobutamine, enoximone echocardiography had higher sensitivity (88% vs. 79%) and negative predictive value (90% vs. 84%) with similar specificity (89% vs. 90%) and positive predictive value (87% for both) for predicting functional recovery. In patients with viable segments supplied by critically stenotic coronary arteries, even low-dose dobutamine can induce ischemia, secondary to increase in heart rate and systolic blood pressure. It has been shown that enoximone does not cause much increase in heart rate and blood pressure and hence can detect viability in critically stenotic segments (where supply and demand are delicately balanced) without inducing ischemia.[22]

## *Strain Rate Measurement*

Hoffmann et al.[14] evaluated the utility of strain rate measurement for evaluation of viability in patients with LV dysfunction undergoing dobutamine stress echocardiography. The peak systolic tissue Doppler velocity and the peak systolic myocardial strain rate were determined at baseline and during low-dose dobutamine stress from the apical views. The standard used for comparison was viability as determined by FDG-PET. Compared to low-dose dobutamine only, strain rate measurement increased both the sensitivity (increased from 75 to 83%) and the specificity (63−84%) for the detection of viability.[14] Thus, strain rate imaging may provide an important adjunct as a quantitative measure of viability especially in identifying subtle improvements in inotropic contractile reserve.

## *Myocardial Contrast Echocardiography*

Myocardial contrast echocardiography evaluates microvascular integrity. Senior et al.[30] evaluated the incremental value of myocardial contrast echocardiography over dobutamine stress echocardiography at predicting the recovery of function following acute myocardial infarction. Addition of myocardial contrast echocardiography to the standard dobutamine stress echocardiography protocol improved sensitivity for the prediction of improvement in contractile function (sensitivity increased from 59% to 79%) in dobutamine nonresponsive segments. Thus, myocardial contrast echocardiography may be an important adjunct to improve the sensitivity of dobutamine stress echocardiography.[30]

## Conclusions

In patients with ischemic left ventricular dysfunction, wall motion abnormalities may be reversible (viable); the presence of viability identifies regions of LV that will improve with revascularization. Dobutamine stress echocardiography is a valuable technique for the assessment of myocardial viability with good sensitivity and excellent specificity even in patients with severe left ventricular dysfunction. It thus has a good positive predictive value and excellent negative predictive value for the detection of viability. Although low-dose dobutamine is the standard protocol for assessing myocardial viability, given the prognostic value of a biphasic response, dobutamine infusion should be carried out to the endpoint whenever possible. The likelihood of improvement of contractile function with revascularization depends on the type of response to dobutamine (biphasic response has the best likelihood for recovery) and the amount of viable myocardium present. Thus, dobutamine stress echocardiography should be routinely considered in patients with ischemic cardiomyopathy for risk stratification, prognosis, and treatment.

## References

1. Massie BM, Shah NB. Evolving trends in the epidemiologic factors of heart failure: rationale for preventive strategies and comprehensive disease management. *Am Heart J.* 1997;133(6):703–712.
2. Wu KC, Lima JA. Noninvasive imaging of myocardial viability: current techniques and future developments. *Circ Res.* 2003;93(12):1146–1158.

3. Bonow RO. The hibernating myocardium: implications for management of congestive heart failure. *Am J Cardiol*. 1995;75(3):17A–25A.

4. Baker DW, Jones R, Hodges J, Massie BM, Konstam MA, Rose EA. Management of heart failure. III. The role of revascularization in the treatment of patients with moderate or severe left ventricular systolic dysfunction. *JAMA*. 1994;272(19):1528–1534.

5. Allman KC, Shaw LJ, Hachamovitch R, Udelson JE. Myocardial viability testing and impact of revascularization on prognosis in patients with coronary artery disease and left ventricular dysfunction: a meta-analysis. *J Am Coll Cardiol*. 2002;39(7):1151–1158.

6. deFilippi CR, Willett DL, Irani WN, Eichhorn EJ, Velasco CE, Grayburn PA. Comparison of myocardial contrast echocardiography and low-dose dobutamine stress echocardiography in predicting recovery of left ventricular function after coronary revascularization in chronic ischemic heart disease. *Circulation*. 1995;92(10):2863–2868.

7. Kim RJ, Wu E, Rafael A, et al. The use of contrast-enhanced magnetic resonance imaging to identify reversible myocardial dysfunction. *N Engl J Med*. 2000;343(20):1445–1453.

8. Tuttle RR, Pollock GD, Todd G, MacDonald B, Tust R, Dusenberry W. The effect of dobutamine on cardiac oxygen balance, regional blood flow, and infarction severity after coronary artery narrowing in dogs. *Circ Res*. 1977;41(3):357–364.

9. Schulz R, Rose J, Martin C, Brodde OE, Heusch G. Development of short-term myocardial hibernation. Its limitation by the severity of ischemia and inotropic stimulation. *Circulation*. 1993;88(2):684–695.

10. Willerson JT, Hutton I, Watson JT, Platt MR, Templeton GH. Influence of dobutamine on regional myocardial blood flow and ventricular performance during acute and chronic myocardial ischemia in dogs. *Circulation*. 1976;53(5):828–833.

11. Nagueh SF, Mikati I, Weilbaecher D, et al. Relation of the contractile reserve of hibernating myocardium to myocardial structure in humans. *Circulation*. 1999;100(5):490–496.

12. Poldermans D, Rambaldi R, Bax JJ, et al. Safety and utility of atropine addition during dobutamine stress echocardiography for the assessment of viable myocardium in patients with severe left ventricular dysfunction. *Eur Heart J*. 1998;19(11):1712–1718.

13. Meza MF, Kates MA, Barbee RW, et al. Combination of dobutamine and myocardial contrast echocardiography to differentiate postischemic from infarcted myocardium. *J Am Coll Cardiol*. 1997;29(5):974–984.

14. Hoffmann R, Altiok E, Nowak B, et al. Strain rate measurement by doppler echocardiography allows improved assessment of myocardial viability inpatients with depressed left ventricular function. *J Am Coll Cardiol*. 2002;39(3):443–449.

15. Ling LH, Christian TF, Mulvagh SL, et al. Determining myocardial viability in chronic ischemic left ventricular dysfunction: a prospective comparison of rest-redistribution thallium 201 single-photon emission computed tomography, nitroglycerin-dobutamine echocardiography, and intracoronary myocardial contrast echocardiography. *Am Heart J*. 2006;151(4): 882–889.

16. Chaudhry FA, Tauke JT, Alessandrini RS, Vardi G, Parker MA, Bonow RO. Prognostic implications of myocardial contractile reserve in patients with coronary artery disease and left ventricular dysfunction. *J Am Coll Cardiol*. 1999;34(3):730–738.

17. Cusick DA, Castillo R, Quigg RJ, Chaudhry FA, Bonow RO. Predictive accuracy of dobutamine stress echocardiography for identification of viable myocardium in patients with severely reduced left ventricular ejection fraction. *J Heart Lung Transplant*. 1997; 15(186S).

18. Bax JJ, Poldermans D, Elhendy A, Boersma E, Rahimtoola SH. Sensitivity, specificity, and predictive accuracies of various noninvasive techniques for detecting hibernating myocardium. *Curr Probl Cardiol*. 2001;26(2):147–186.

19. Afridi I, Kleiman NS, Raizner AE, Zoghbi WA. Dobutamine echocardiography in myocardial hibernation. Optimal dose and accuracy in predicting recovery of ventricular function after coronary angioplasty. *Circulation*. 1995;91(3):663–670.

20. Yao SS, Chaudhry FA. Assessment of myocardial viability with dobutamine stress echocardiography in patients with ischemic left ventricular dysfunction. *Echocardiography*. 2005;22(1):71 83.

21. Meluzin J, Cerny J, Frelich M, et al. Prognostic value of the amount of dysfunctional but viable myocardium in revascularized patients with coronary artery disease and left ventricular dysfunction. Investigators of this Multicenter Study. *J Am Coll Cardiol*. 1998;32(4):912–920.

22. Arnese M, Cornel JH, Salustri A, et al. Prediction of improvement of regional left ventricular function after surgical revascularization. A comparison of low dose dobutamine echocardiography with [201]Tl single-photon emission computed tomography. *Circulation*. 1995;91(11):2748–2752.

23. Bonow RO. Identification of viable myocardium. *Circulation*. 1996;94(11):2674–2680.

24. Bonow RO, Dilsizian V, Cuocolo A, Bacharach SL. Identification of viable myocardium in patients with chronic coronary artery disease and left ventricular dysfunction. Comparison of thallium scintigraphy with reinjection and PET imaging with 18F-fluorodeoxyglucose. *Circulation*. 1991;83(1):26–37.

25. Perrone-Filardi P, Bacharach SL, Dilsizian V, Maurea S, Frank JA, Bonow RO. Regional left ventricular wall thickening. Relation to regional uptake of 18 fluorodeoxyglucose and [201]Tl in patients with chronic coronary artery disease and left ventricular dysfunction. *Circulation*. 1992;86(4):1125–1137.

26. Helfant RH, Pine R, Meister SG, Feldman MS, Trout RG, Banka VS. Nitroglycerin to unmask reversible asynergy. Correlation with post coronary bypass ventriculography. *Circulation*. 1974;50(1):108–113.

27. Martinez RR, Bennett J, Eikman EA, Fontanet HL, Sayad DE. Comparison of nitroglycerin magnetic resonance imaging with dobutamine echocardiography for predicting recovery of function after revascularization. *Am J Cardiol*. 2000;85(10):1250–1252.

28. Fujita M, Yamanishi K, Hirai T, et al. Significance of collateral circulation in reversible left ventricular asynergy by nitroglycerin in patients with relatively recent myocardial infarction. *Am Heart J*. 1990;120(3):521–528.

29. Greco C, Tanzilli G, Ciavolella M, et al. Nitroglycerin-induced changes in myocardial sestamibi uptake to detect tissue viability: radionuclide comparison before and after revascularization. *Coron Artery Dis*. 1996;7(12):877–884.

30. Senior R, Swinburn JM. Incremental value of myocardial contrast echocardiography for the prediction of recovery of function in dobutamine nonresponsive myocardium early after acute myocardial infarction. *Am J Cardiol*. 2003;91(4):397–402.

31. Bax JJ, Wijns W, Cornel JH, et al. Accuracy of currently available techniques for prediction of functional recovery after revascularization in patients with left ventricular dysfunction due to chronic coronary artery disease: comparison of pooled data. *J Am Coll Cardiol*. November 15, 1997;30(6):1451–1460.

32. Cornel JH, Bax JJ, Elhendy A, et al. Biphasic response to dobutamine predicts improvement of global left ventricular function after surgical revascularization in patients with stable coronary artery disease. *J Am Coll Cardiol*. 1998;31:1002–1010.

# Chapter 25
# Pathway for the Management of Heart Failure Complicating Acute Coronary Syndrome

David Wild, Eyal Herzog, Emad Aziz, and Marrick Kukin

Patients presenting to the emergency department, with acute heart failure (AHF), pose a major health care problem.[1] Acute heart failure accounts for over 1,000,000 hospitalization in the United States with an in-hospital morality rate of 4.1%, and a mean length of stay of 6.5 days. Whether due to inadequate in-hospital treatment, refractory disease, noncompliance with diet or medications, or co-morbidities, there is a hospital readmission rate of 20% within 30 days, and 50% during the next 6–12-month interval. Additionally, there is a 10% mortality rate at 30 days, which increases to 20–40% at 12 months.[2]

Heart failure can occur in the setting of ACS (acute coronary syndrome) and acute MI (myocardial infarction). Other chapters in this book focus on the primary care of these conditions (i.e., angioplasty/revascularization) and treatment of mechanical complications associated with acute MI and heart failure. In this chapter, we will focus on the medical diagnosis and therapy of acute decompensated heart failure – both in the setting of ACS and in chronic heart failure patients with acute heart failure decompensation.

The American College of Cardiology and the American Heart Association have recently published revised guidelines for the management of chronic heart failure in adults.[2] The European Society of Cardiology has also developed guidelines for chronic heart failure.[3] Both sets of guidelines focus on outpatient management of chronic heart failure; treatment options for acutely decompensated heart failure (ADHF) and new onset heart failure are not addressed. To address this deficiency, we have developed a unified pathway for the management of patients presenting with AHF to the emergency department. This pathway is simple, yet comprehensive and covers the entire spectrum of patient care, from the time of ER presentation through their admission and the discharge plan (Fig. 25.1)

This pathway is not describing new treatments for heart failure. Rather it is an attempt to incorporate, in a user friendly format, the keys to initial diagnosis and management of heart failure. This is followed by a comprehensive guideline to therapy with a goal of shortening length of stay (LOS) without compromising on

D. Wild (✉)
Cardiovascular Associates; Teaneck, NJ, USA
e-mail: david.wild1@gmail.com

E. Herzog, F.A. Chaudhry (eds.), *Echocardiography in Acute Coronary Syndrome*,
DOI 10.1007/978-1-84882-027-2_25, © Springer-Verlag London Limited 2009

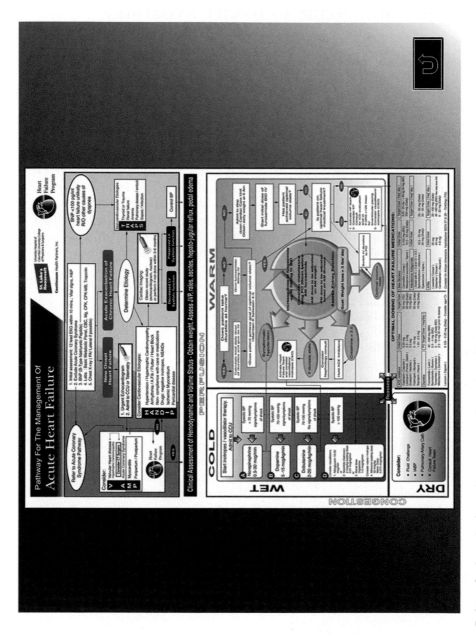

**Fig. 25.1** Pathway for the evaluation and management of acute heart failure

medical stabilization, optimal diuresis, and implementation of outpatient therapies based on the proven results of clinical trials. While the use of aggressive loop diuretics with daily weight monitoring is empirically derived from our clinical experience, the usage and dosing of the other medications are derived from clinical trials[2] and published ACLS guidelines.[4]

The ESCAPE trial[5] evaluated the use of the pulmonary artery catheter in patients admitted with decompensated heart failure. The results demonstrated that outcomes are not improved by invasive hemodynamic monitoring for the patients that would generally be eligible for the pathway described herein. A careful history and physical exam combined with clinical judgment and incorporation of clinically proven therapies are the guiding principles in the development of this pathway.

## Diagnosis

The first step in the management of the patient with heart failure is a rapid but thorough evaluation of the patient in the emergency department. This includes a 12-lead EKG within 10 min, vital signs, H&P, Labs, and Chest X-ray. The primary goal is to exclude an acute coronary syndrome which would lead to different, more aggressive therapy. In addition, one can obtain a BNP level to exclude noncardiovascular causes of dyspnea[6] when the diagnosis of heart failure may be in doubt (Fig. 25.2).

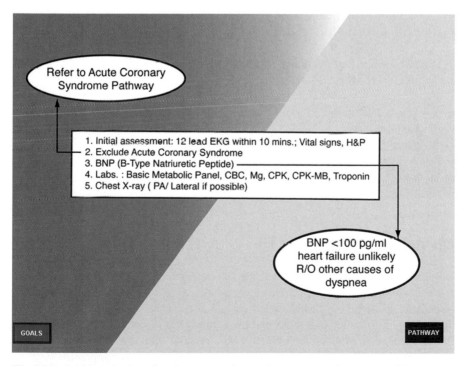

**Fig. 25.2**  Initial evaluation of patients presenting to the emergency department with suspected acute heart failure (AHF)

The development of assays for the natriuretic peptides (NPs), brain NP (BNP), and *N*-terminal pro-BNP (NT-proBNP) has become increasingly important for the evaluation of dyspneic patients, and depending on the results of clinical trials it may prove useful to guide treatment of congestive heart failure.

## New Onset HF vs. Acute Exacerbation of Chronic HF

The next diagnostic step would be to differentiate between new onset heart failure and acute exacerbations of chronic heart failure. This early recognition emphasizes that new onset heart failure is an urgent situation, which may require cardiothoracic surgery involvement for reversible causes. If the heart failure is felt to be new onset, the patient should have an urgent echocardiogram. If the heart failure is felt to be an exacerbation of chronic heart failure, it is necessary to determine the etiology of the decompensation by considering causes with the reminder acronym, **HANDIP:**

- H – Hypertension
- A – Arrhythmias: atrial fibrillation, atrial flutter, heart block
- N – Noncompliance with care (i.e., diet, fluid excess) or medications
- D – Drugs: negative inotropes (i.e., calcium channel blockers), nonsteroidals (NSAIDs), alcohol, illicit drug use
- I – Ischemic myocardium
- P – Pericardial disease

In addition, noncardiovascular causes of heart failure should be considered using the acronym, **TRAPS** as a guide:

- T – Thyroid or trauma
- R – Renal failure
- A – Anemia
- P – Pulmonary disease, pulmonary emboli
- S – Sepsis, infection

## The Role of Echo in Acute HF

Patients with new onset heart failure must have an echocardiogram to rule out emergent reversible causes. The primary emergent etiologies to exclude are valvular diseases, such as a flail mitral leaflet and critical aortic stenosis. In addition, in acute coronary syndrome patients who exhibit hemodynamic collapse, an echocardiogram is needed to evaluate for ischemic MR, papillary muscle rupture, ventricular septal defect, or free wall rupture. These complications are all generally surgical

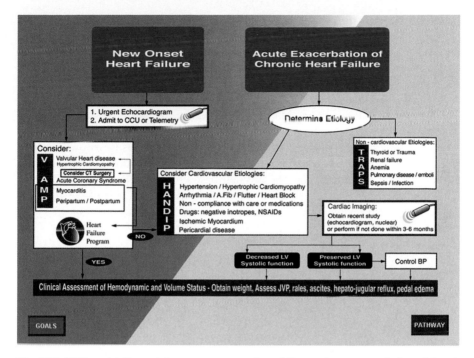

**Fig. 25.3** Differential diagnosis between new onset heart failure and acute exacerbation of chronic heart failure with timing of imaging and consideration of precipitating pathophysiology

indications. Nonemergent etiologies such as myocarditis and peripartum cardiomyopathy can also be confirmed by echocardiogram under the appropriate clinical circumstances (Fig. 25.3).

## The Role of Cardiac Catheterization in New Onset Heart Failure

For newly diagnosed heart failure, is routine cardiac catheterization indicated? In the absence of angina, diagnostic electrocardiogram of ischemia, or multiple coronary risk factors, the answer is not clear. Certainly, when there is an index of suspicion, all reversible causes of heart failure, such as ischemia, must be considered. However, in a young patient with no coronary risk factors, the risks of cardiac catheterization must be carefully weighed against the low probability of finding coronary artery disease. When in doubt, we would err on the side of performing a cardiac catheterization. However, in the absence of anginal symptoms or multiple risk factors, the majority of these procedures document clean coronaries. A second procedure often debated is endomyocardial biopsy.[2] This is not recommended in the practice guidelines (level of evidence = C).

## Bedside Assessment

Cardiac imaging is utilized to determine whether LV function is decreased or preserved as this distinction effects therapy. Once the etiology has been established
the next phase of management is rapid clinical assessment of hemodynamics based
on perfusion and congestion.[7,8] This assessment is based on bedside examination:
whether the clinical symptoms indicate the adequacy of filling pressure/perfusion
(warm or cold) and the volume status of the patient based on history and physical
exam (wet or dry) (Fig. 25.4). The sizing of the four quadrants (warm-wet, warm-
dry, cold-wet, cold-dry) is not equal, reflecting the actual proportionate distribution
of these patient admissions into the hospital based on their clinical presentation.[8]
Thus, the group of warm-wet patients is visually the largest part of the pathway
emphasizing their relative frequency compared to all HF admissions (Fig. 25.4).

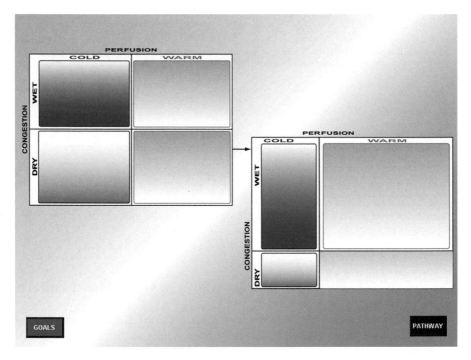

**Fig. 25.4** Depiction of perfusion and congestion concept with consideration of disproportionate
group size of each quadrant

## Therapy

The determination of volume status will have implications in the pharmacologic
management of the patient. Most patients admitted with symptomatic heart failure
will have warm-wet physiology and the key in their management will be aggressive

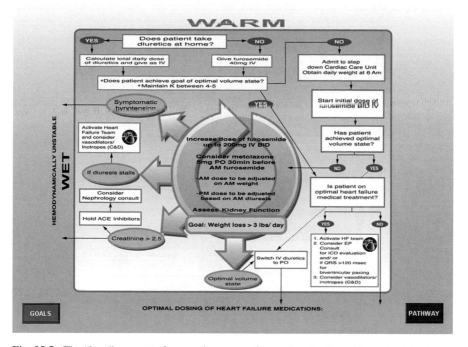

**Fig. 25.5**  The "loop" concept of aggressive usage of loop diuretics to rapidly and safely diurese patients, shorten length of stay (LOS) and transition to oral therapy upon successful completion of diuresis

loop diuretic management (Fig. 25.5). This recognition and early aggressive treatment are the keys to decreasing the length of in-hospital stay. Three major decisions regarding pharmacological treatment need to be addressed based on the hemodynamic assessment: What regimen of diuretic should be used? If the patient is on chronic therapy with beta blockers, should it be discontinued or reduced? Does the patient require inotropes? In Fig. 25.5, the algorithm shows the optimal method of deciding appropriate diuretic doses. If the patient has been taking oral diuretics as an outpatient, that total daily dose should be given intravenously as a bolus infusion. If the patient has not been taking diuretics, the patient should be given an intravenous loop diuretic (i.e., furosemide 40 mg).

Once an optimal volume state is achieved then the patient can be changed to oral therapy and begun on a chronic heart failure regimen. If the patient does not initially achieve a euvolemic state, then the patient should be admitted to a monitored setting and have the diuretic dose doubled and given twice daily. If this still does not work, the dose of diuretic can be increased and consideration given to adding other diuretics, such as metolazone. If there is difficulty in achieving a euvolemic state or if the patient develops symptomatic hypotension or a significant increase in serum creatinine, which together can signify a low-flow state, the patient should be started on appropriate inotropic therapy (Fig. 25.6). Guidelines of management of

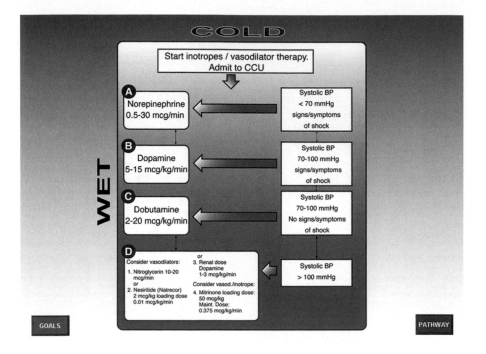

**Fig. 25.6** Management of hemodynamically unstable heart failure patients adapted from ACLS guidelines

hemodynamically unstable patients are based on the ACLS Guidelines, incorporating vasodilators and inotropic infusions.[4] In these circumstances it is appropriate to activate the heart failure team (if there is one present at the institution).

## Beta Blockers

The next question is what to do if the patient is chronically being treated with beta blockers. The use of beta blockers in chronic heart failure has been well established in multiple randomized trials.[9–11] However, the majority of heart failure patients we encounter in the hospital are in decompensated heart failure. It is in these patients where there is ambiguity as to the role of beta blockers. There are no clear guidelines as to whether to stop or reduce the dose of the beta blocker.

There are two major questions yet to be answered regarding beta blockers and acutely decompensated heart failure: (1) In patients currently taking beta blockers should the beta blocker be held completely or have the dose reduced when these patients are admitted with fluid overloaded states? (2) In these patients who are admitted with acute exacerbations of heart failure who have not been on chronic beta blocker therapy, when is it safe to start a beta blocker?

The theoretical concern with continuing beta blockers in decompensated heart failure is that administration of a beta blocker may exacerbate the fluid overload state due to its negative inotropic effects. However, there is no data to suggest that this is true. On the other hand it may be desirable to continue beta blockers because doing so may help avoid the long process of having to uptitrate the medications and may decrease the delay of ultimately reaching target doses. In addition there is data suggesting that patients with systolic dysfunction have poorer outcomes after stopping beta blocker therapy.[12,13] Recently, two studies have examined the safety of continuing beta blocker therapy in patients admitted with acutely decompensated heart failure.[14,15] These studies examined two large data bases of heart failure patients admitted with fluid overload, the OPTIME-CHF and ESCAPE databases. However, these studies have shown that continuing beta blockers during the hospitalization is not associated with an increase in adverse outcomes, and even suggest that there may be improved outcomes in patients in whom the beta blockers are continued. These studies were observational and nonrandomized and therefore cannot be used as definitive evidence.

In view of these recent developments and lack of randomized studies examining beta blocker therapy in this group of patients, we recommend the following: In patients who are "Warm and Wet" upon hospitalization with no evidence of poor perfusion or low-flow state, such as pre-renal azotemia, and not requiring intubation or bipap for respiratory distress, the beta blocker should be continued at the same dose as outpatient. However, if there is difficulty after 24−48 h in achieving a euvolemic state, then the dose should be reduced to 50% or stopped entirely. In the very small population of "cold and wet" patients requiring inotropic therapy for low-flow state, the beta blocker should be discontinued altogether until there is significant improvement in the fluid status. Thought should be given to the choice of inotropic therapy because of differential effects of the various inotropes depending on which beta blocker the patient was on chronically. Data suggest that patients on carvedilol do not respond as well to dobutamine as to milrinone, a phosphodiesterase inhibitor.[16–18]

In patients admitted with decompensated heart failure who are not already taking beta blockers, there is controversy regarding the appropriate time to initiate therapy. HFSA guidelines recommend that beta blockers should not be initiated during a hospitalization for an exacerbation of heart failure.[19] However, in the IMPACT-HF trial published in 2004, they conclude that predischarge initiation of beta blockers improves the probability of use of beta blockers at subsequent visits without increasing side effects or length of stay.[20] We recommend starting therapy with an approved beta blocker at the lowest dose once patients are felt to be euvolemic. Outpatient uptitration as tolerated to target doses as established in mortality trials should follow.

## Oral Medications

Once patients are stabilized and are felt to be euvolemic, attention should be given to placing the patient on an optimal medical regimen (Fig. 25.7).[21] Although representative, not all medications in some categories are included in the chart due

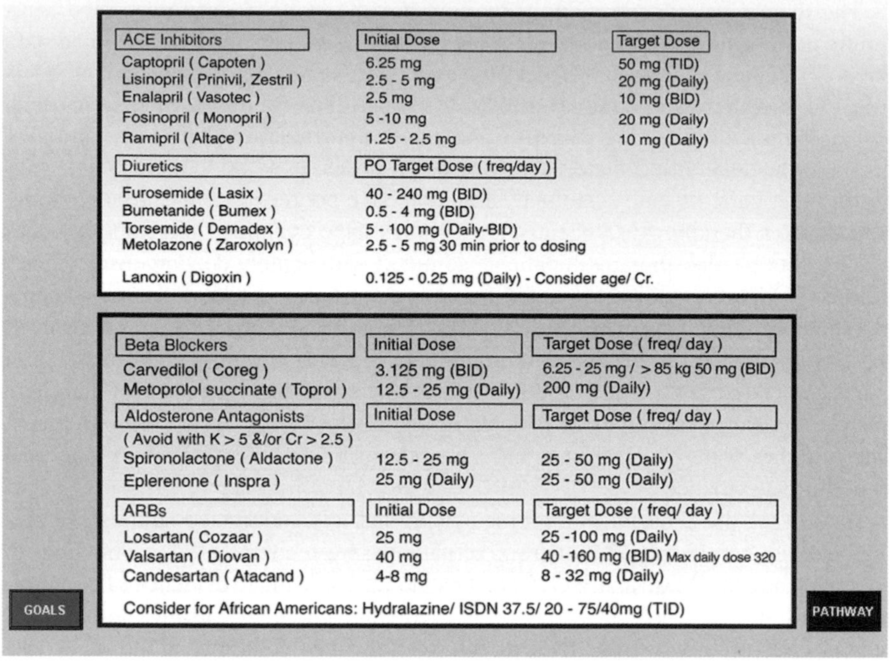

| ACE Inhibitors | Initial Dose | Target Dose |
|---|---|---|
| Captopril ( Capoten ) | 6.25 mg | 50 mg (TID) |
| Lisinopril ( Prinivil, Zestril ) | 2.5 - 5 mg | 20 mg (Daily) |
| Enalapril ( Vasotec ) | 2.5 mg | 10 mg (BID) |
| Fosinopril ( Monopril ) | 5 -10 mg | 20 mg (Daily) |
| Ramipril ( Altace ) | 1.25 - 2.5 mg | 10 mg (Daily) |

| Diuretics | PO Target Dose ( freq/day ) |
|---|---|
| Furosemide ( Lasix ) | 40 - 240 mg (BID) |
| Bumetanide ( Bumex ) | 0.5 - 4 mg (BID) |
| Torsemide ( Demadex ) | 5 - 100 mg (Daily-BID) |
| Metolazone ( Zaroxolyn ) | 2.5 - 5 mg 30 min prior to dosing |
| Lanoxin ( Digoxin ) | 0.125 - 0.25 mg (Daily) - Consider age/ Cr. |

| Beta Blockers | Initial Dose | Target Dose ( freq/ day ) |
|---|---|---|
| Carvedilol ( Coreg ) | 3.125 mg (BID) | 6.25 - 25 mg / > 85 kg 50 mg (BID) |
| Metoprolol succinate ( Toprol ) | 12.5 - 25 mg (Daily) | 200 mg (Daily) |

| Aldosterone Antagonists | Initial Dose | Target Dose ( freq/ day ) |
|---|---|---|
| ( Avoid with K > 5 &/or Cr > 2.5 ) | | |
| Spironolactone ( Aldactone ) | 12.5 - 25 mg | 25 - 50 mg (Daily) |
| Eplerenone ( Inspra ) | 25 mg (Daily) | 25 - 50 mg (Daily) |

| ARBs | Initial Dose | Target Dose ( freq/ day ) |
|---|---|---|
| Losartan( Cozaar ) | 25 mg | 25 -100 mg (Daily) |
| Valsartan ( Diovan ) | 40 mg | 40 -160 mg (BID) Max daily dose 320 |
| Candesartan ( Atacand ) | 4-8 mg | 8 - 32 mg (Daily) |

GOALS    Consider for African Americans: Hydralazine/ ISDN 37.5/ 20 - 75/40mg (TID)    PATHWAY

**Fig. 25.7** Initiation and target dosages of oral heart failure medications

to space constraints. Early ambulation of these patients during their hospital stay and exercise regiments are encouraged. In addition, for appropriate patients, a heart failure and or an EPS (electrophysiology) consult should be considered because current therapy for heart failure now encompasses electrical devices and close collaboration with electrophysiologists. Incorporated into the pathway is the timing and consideration of biventricular pacemakers (BIVPM) in patients with wide QRS complexes and the consideration of implantable defibrillators (ICD) based on MADIT-2,[22] SCD-HEFT,[23] and COMPANION[24] criteria (Fig. 25.5).

This acute heart failure pathway flows as the patient progresses toward the warm/dry group which is a segue to outpatient management of heart failure. The AHA/ACC[2] and European guidelines[3] detail the major trials and dosing of the appropriate heart failure medications. The key point in this algorithm is that upon discharge, all HF patients should be on, at a minimum, starting doses of ACEI and β-blockers, unless contraindicated. Angiotensin receptor blockers (ARBs) should be used instead of ACEI when ACEI cannot be given, (i.e., ACEI-induced cough). In certain instances it may be appropriate to combine an ACEI and ARB.[25] Data from RALES[26] and EPHESUS[27] would support the addition of aldosterone antagonists with the precaution of monitoring potassium and creatinine levels on therapy.[28]

With the recent publication of the results of A-HeFT,[29] consideration should be given to the addition of hydralazine/isosorbide dinitrate in African Americans. Most

US physicians use digoxin for patients with NYHA class III/IV heart failure with an age/creatinine nomogram. Dosages of oral diuretics should be adjusted to maintain the euvolemic state achieved during the hospitalization, along with adherence to a 2 g sodium diet and daily weight monitoring. A motivated patient with a home scale can be taught to self adjust diuretics based on his/her morning weight.

# References

1. Fonarow GC, Weber JE. Rapid clinical assessment of hemodynamic profiles and targeted treatment of patients with acutely decompensated heart failure. *Clin. Cardiol.* 2004;27 (suppl V):V-1–V-9.
2. Hunt SA, Baker DW, Chin MH, et al. ACC/AHA Guidelines for the Evaluation and Management of Chronic Heart Failure in the Adult: A report of American College of Cardiology/American Heart Association Task Force on Practice Guidelines (Committee to Revise the 1995 Guidelines for the Evaluation and Management of Heart Failure) 2001. American College of Cardiology website. Available at: http://www.heartfailureguideline.org  *J Am Coll Cardiol.* 2001;38:2101–2113.
3. Remme WJ, Swedberg K. Comprehensive guidelines for the diagnosis and treatment of chronic heart failure. Task force for the diagnosis and treatment of chronic heart failure of the European Society of Cardiology. *Eur J Heart Fail.* January 2002;4(1):11–22.
4. Mary FH, Richard OC, John MF. *AHA 2000 Handbook of Emergency Cardiovascular Care for Healthcare Providers.* Dallas, TX: American Heart Association.
5. Shah MR, Stevenson LW. *Evaluation Study of Congestive Heart Failure and Pulmonary Artery Catheterization Effectiveness (ESCAPE).* New Orleans, LA: American Heart Association Scientific Sessions, September 11, 2004.
6. Maisel SA, Krishnaswamy P, Nowak, RM, et al. Rapid measurement of B-Type natriuretic peptide in the emergency diagnosis of heart failure. *N Engl J Med.* 2002;347:161–167.
7. Stevenson LW. Tailored therapy of hemodynamic goals for advanced heart failure. *Eur J Heart Fail.* 1999;1:252–257.
8. Nohria A, Tsang SW, Fang JC, et al. Clinical assessment identifies hemodynamic profiles that predict outcomes in patients admitted with heart failure. *J Am Coll Cardiol.* 2003;41: 1797–1804.
9. Packer M, Coats AJ, Fowler MB, et al. Effect of carvedilol on survival in severe chronic heart failure. *N Engl J Med.* 2001;344:1651–1658.
10. Metoprolol CR/XL. Randomised intervention trial in congestive heart failure (MERIT-HF). *Lancet.* 1999;353:2001–2007.
11. Packer M, Bristow MR, Cohn JN, et al. The effect of carvedilol on morbidity and mortality in patients with chronic heart failure. U.S. Carvedilol Heart Failure Study Group. *N Engl J Med.* 1996;334:1349–1355.
12. Morimoto S, Shimizu K, Yamada K, Hiramitsu S, Hishida H. Can beta-blocker therapy be withdrawn from patients with dilated cardiomyopathy? *Am Heart J.* 1999;138:456–459.
13. Waagstein F, Caidahl K, Wallentin I, Bergh CH, Hjalmarson A. Long term beta blockade in dilated cardiomyopathy. Effects of short- and long-term metoprolol treatment followed by withdrawal and readministration of metoprolol. *Circulation.* 1989;80:551–563.
14. Gattis WA, O'Connor CM, Leimberger JD, Felker GM, Adams KF, Gheorghiade M. Clinical outcomes in patients on beta-blocker therapy admitted with worsening chronic heart failure. *Am J Cardiol.* 2003;91:169–174.
15. Butler J, Young JB, Abraham WT, et al. Beta-blocker use and outcomes among hospitalized heart failure patients. *J Am Coll Cardiol.* 2006;47:2462–2469.
16. Lowes BD, Tsvetkova T, Eichhorn EJ, Gilbert EM, Bristow MR. Milrinone versus dobutamine in heart failure subjects treated chronically with carvedilol. *Int J Cardiol.* 2001;81:141–149.

17. Metra M, Nodari S, D'Aloia A, et al. Beta-Blocker therapy influences the hemodynamic response to inotropic agents in patients with heart failure: a randomized comparison of dobutamine and enoximone before and after chronic treatment with metoprolol or carvedilol. *J Am Coll Cardiol.* 2002;40:1248–1258.

18. Bollano E, Tang MS, Hjalmarson A, Waagstein F, Andersson B. Different responses to dobutamine in the presence of carvedilol or metoprolol in patients with chronic heart failure. *Heart.* 2003;89:621–624.

19. Heart Failure Society of America Guideline Committee. HFSA guidelines for the management of patients with heart failure caused by left ventricular systolic dysfunction: pharmacologic approaches. *J Card Fail.* 1999;5:357–382.

20. Gattis WA, O'Connor CM, Gallup DS, Hasselblad V, Gheorghiade M, IMPACT-HF Investigators and Coordinators. Predischarge initiation of carvedilol in patients hospitalized for decompensated heart failure: results of the Initiation Management Predischarge: process for Assessment of Carvedilol Therapy in Heart Failure (IMPACT-HF) trial. *J Am Coll Cardiol.* 2004;43:1534–1541.

21. Bukharovich IF, Kukin ML. Optimal medical therapy for heart failure. *Prog Cardiovasc Dis.* 2005; In press.

22. Moss AJ, Zareba W, Hall WJ, et al. Prohylactic implantation of a defibrillator in patients with myocardial infraction and reduced ejection fraction. *N Engl J Med.* 2002;346:877–883.

23. Bardy GH, Lee KL, Mark DB, et al. Amiodarone or an implantable cardioverter-defibrillator for congestive heart failure. *N Engl J Med.* 2005;352:225–237.

24. Bristow MR, Saxon LA, Boehmer J, et al. Cardiac-resynchronization therapy with or without an implantable defibrillator in advance chronic heart failure. *N Eng J Med.* 2004;350:2140–2150.

25. McMurray JJV, Östergren J, Sweedberg K, et al. Effects of candesartan in patients with chronic heart failure and reduced left-ventricular systolic function taking angiotensin-converting-enzyme inhibitors; the CHARM-Added trial. *Lancet.* 2003;362:767–771.

26. Pitt B, Zannad F, Remme WJ, et al. The effect of spironolactone on morbidity and mortality in patients with severe heart failure. *N Engl J Med.* 1999;341:709–717.

27. Pitt B, Willem R, Zannad F, et al. Eplerenone, a selective aldosterone blocker, in patients with ventricular dysfunction after myocardial infraction. *N Engl J Med.* 2003;348:1309–1321.

28. Juurklink D, Mamdani MM, Lee DS, et al. Rates of hyperkalemia after publication of the randomized aldactone evaluation study. *N Engl J Med.* 2004;351:543–551.

29. Taylor AL, Ziesche S, Yancy C, et al. Combination of isosorbride dinitrate and hydralazine in blacks with heart failure. *N Engl J Med.* 2004;351:2049–2057.

# Chapter 26
# Echocardiography for the Management of End Stage Ischemic Heart Disease and as a Tool for Resynchronization Therapy

**Ajay S. Shah, Farooq A. Chaudhry, Rawa Sarji, and Bilal Ayub**

**Abbreviation** CRT, cardiac resynchronization therapy; EF, ejection fraction; HF, heart failure; ICD, implantable cardioverter-defibrillator; LV, left ventricle/ventricular; LVEDP, left ventricular end-diastolic pressure; LVOT, left ventricular outflow tract; TDI, tissue Doppler imaging; SF, systolic fraction of pulmonary venous forward flow; VAD, ventricular assist device; Vp, flow propagation slope of early diastolic left ventricular filling

## Introduction

This chapter will discuss: (1) the clinical uses of echocardiography in HF after acute coronary syndrome and its prognostic value; (2) the use of echocardiography to guide treatment in HF patients; and (3) promising future techniques for echocardiographic-based imaging in HF. In addition, we will highlight some of the limitations of echocardiography.

According to the recently released American College of Cardiology/American Heart Association (ACC/AHA) guidelines for the diagnosis and management of heart failure (HF), "Echocardiography is the single most useful diagnostic test in the evaluation of patients with HF…," because of its ability to accurately and noninvasively provide measures of ventricular function, assess causes of structural heart disease[1] define the hemodynamic and morphologic changes in heart failure (HF), and guide therapy. An estimated five million people have HF, and their ranks are increased by an estimated 550,000 each year.[2] Heart failure hospital stays have increased 150% over the last 20 years.[2] The lifetime risk of developing HF has been estimated at 20% for the U.S. population. And, although ischemic heart disease is the most common cause of HF, up to 11% of the population without evidence for coronary artery disease will also develop HF.[3]

A.S. Shah (✉)
Cardiology, St Luke's-Roosevelt Hospital Center, New York, NY, USA
e-mail: ashah@chpnet.org

E. Herzog, F.A. Chaudhry (eds.), *Echocardiography in Acute Coronary Syndrome*, DOI 10.1007/978-1-84882-027-2_26, © Springer-Verlag London Limited 2009

Heart failure is classically described as left ventricular (LV) dysfunction leading to congestion and reduced systemic perfusion, most often manifesting symptomatically as dyspnea and fatigue. After an insult to the myocardium like acute coronary syndrome, the LV progressively dilates or hypertrophies, a process followed by spherical remodeling. These morphologic changes cause further stress on the myocardium by increasing wall tension and cause or exacerbate mitral regurgitation, which, in turn, results in further dilatation and contractile dysfunction in a vicious cycle.[1] Such remodeling is often the final common pathway for many although not all etiologies of HF.

Because this morphologic process begins before the onset of symptoms, the recent HF guidelines place special emphasis on detecting subclinical LV systolic and diastolic dysfunction.[1,4] Several studies have emphasized that standard physical examination maneuvers are suboptimal in detecting either systolic or diastolic LV dysfunction, especially in the preclinical phase. Similarly, physical examination is limited in its ability to accurately characterize the volume and cardiac output status in patients with LV dysfunction.[5,6] As a rapid and accurate modality, echocardiography can improve the noninvasive detection and definition of the hemodynamic and morphologic changes in HF. Echocardiography might also be equivalent to catheter-based techniques in guiding therapy and improving outcomes, without the risks and cost of invasive measures.[5] The 2D-derived measurements of volume and chamber dimensions of both right and left ventricle are quick and easily measurable online and have immense prognostic implication. They are limited by image quality, overestimated due to foreshortening, and require geometric assumptions. They may not correlate with clinical status. They have considerable inter and intraobserver variability. The Doppler-derived hemodynamics are quick and easy to measure online; however, it may be limited particularly in critical patients due to inability to obtain a parallel alignment of Doppler beam. The signals of pulmonary and tricuspid valve flow may be difficult to obtain. The stroke volume may be overestimated with associated valvular pathology like aortic regurgitation. Similarly, Doppler-derived diastolic parameters are heart rate and load dependent.

The real-time 3D for EF and volume measurement eliminates foreshortening, geometric assumptions not required and simultaneous assessment of all wall segments can be done with a multiplane probe. They are limited by image quality, expense of software and probe, incremental value over 2D not well established, technical expertise and training required and it is not widely available. Tissue Doppler, strain, and strain rate have been shown to have prognostic value, most parameters load independent, widely available (tissue velocity), and less dependent on image quality. However it is also angle dependent, requires off-line analysis and has low signal/noise ratio. The tissue tracking or velocity vector imaging is not angle dependent and able to assess torsional mechanics. However it requires extra expense of software, incremental value over TDI not well established, speckles move in and out of plane (requires mathematical assumptions to compensate), requires off-line analysis, and is not widely available.

## Clinical Measurements and Prognosis

Used for many years to provide structural correlates to the clinical picture of HF, echocardiography can also measure multiple clinically important parameters of cardiac function, including hemodynamic status and LV ejection fraction (EF), volumes, and mass.

## *Hemodynamics*

Intracardiac pressure measurements have traditionally required invasive methods. This limitation, which also precludes serial measurements outside of the intensive care context, can often be circumvented with the use of echocardiographic techniques. In selected patients, echocardiography might be a noninvasive surrogate (Fig. 26.1). Stroke volume and cardiac output can be estimated from the velocity–time integral obtained by pulse wave Doppler recordings in the left ventricular outflow tract (LVOT), multiplied by the LVOT area. Figure 26.1 illustrates the echocardiographic estimates of right atrial pressure, right ventricular systolic pressure/pulmonary artery systolic pressure, and pulmonary artery mean and diastolic pressures.[7–9] All of these measurements require adequate imaging windows and parallel alignment of the Doppler cursor with blood flow to avoid underestimation of Doppler jet velocity and calculated pressure. Stroke volume as measured in the LVOT is overestimated in the presence of significant aortic insufficiency. Small errors in the measurement of LVOT diameter lead to large errors in the calculation of LVOT area. Pulmonary artery pressure estimates require the presence of tricuspid valve regurgitation for systolic pressure and pulmonic valve regurgitation for mean and diastolic pressures as well as an accurate estimate of right atrial pressure.[10]

A variety of echocardiographic techniques can determine abnormal diastolic function, increased left atrial pressure, and left ventricular end-diastolic pressure (LVEDP). These measurements have demonstrated considerable prognostic value in symptomatic and asymptomatic patients with either preserved or abnormal LV systolic function.[11] The adverse prognosis associated with systolic dysfunction is well described, but isolated diastolic HF also carries a poor prognosis, including future development of systolic HF.[12]

Diastolic function can be characterized according to severity. Mild diastolic dysfunction – abnormal LV relaxation – can be detected via a decrease in early diastolic flow velocity (E-wave) and a greater reliance on atrial contraction (A-wave) to fill the LV (E/A <1). Moderate diastolic dysfunction – "pseudo normalization" – reflects increasing left atrial pressure at the onset of diastole and an increase in early diastolic flow velocity to a level near that of normal filling (E/A 1–1.5). Severe diastolic dysfunction – restrictive filling – occurs when left atrial pressure is further elevated such that early diastolic flow is extremely rapid and left atrial and LV pressures equalize quickly during early diastole (E/A >2, DT <115–150 ms). Reduction in preload with the Valsalva maneuver can unmask diastolic dysfunction by

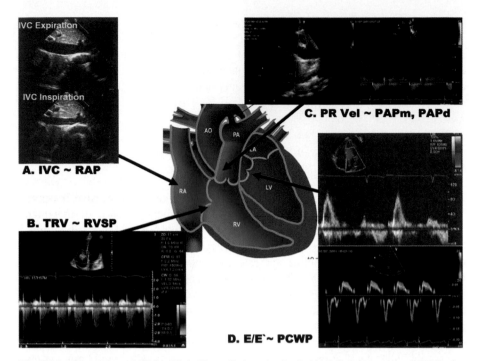

**Fig. 26.1**  Illustration of "Echo Right Heart Catheterization". (**A**) Inferior vena caval (IVC) size and degree of collapse yield a range of right atrial pressure (RAP): <1.5 cm with full collapse = RAP 0–5 mmHg; 1.5–2.5 cm with >50% collapse = RAP 6–10 mmHg; 1.5–2.5 cm with <50% collapse = RAP 11–15 mmHg; >2.5 cm with >50% collapse = RAP 16–20 mmHg; and >2.5 cm with <50% collapse = RAP >20 mmHg. (**B**) The tricuspid regurgitant velocity (TR Vel) is used to estimate the systolic right ventricle–right atrium gradient (and the pulmonary artery systolic pressure, in the absence of pulmonic stenosis). (**C**) The maximal pulmonic valve regurgitant velocity is used to estimate the mean pulmonary artery pressure (PAPm). The end-diastolic pulmonic regurgitant velocity is used to estimate diastolic pulmonary artery pressure (PAPd). (**D**) The early mitral inflow (E-wave)/early diastolic mitral valve annular motion (E'-wave) ratio <8 or >15 is calculated to assess PCWP <15 mmHg or >15 mmHg, respectively. E/E' = ratio of early diastolic mitral inflow velocity to early diastolic velocity of the mitral valve annulus; IVC = inferior vena cava; PCWP = pulmonary capillary wedge pressure; PR Vel. = pulmonic valve regurgitant velocity; RVSP = right ventricular systolic pressure (Source: Kirkpatrick J. Echocardiography in Heart Failure. *Journal of the American College of Cardiology*. 2007;50(5): 381–396)

changing a pseudo normalized pattern to an abnormal relaxation pattern or a restrictive pattern to a pseudo normalized one.[13,14] Persistence of a restrictive filling pattern during the Valsalva maneuver or on follow-up echocardiogram after HF therapy portends a particularly grim prognosis, as shown by Pinamonti et al.[15] and others. These traditional techniques, however, are dependent on heart rate and loading conditions and lack validity in patients with preserved EF.

Additional parameters such as (1) an abnormal ratio of the systolic and diastolic velocities of pulmonary venous inflow (S/D <1); (2) a systolic fraction of pulmonary venous forward flow (SF) of <40%; and (3) an early LV filling flow propagation slope (Vp) of <45 cm/s are less dependent on loading conditions and heart rate and have been shown to be robust predictors of high LV filling pressures and cardiovascular mortality.[16,17] These measures are limited by inability to adequately image the pulmonary veins in some patients and by the limited reproducibility of Vp. A ratio of peak early mitral inflow velocity (E) to peak early diastolic myocardial velocity (E′) of = 8 predicts an LVEDP of <15 mmHg, whereas a ratio of >15 predicts an elevated LVEDP (− 15 mmHg) (Fig. 26.1D).[11] The ratio of peak early mitral inflow velocity to slope of the propagation velocity (E/Vp) of = 1.5 predicts an LVEDP >15 mmHg and has been shown to have prognostic value in post-myocardial infarction patients.[18] Increased left atrial volumes (>32 ml/m$^2$), which are usually larger in diastolic compared with systolic HF, have been shown to predict morbidity.[19] Among multiple diastolic parameters in patients with a broad range of EF and degrees of mitral regurgitation, Rossi et al.[20] have demonstrated that a >30-ms difference between pulmonary vein atrial flow reversal and mitral A-wave durations was the most sensitive predictor of elevated LVEDP >18 mmHg. Interestingly, E/E′ has proven superior to brain natriuretic peptide (BNP) levels in diagnosing volume overload, even in patients with preserved systolic function.[21,22] Tables 26.1 and 26.2 list patient population,[23] Doppler modality, cutoff values, and outcome measures used in a variety of prognostic studies of diastolic function and filling pressures.[12,15,16,19,24–42] Figure 26.2A and B depicts strategies for using Doppler techniques to noninvasively estimate filling pressures and characterize the severity of diastolic dysfunction in patients with reduced EF. The strategies reflect the fact that synthesis of multiple parameters is often required to give an assessment of filling dynamics, particularly when poor acoustic windows might limit the ability to make every measurement.

## The Myocardial Performance Index

The myocardial performance index (better known as the Tei index) is a simple Doppler parameter that provides global assessment of systolic and diastolic function. The Tei index consists of the ratio of the isovolumic contraction + isovolumic relaxation times/the ejection time – all parameters that can be obtained from Doppler interrogation. The Tei index is independent of heart rate and blood pressure, applies to left and right ventricular systolic and diastolic dysfunction, does not rely on geometric assumptions, and is highly reproducible, although normal values vary with age.[43,44] It has been correlated with invasively measured changes in LV dP/dt.[45] The prognostic value of the Tei index was initially tested in patients with infiltrative cardiomyopathy and pulmonary hypertension.[46] It has subsequently been validated in patients with dilated cardiomyopathy, with a value of >0.77 proving superior to EF in predicting cardiac death and disease severity.[47] The Tei index also proved beneficial in predicting the development of HF in a cohort of elderly men without baseline LV dysfunction[48] and in predicting the lack of clinical response to medical treatment in a study including both patients with systolic HF and HF with preserved systolic function.[49] Because adequate Doppler images can often be acquired when

**Table 26.1** Prognostic significance of echocardiographic diastolic dysfunction measures: single component studies

| Modality | Patient population | Cutoff values | Outcome |
|---|---|---|---|
| **Mitral inflow Doppler** | | | |
| E/A | 2,671 Elderly patients, no CVD | <0.7 or >1.5 | Incident HF |
| E/A | 1,839 Hypertensive patients | Age- and heart rate-adjusted ratio below median | Cardiovascular events |
| E/A | 3,008 Native Americans | <0.6 or >1.5 | Death or cardiac death |
| DT | 110 Patients, EF <50%, no CAD | <115 ms, persisting after 3 months' HF treatment | Death or transplant at 4 years |
| Peak E | 2,671 Elderly, no CVD | Continuous | Incident HF |
| DT | 571 Patients post-AMI | <130 ms | Death at 4 years |
| DT | 79 HF patients, no CAD | <115 ms | Death or transplant |
| **M-mode IVRT** | 185 Elderly HF patients | ≤ 30 ms | Death |
| **Pulmonary vein Doppler** | | | |
| PV AR dur–MV A dur | 145 LV dysfunction patients | ≥30 ms | Cardiac death or hospital stay |
| S/D | 115 Patients, EF <45% | <1 | HF hospital readmission or HF death at 1 year |
| **Tissue Doppler** | | | |
| E/E' | 250 Patients post-AMI | >15 | Death |
| E/E' | 45 Patients, NYHA functional class III or IV HF | Continuous | Predictor of NYHA functional class, HF hospital stay, cardiac death |
| E/E' | 130 Chronic HF patients | >12.5 | Composite: cardiac death, HF hospital stay, urgent transplant |
| E/E' | 110 Patients hospitalized with HF | ≥ 15 | Cardiac death or hospital readmission for HF |
| E', E/E' | 518 Patients referred for echocardiography | E' <3 or 3–5 cm/s, E/E' >20 | Cardiac death |
| Systolic mitral annular velocity | 185 Patients, EF <45% | Continuous | Death or transplant |
| LA volume | 1,375 Elderly patients with preserved EF | ≥ 32 ml/m$^2$ | Incident HF |
| **Flow propagation** | | | |
| E/Vp | 67 Post-MI patients | E/Vp ≥ 1.5 | Death and HF readmission |
| Vp | 125 Post-MI patients | Vp <45 cm/s | Cardiac death |

A = atrial filling velocity; AMI = acute myocardial infarction; CAD = coronary artery disease; CVD = cardiovascular disease; D = diastolic pulmonary vein wave; DT = deceleration time of E-wave; E = early diastolic filling velocity; E' = tissue Doppler early filling velocity; EF = ejection fraction; IVRT = interventricular relaxation time; LA = left atrium; LV = left ventricle; MV A dur = mitral valve atrial wave duration; NYHA = New York Heart Association; PV AR dur = pulmonary vein atrial reversal duration; S = systolic pulmonary vein wave; Vp = flow propagation velocity slope. New onset event = myocardial infarction, sudden cardiac death, unstable angina, revascularization, stroke/transient ischemic attack, hospital stay for heart failure (HF), symptomatic aorto-iliac disease, end-stage renal disease.
Source: Kirkpatrick J. Echocardiography in Heart Failure. *Journal of the American College of Cardiology.* 2007;50(5): 381–396.

**Table 26.2** Prognostic significance of echocardiographic diastolic dysfunction measures: composite studies

| Composite study | Patient population | Components | Outcome | Degree of predictive significance |
|---|---|---|---|---|
| Mild diastolic dysfunction vs. normal | 2,042 Patients >45 years | E/A <0.75, E/A Valsalva <0.5, E/E' <10, S >D, PV AR cur >MV A dur | Death | HR 8.31 |
| Moderate or severe diastolic dysfunction vs. normal | 2,042 Patients >45 years | E/A 0.75–1.5, DT >140 ms, E/A Valsalva ≥ 0.5, E/E' ≥ 10, S <D, PV AR dur–MV A dur >30 ms | Death | HR 10.17 |
| | | E/A >1.5, DT <140 ms, E/A Valsalva <0.5, E/E' ≥ 10, S <D, PV AR dur–MV A dur >30 ms | | |
| Restrictive vs. nonrestrictive | 311 HF patients evaluated for transplant | E/A >2 or DT ≤ 140 ms | Death or transplant | RR 2.4 |
| Restrictive vs. nonrestrictive | 98 Chronic HF patients | E/A >1 and DT ≤ 130 ms | Cardiac death or transplant | NA |
| Restrictive vs. nonrestrictive | 100 Patients, EF <40% | E/A–2 or 1–2 plus DT <140 ms | Cardiac death at 2 years | RR 8.6 |
| Restrictive vs. nonrestrictive | 193 HF patients, EF <45% | E/A >2, DT <150 ms, E' <8 cm/s | Cardiac death or early transplant | RR 6.62 |
| Restrictive vs. nonrestrictive | 63 Patients with amyloid cardiomyopathy | E/A >1 and DT <150 ms | Cardiac death at 1 year | RR 4.87 |
| AR vs. PN vs. RFP | 115 Patients admitted with HF | E/A <1 or >2, DT <140 or >230 ms, PV AR dur/MV A dur >1.2 | Death, HF hospital readmission | PN and RFP more predictive of outcomes than AR |

AR = abnormal relaxation; HR = hazard ratio; PN = pseudo normal; RFP = restrictive filling pattern; RR = relative risk; other abbreviations as in Table 26.1.
Source: Kirkpatrick J. Echocardiography in Heart Failure. *Journal of the American College of Cardiology*. 2007;50(5): 381–396.

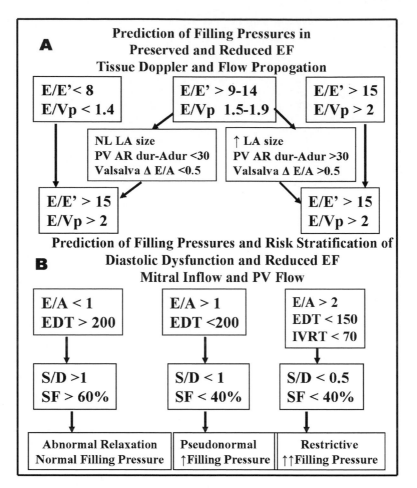

**Fig. 26.2** Diastolic filling parameters and the prediction of normal vs. elevated filling pressure. (**A**) Prediction of normal vs. elevated filling pressure. In patients with preserved and reduced left ventricular ejection fraction (LVEF), normal filling pressures are predicted by normal mitral inflow E-wave to tissue Doppler E′-wave ratio (E/E′) and mitral inflow E-wave to flow propagation ratio (E/Vp) values or intermediate values with normal left atrium (LA) size, normal pulmonary vein atrial reversal duration minus mitral inflow A-wave duration (AR dur–A dur), and a minimal change in the E/A wave ratio with Valsalva. Elevated filling pressures are predicted by elevated E/E′ and E/Vp values or intermediate values with elevated LA size, prolonged AR dur–A dur, a substantial change in the E to A valve with Valsalva, or a prolonged pulmonary vein D-wave deceleration time (DDT). (**B**) Degree of diastolic dysfunction. In patients with reduced LVEF, mitral inflow E/A, mitral inflow E-wave deceleration time (EDT), and isovolumic relaxation time (IVRT) parameters, confirmed by pulmonary vein S to D ratio (S/D), systolic fraction of pulmonary venous forward flow (SF), and DDT can further define filling dynamics by stratifying diastolic function into "abnormal relaxation" (normal filling pressures), "pseudonormal" (elevated filling pressures), and "restrictive" (very high filling pressures) categories. Valsalva $\Delta$E/A = change in mitral inflow E to A-wave ratio with Valsalva maneuver. (Modified from Nagueh and Zoghbi[146]) (Source: Kirkpatrick J. Echocardiography in Heart Failure. *Journal of the American College of Cardiology*. 2007;50(5): 381–396)

two dimensional (2D) image quality is suboptimal, the Tei index might be particularly useful when other measures of left and right ventricular function are obscured or indeterminate.

## EF and Dimensions

Traditionally, EF measurements have been visually estimated with important limitations of subjectivity and dependence on highly trained expert interpretation for accuracy. Although symptoms guide the majority of HF management decisions, precise and reproducible EF measurements play an increasingly important role in guiding important interventions. Consequently, quantified, objective measurements of LV systolic function should become standard practice in echocardiography. Although fractional shortening measured from M-mode tracings can quantify LV function, it is valid only in a symmetrically contracting heart without regional variability and is therefore inappropriate for the remodeled ventricles of many HF patients. The new guidelines from the American Society of Echocardiography (ASE) advocate the biplane method of discs for EF quantification and discourage the use of M-mode measurements that rely on geometric assumptions to convert linear measurements to three-dimensional (3D) volumes.[50] An alternative method for volume calculation, useful when the endocardium is not well defined, is the area–length method. This method assumes a bullet-shaped ventricle and involves planimetry of the mid-ventricle short-axis area and the annulus-to-apex length in systole and diastole. With either 2D method, the new ASE guidelines define an abnormal EF as <55%, with the cutoffs for moderately abnormal and severely abnormal at 44 and 30%, respectively. The reference ranges for LV dimensions are best indexed to body surface area, with reference ranges 2.4–3.2 cm/m$^2$ and cutoff values of 3.5 and 3.8 cm/m$^2$ for moderate and severe dilation, respectively.[50]

Image quality in patients with poor acoustic windows has traditionally played a major role in limiting the accuracy of quantification of LV volumes and EF. Tissue harmonic imaging with and without echocardiographic contrast for LV cavity opacification has improved the accuracy and reproducibility of EF measurements.[51,52] This method has enabled the accurate assessment of LV function in nearly all patients, irrespective of body habitus, chest wall deformities, or pulmonary diseases [53–55] (Fig. 26.3). Two-dimensional echocardiography, even when employing these methods, lacks accuracy compared with the gold standards of magnetic resonance imaging (MRI) or radionuclide ventriculography for quantification of EF and volumes.[56] The reasons for the consistent underestimation of LV volumes and EF involve reliance on geometric assumptions, combined with foreshortening of the LV from transducer positioning errors. This underestimation might be overcome with the use of 3D echocardiography.[57]

Although EF and LV dimensions do not correlate with HF symptoms, exercise capacity, or myocardial oxygen consumption,[58,59] they do provide crucial prognostic information.[60] Morbidity and mortality are closely linked to both EF and LV

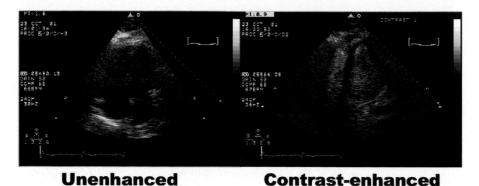

**Unenhanced**                    **Contrast-enhanced**

**Fig. 26.3**   Contrast opacification of the left ventricular cavity. (**A**) Apical four-chamber view with poor endocardial definition. (**B**) The same view with improved endocardial definition after echocardiographic contrast administration

volumes in HF patients in multicenter trials.[61,62] Although influenced by a myriad of demographic and clinical factors, post-myocardial infarction prognosis is most powerfully predicted by EF and LV size. Early studies of acute myocardial infarction survivors using cineangiography and radionuclide ventriculography demonstrated EF <40% and increased LV volumes to be predictors of subsequent cardiovascular mortality and sudden death.[63–66] More recent studies using echocardiography have also found EF and LV volumes to be powerful prognosticators for major adverse cardiac events.[67,68] The ability of echocardiography to assess global dysfunction and regional wall motion has aided in the assessment of the size of myocardial infarctions (Fig. 26.4). This measurement predicts cardiogenic shock (if >40% of the myocardium is involved), development of chronic HF, and mortality, despite the fact that myocardial stunning and hibernation complicate the prediction of eventual infarct size.[69,70]

## LV Mass

Although LV mass has received less attention in clinical cardiology than EF, it is an important prognostic marker in HF in patients with and without coronary artery disease.[71] This observation in smaller studies was confirmed in the echocardiographic substudy of the SOLVD registry and trials, in which investigators examined the effect of LV hypertrophy on clinical outcomes and found that increased LV mass was associated with high mortality and rate of cardiovascular hospital stays, independent of EF.[72] Because population studies suggest that the etiology of HF in African-American patients is more likely to be hypertensive than ischemic,[73] the routine and accurate measurement of LV mass and its prognostic significance might be even more salient in this population.

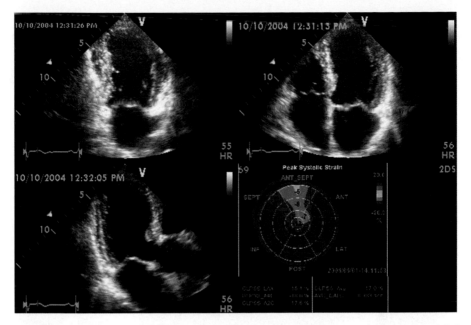

**Fig. 26.4** Automated ejection fraction calculation through a multiplanar probe, providing global and regional ejection fraction on a bull's eye plot

Left ventricular mass assessment is subject to the same limitations in reproducibility and accuracy as measurement of LV dimensions.[74] The current ASE guidelines recommend mass calculation from linear dimensions with the cubed formula, modeling the LV as a prolated ellipse, because this method has been validated in multiple studies with pathologic correlation. The cubed formula lacks precision, however, when applied to many HF patients, because it involves geometric assumptions that are invalid in an asymmetrically contracting, remodeled ventricle. 2D methods, including the truncated ellipsoid and the area–length formula, might be more appropriate for distorted ventricles with regional wall motion abnormalities. These methods, however, rely heavily on geometric assumptions. Furthermore, as mentioned, these methods are subject to inaccuracies from foreshortening.

Unlike EF and LV dimensions, LV mass has different cutoff values for men and women and for linear and 2D methods. The reference ranges for women are 67–162 g and 66–150 g for the linear and 2D methods, respectively. Indexed to body surface area, these ranges are 43–95 g/m² and 44–88 g/m². For men, the reference ranges are 88–224 g and 96–200 g, and 49–115 g/m² and 50–102 g/m².[50]

The LV mass increases in the remodeled, failing heart, either from increased volumes with myocardial thinning or from wall hypertrophy in patients with hypertensive cardiomyopathy.[75] Despite its limitations, the assessment of LV mass provides not only an important research tool to evaluate remodeling but also a precise and prognostically powerful way to characterize clinical status.

## Viability Assessment

LV contractile reserve and myocardial viability, as assessed by low-dose dobutamine stress echocardiography (DSE), significantly influence prognosis in patients with chronic LV dysfunction. Patients with contractile reserve who undergo myocardial revascularization have an excellent outcome. The presence and the extent of viable myocardium are important determinants of prognosis in patients with LV dysfunction and that both survival and symptomatic status are enhanced by revascularization in patients with systolic dysfunction who manifest myocardial contractile reserve (Fig. 26.5).[76–78]

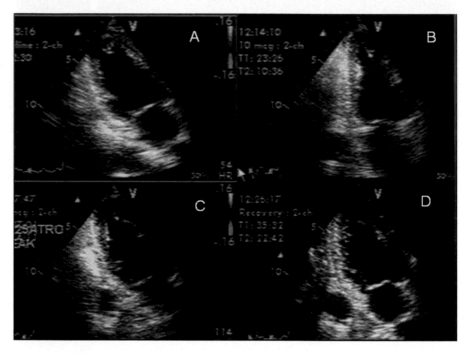

**Fig. 26.5**    Four stages of dobutamine stress echocardiography. (**A**) Resting. (**B**) Low dose. (**C**) Peak, and (**D**) Recovery stage

## Therapeutic Guidance

Echocardiography not only provides clinical measures and prognostic assessments in patients with HF but can also supply information to guide application of HF therapies.

## Medications

In addition to the demonstrated benefit of angiotensin-converting enzyme (ACE) inhibitors for patients with both symptomatic and asymptomatic LV dysfunction,[79] beta-blocker drugs are beneficial for almost all well-compensated patients with LV systolic dysfunction,[80,81] and aldosterone antagonists reduce mortality in New York Heart Association functional class III and IV patients hospitalized for HF with EF = 35% and in post-myocardial infarction patients with EF <40%.[82,83] Not only does echocardiographic EF measurement commonly establish an indication for these medications but also improvements in EF and LV volumes by echocardiography are used as standard measures of therapeutic effect in many clinical trials of HF medications.[79,84] Conversely, echocardiography also supplies an assessment tool for the detrimental effects on LV function of cardiotoxic medications, such as anthracycline chemotherapeutic agents. The EF decrements while taking these medications are often an indication for discontinuation.[85,86]

The strategy of combining echocardiographic assessment of filling pressures with BNP measurement has definite prognostic value and might prove one of the most accurate ways to noninvasively guide fluid management. In a study by Dokainish et al.,[32] an E/E′ value >15, combined with BNP = 250 pg/ml, measured on the day before discharge, had incremental power in predicting readmission or cardiac death compared with traditional clinical risk factors. If proven to be cost-effective, echocardiography with BNP might become an important strategy for triaging HF patients in acute care settings, for assessing suitability for discharge, or for identifying patients who need more intensive outpatient management.

## Implantable Cardioverter-Defibrillators (ICDs)

Recent studies have demonstrated the benefit of prophylactic ICD for the primary prevention of sudden death in patients with reduced EF.[87,88] Reimbursement strategies for ICDs therefore rely on EF as a common parameter for placement of these devices in HF patients, and echocardiography is often employed to assess EF.[1] Repeat EF assessment at 30–40 days after myocardial infarction and after initiation of optimal HF medical therapy is necessary to determine the candidacy for ICD. Many patients' EF rise above 30–35% cutoff after a month on an appropriate medical regimen, and premature ICD implantation has shown no benefit.[89]

## Cardiac Resynchronization Therapy (CRT)

Many HF patients lack coordinated contraction of the LV walls (intraventricular dyssynchrony) and between the right and left ventricles (interventricular dyssynchrony). Cardiac resynchronization therapy can restore coordinated contraction with demonstrated improvement in symptoms and survival.[90] Current recommendations and reimbursement strategies advocate that only patients with EF = 35%, moderate-to-severe HF symptoms, a widened QRS interval, and sinus rhythm should undergo CRT.[1] Nevertheless, it is now clear that not all patients meeting these criteria will respond to CRT; furthermore, it has been recently shown that a subgroup of patients lacking these criteria could benefit from CRT.[91] Echocardiographic measurement of dyssynchrony can accurately predict beneficial response in the form of reverse remodeling (reduction in LV volumes, improved EF, and reduced mitral regurgitation)[92] and echocardiographically demonstrated reverse remodeling predicts improved survival.[93,94] Currently, different techniques are used to assess dyssynchrony, some of which are discussed in the following text.[95] It remains to be seen which measurement or combination of measurements will prove most accurate in predicting beneficial response to CRT. This is an area of active investigation in the PROSPECT (predictors of response to cardiac resynchronization therapy) trial and other studies.[96]

## Mitral Valve Surgery

So-called "functional" mitral regurgitation in HF has traditionally been ascribed to stretching of the mitral annulus and malcoaptation of the mitral valve leaflets. More recent echocardiographic and pathologic investigations have described tethering of the mitral valve leaflets from remodeling-induced displacement of one or both papillary muscles and structural changes of the mitral valve itself. These mechanisms rather than annular dilatation might be the main determinants of functional mitral regurgitation.[97,98]

The rationale behind repair or replacement of the mitral valve has been the traditional perspective on functional mitral regurgitation; nonetheless, surgery has demonstrated efficacy, even in advanced HF.[99] But it is not always clear whether repair or replacement is indicated. Furthermore, the severity of functional mitral regurgitation can be reduced by CRT and by ACE inhibitor therapy without surgery, presumably owing to the effects of reverse remodeling.[100]

Traditional echocardiographic evaluation of mitral regurgitation has significant limitations. The mitral valve annulus is saddle-shaped and cannot be fully visualized in 2D imaging planes.[101] The mitral valve regurgitant jet, especially when eccentric, is also incompletely visualized in traditional imaging planes, leading to misclassification of mitral regurgitation severity. Similarly, the geometric assumptions involved in calculating mitral regurgitation severity with Doppler flow and color Doppler (e.g., calculations of effective regurgitant orifice area) lead to inaccuracies in noncentral jets.[102,103]

## Ventricular Reconstruction Surgery

A number of ventricular reconstruction surgeries have been proposed for patients with ischemic HF and apical dyskinesis or LV aneurysms.[104,105] These surgical mechanical techniques reduce ventricular remodeling and have improved both morbidity and mortality in HF patients in small studies,[106,107] but definitive conclusions await the results of ongoing trials.[108] Decision making for these surgical procedures relies heavily on accurate determination of dyskinesis or akinesis, thinning of the apical segment, depressed EF, coexistence of mitral regurgitation, and volumetric measurement.[109,110] An elevated LV end systolic volume index >60 ml/m$^2$, in particular, portends poor postoperative survival.[111] Echocardiography provides accurate preoperative modeling to guide the amount of myocardium to be excluded or resected.[112] And echocardiography provides an important way to judge the efficacy of these procedures in improving ventricular remodeling, hemodynamic status, and EF.

## Ventricular Assist Devices

Ventricular assist devices (left ventricular assist device = LVAD, bi-ventricular assist device = bi-VAD) are commonly used as bridges to heart transplantation or ventricular recovery and, more recently, have demonstrated both mortality and quality of life benefit as "destination therapy" in patients for whom heart transplantation is not an option.[113] Candidates for VAD placement, however, require careful preoperative consideration. Significant intracardiac shunts, such as an atrial septal defect, will be exacerbated by LVAD placement, leading to significant hypoxia.[114] Furthermore, significant valvular disease, especially significant aortic stenosis or aortic regurgitation, must be detected to allow valve repair or replacement before VAD implant. Decreased right ventricular function and high pulmonary pressures often necessitate placement of a bi-VAD. Preoperative echocardiography can detect all of these disorders. After implantation, echocardiography can detect thrombus formation within the VAD[115] or other causes of inflow cannula obstruction. Doppler and color Doppler imaging can also detect significant inflow and outflow cannulae regurgitation and also assess aortic valve opening and insufficiency.[116]

## New Horizons for Advanced Echocardiographic Techniques in HF

Echocardiographic techniques applicable to HF patients are advancing rapidly. New techniques have been developed to image myocardial mechanics and provide more precise measurements to guide therapeutic decisions. Although MRI is an established technique for measuring myocardial mechanics and obtaining highly accurate measurements of cardiac size and structures, the evaluation of these parameters by echocardiography is considerably more feasible for clinical use, because it is widely available and repeat assessment can be readily performed.

## *Myocardial Motion, Strain, and Strain Rate*

One of the most promising techniques, already used in daily clinical practice, is tissue Doppler imaging (TDI). Tissue Doppler imaging has been used with M-mode, 2D, and pulse wave Doppler.[117] The peak systolic myocardial velocity, reflective of longitudinal myocardial fiber shortening, has been used to assess systolic function in HF. Yip et al.[118] and Yu et al.[119] noted systolic abnormalities (Sm <4.4 m/s) with TDI in 38–52% of HF patients with normal EFs. Their findings suggest that systolic myocardial velocity might provide a more accurate measure of systolic dysfunction than EF. Many HF patients with normal EF might have systolic as well as diastolic HF. In this setting, tissue velocity measures have demonstrated incremental[120,121] and, in a recent study, superior[122] prognostic ability compared with standard echocardiographic measures, including EF.

Tissue velocity measurements are susceptible to artifact from tethering and translational motion (i.e., displacement of the entire heart is recorded as tissue motion of the specific segment being measured). Strain imaging, derived from tissue velocity measurements, overcomes this limitation by measuring actual deformation of the myocardium (expressed as a percentage) in systole and diastole. Strain rate is the inverse of the time to deformation. As measured in the longitudinal direction (base to apex in the apical views), the normal values for strain are 15–25% and for strain rate are 1–1.5/s.[123] This could be decreased or positive in patients with regional wall motion abnormalities (Fig. 26.6A and B). Like tissue velocity measures, strain and strain rate imaging detect abnormalities of systolic and diastolic function in patients with infiltrative cardiomyopathies.[124] In addition, Palka et al.[125] described the use of strain rate to differentiate restrictive cardiomyopathy (reduced early diastolic strain rate compared with normal hearts) from constrictive physiology (increased early diastolic strain rate).

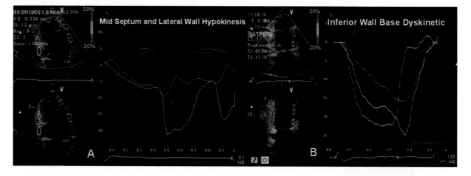

**Fig. 26.6** Regional wall motion abnormality as assessed using strain. (**A**) Mid septum and lateral wall hypokinesis following LAD infarct. (**B**) Inferior wall dyskinesis following RCA infarct (*red sample*)

The identification and measurement of dyssynchrony is one of the most widely published uses of tissue velocity, strain, and strain rate imaging in HF. The TDI techniques predict echocardiographic and clinical response to bi-ventricular pacing with high sensitivity and specificity. Several parameters have been used, such as an intersegmental delay in peak systolic longitudinal motion between segments (abnormal >60–65 ms), the SD of time to peak velocity of 12 segments (abnormal >30–31 ms), and intersegmental delay in peak systolic radial contraction as assessed by Speckled tracking 2D Strain[126,127] (Fig. 26.7). Tissue Doppler imaging can identify the specific regions involved in dyssynchrony as well as the magnitude of dyssynchronous contraction. This information can be available to guide specific placement of bi-ventricular pacing leads and assess response during long-term follow-up. Furthermore, as bi-ventricular pacemakers can be set with a delay between right ventricular and LV activation, dyssynchrony measures can been used to optimize these settings, improving intraventricular and interventricular synchrony, and hemodynamic status.[128]

## Tissue Tracking

The major limitations to TDI are Doppler angle dependency and problems in assessing regional LV torsional dynamics. In particular, the rotational component of cardiac contraction plays a significant role in LV ejection and relaxation and is poorly imaged by most TDI techniques.

Newer techniques such as "speckle tracking" algorithms involve identification of multiple unique patterns of echocardiographic pixel intensity that are automatically tracked throughout the cardiac cycle. The angular displacement of these pixels can be plotted over time for the apex, mid ventricle, and basal segments. Each pixel's angular displacement is averaged to provide a measurement of both degree and direction of rotational motion for each segment. This method is not limited by angle dependency and compares favorably with MRI.[129,130]

Although the prognostic significance of abnormal ventricular torsion has not been validated in large studies, measurement of rotational motion has shown promise as a sensitive marker for cardiac ischemia[131] and loading conditions[132] and might prove beneficial as a refined measure of LV dysfunction in HF and regional and global dyssynchrony.[133] As such, it might become an important marker of the functional significance of remodeling and reverse remodeling in HF patients.[134] It might also be able to detect early allograft rejection in transplant patients, potentially circumventing the need for frequent myocardial biopsies. In fact, when combined with 3D imaging techniques, it might prove to be a more sensitive marker for occult LV dysfunction.

## 3D Echocardiography

Previously hampered by the need for cumbersome off-line reconstruction of images, 3D echocardiography has benefited from the development of new matrix array transducers that acquire full volume data sets to allow real-time imaging.[135] The ability to visualize all LV walls contemporaneously prevents foreshortening of the LV cavity

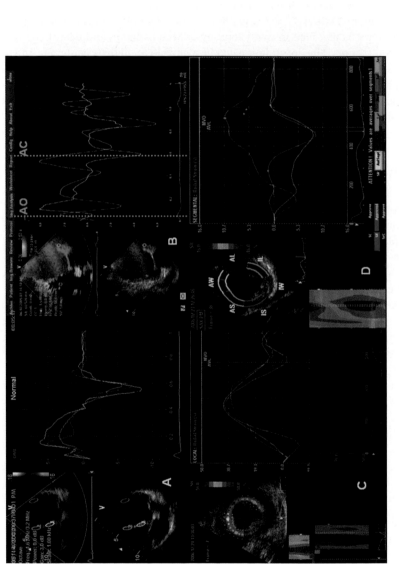

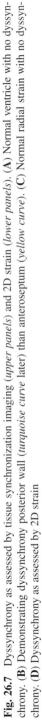

**Fig. 26.7** Dyssynchrony as assessed by tissue synchronization imaging (*upper panels*) and 2D strain (*lower panels*). (**A**) Normal ventricle with no dyssynchrony. (**B**) Demonstrating dyssynchrony posterior wall (*turquoise curve* later) than anteroseptum (*yellow curve*). (**C**) Normal radial strain with no dyssynchrony. (**D**) Dysssynchrony as assessed by 2D strain

and allows analysis of regional myocardial function. No geometric assumptions are required in calculating volumes from a 3D image. In recent studies, 3D echocardiography demonstrated accurate global and regional assessments of LV size and function compared with the gold standard of MRI as well as lower intra and inter-observer variability than traditional techniques.[136] Sugeng et al.[137] showed 3D imaging to be superior to cardiac computed tomography in EF and volumes assessment. Application of new endocardial border detection techniques to 3D images might allow direct calculation of LV volumes and EF, leading to improved reproducibility[138] (Fig. 26.8). Mor-Avi et al.[139] demonstrated that, as in volumetric assessments, 3D echocardiography is more accurate and reproducible than methods for LV mass calculation, compared with the gold standard of MRI.

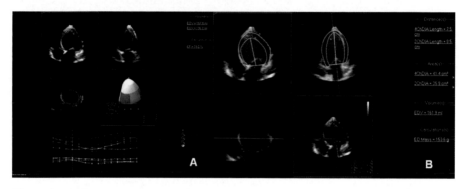

**Fig. 26.8**   Online 3D echocardiography depicting (**A**) global and regional ejection fraction and dyssynchrony assessment (**B**) Volumes and mass assessment

The 3D imaging of global and regional function and LV volumes has not yet translated into clear improvements in or predictions of clinical outcomes. 3D echocardiography might, in the future, prove beneficial in several areas. The improved precision in measuring EF might guide more appropriate selection of patients for ICD and CRT therapy. Like TDI, 3D echocardiography can assess segmental myocardial motion over time, thereby detecting and characterizing dyssynchrony. 3D echocardiography has been used in the functional assessment of mitral annular size and tenting volume and improves the echocardiographic measurement of mitral regurgitation.[140] A recent review discusses these and other applications of 3D echocardiography in imaging HF patients, such as assessments of atrial size and of right ventricular size and function.[141]

## Conclusions

Echocardiography is well qualified to meet the growing need for noninvasive imaging in the HF population. Because HF patients often have more than one structural and/or functional abnormality contributing to their disease state, echocardiography's versatility in detecting valvular and pericardial pathology along with myocardial disorders yields obvious benefits. Doppler measurements provide important information to direct management of volume status, diagnose and characterize HF with preserved systolic function, and identify patients at high risk for cardiovascular morbidity and mortality. Not surprisingly, the underuse of echocardiography in populations at significant risk for HF is associated with adverse cardiovascular outcomes.[142,143] Assessment of LVEF in clinical HF is one of the primary measures in a number of cardiovascular quality improvement initiatives, including the AHA's "Get with the Guidelines" and the ACC's "Guidelines Applied in Practice".[144,145] Echocardiography is well suited to repeated measurements of EF and LV mass in clinical trials and routine patient care. In fact, the new HF guidelines recommend repeat echocardiography for HF patients with changes in symptoms, a clinical event, or a treatment likely to affect cardiac function.[1] Echocardiography provides important data for therapeutic decision-making, including defining candidacy for medications, implantable cardiac devices, and surgical procedures. New techniques for the characterization of ventricular mechanics and recent developments in 3D echocardiography hold great promise for improving the quality of care to the growing population of HF patients.

# References

1. Hunt SA, Abraham WT, Chin MH, et al. ACC/AHA 2005 Guideline Update for the Diagnosis and Management of Chronic Heart Failure in the Adult: a report of the American College of Cardiology/American Heart Association Task Force on Practice Guidelines (Writing Committee to Update the 2001 Guidelines for the Evaluation and Management of Heart Failure): developed in collaboration with the American College of Chest Physicians and the International Society for Heart and Lung Transplantation: endorsed by the Heart Rhythm Society. *Circulation.* 2005;112:e154–e235.
2. American Heart Association ASA. Heart disease and stroke statistics: 2005 update. Available at: http://www.americanheart.org/downloadable/heart/1072969766940HSStats2004 Update.pdf
3. Lloyd-Jones DM, Larson MG, Leip EP, et al. Lifetime risk for developing congestive heart failure: the Framingham Heart Study. *Circulation.* 2002;106:3068–3072.
4. Ho KK, Anderson KM, Kannel WB, Grossman W, Levy D. Survival after the onset of congestive heart failure in Framingham Heart Study subjects. *Circulation.* 1993;88:107–115.
5. Capomolla S, Ceresa M, Pinna G, et al. Echo-Doppler and clinical evaluations to define hemodynamic profile in patients with chronic heart failure: accuracy and influence on therapeutic management. *Eur J Heart Fail.* 2005;7:624–630.
6. Badgett RG, Lucey CR, Mulrow CD. Can the clinical examination diagnose left-sided heart failure in adults? *JAMA.* 1997;277:1712–1719.
7. Nagueh SF, Kopelen HA, Zoghbi WA. Relation of mean right atrial pressure to echocardiographic and Doppler parameters of right atrial and right ventricular function. *Circulation.* 1996;93:1160–1169.
8. Masuyama T, Kodama K, Kitabatake A, Sato H, Nanto S, Inoue M. Continuous-wave Doppler echocardiographic detection of pulmonary regurgitation and its application to non-invasive estimation of pulmonary artery pressure. *Circulation.* 1986;74:484–492.
9. Berger M, Haimowitz A, Van Tosh A, Berdoff RL, Goldberg E. Quantitative assessment of pulmonary hypertension in patients with tricuspid regurgitation using continuous wave Doppler ultrasound. *J Am Coll Cardiol.* 1985;6:359–365.

10. Sorrell VL, Reeves WC. Noninvasive right and left heart catheterization: taking the echo lab beyond an image-only laboratory. *Echocardiography*. 2001;18:31–41.
11. Franklin KM, Aurigemma GP. Prognosis in diastolic heart failure. *Prog Cardiovasc Dis*. 2005;47:333–339.
12. Aurigemma GP, Gottdiener JS, Shemanski L, Gardin J, Kitzman D. Predictive value of systolic and diastolic function for incident congestive heart failure in the elderly: the cardiovascular health study. *J Am Coll Cardiol*. 2001;37:1042–1048.
13. Nagueh SF. Noninvasive evaluation of hemodynamics by Doppler echocardiography. *Curr Opin Cardiol*. 1999;14:217–224.
14. Ommen SR, Nishimura RA, Appleton CP, et al. Clinical utility of Doppler echocardiography and tissue Doppler imaging in the estimation of left ventricular filling pressures: a comparative simultaneous Doppler-catheterization study. *Circulation*. 2000;102:1788–1794.
15. Pinamonti B, Zecchin M, Di Lenarda A, Gregori D, Sinagra G, Camerini F. Persistence of restrictive left ventricular filling pattern in dilated cardiomyopathy: an ominous prognostic sign. *J Am Coll Cardiol*. 1997;29:604–612.
16. Dini FL, Dell'Anna R, Micheli A, Michelassi C, Rovai D. Impact of blunted pulmonary venous flow on the outcome of patients with left ventricular systolic dysfunction secondary to either ischemic or idiopathic dilated cardiomyopathy. *Am J Cardiol*. 2000;85:1455–1460.
17. Garcia MJ, Smedira NG, Greenberg NL, et al. Color M-mode Doppler flow propagation velocity is a preload insensitive index of left ventricular relaxation: animal and human validation. *J Am Coll Cardiol*. 2000;35:201–208.
18. Garcia MJ, Ares MA, Asher C, Rodriguez L, Vandervoort P, Thomas JD. An index of early left ventricular filling that combined with pulsed Doppler peak E velocity may estimate capillary wedge pressure. *J Am Coll Cardiol*. 1997;29:448–454.
19. Takemoto Y, Barnes ME, Seward JB, et al. Usefulness of left atrial volume in predicting first congestive heart failure in patients > or = 65 years of age with well-preserved left ventricular systolic function. *Am J Cardiol*. 2005;96:832–836.
20. Rossi A, Loredana L, Cicoira M, et al. Additional value of pulmonary vein parameters in defining pseudonormalization of mitral inflow pattern. *Echocardiography*. 2001;18: 673–679.
21. Mottram PM, Leano R, Marwick TH. Usefulness of B-type natriuretic peptide in hypertensive patients with exertional dyspnea and normal left ventricular ejection fraction and correlation with new echocardiographic indexes of systolic and diastolic function. *Am J Cardiol*. 2003;92:1434–1438.
22. Dokainish H, Zoghbi WA, Lakkis NM, Quinones MA, Nagueh SF. Comparative accuracy of B-type natriuretic peptide and tissue Doppler echocardiography in the diagnosis of congestive heart failure. *Am J Cardiol*. 2004;93:1130–1135.
23. Kirkpatrick JN, Vannan MA, Narula J, Lang RM. Echocardiography in heart failure: applications, utility, and new horizons. *J Am Coll Cardiol*. 2007;50:381–396.
24. Schillaci G, Pasqualini L, Verdecchia P, et al. Prognostic significance of left ventricular diastolic dysfunction in essential hypertension. *J Am Coll Cardiol*. 2002;39:2005–2011.
25. Bella JN, Palmieri V, Roman MJ, et al. Mitral ratio of peak early to late diastolic filling velocity as a predictor of mortality in middle-aged and elderly adults: the Strong Heart Study. *Circulation*. 2002;105:1928–1933.
26. Temporelli PL, Giannuzzi P, Nicolosi GL, et al. Doppler-derived mitral deceleration time as a strong prognostic marker of left ventricular remodeling and survival after acute myocardial infarction: results of the GISSI-3 echo substudy. *J Am Coll Cardiol*. 2004;43:1646–1653.
27. Pinamonti B, Di Lenarda A, Sinagra G, Camerini F. Restrictive left ventricular filling pattern in dilated cardiomyopathy assessed by Doppler echocardiography: clinical, echocardiographic and hemodynamic correlations and prognostic implications. Heart Muscle Disease Study Group. *J Am Coll Cardiol*. 1993;22:808–815.
28. Florea VG, Henein MY, Cicoira M, et al. Echocardiographic determinants of mortality in patients >67 years of age with chronic heart failure. *Am J Cardiol*. 2000;86:158–161.

29. Hillis GS, Moller JE, Pellikka PA, et al. Noninvasive estimation of left ventricular filling pressure by E/E′ is a powerful predictor of survival after acute myocardial infarction. *J Am Coll Cardiol*. 2004;43:360–367.

30. Hamdan A, Shapira Y, Bengal T, et al. Tissue Doppler imaging in patients with advanced heart failure: relation to functional class and prognosis. *J Heart Lung Transplant*. 2006;25:214–218.

31. Acil T, Wichter T, Stypmann J, et al. Prognostic value of tissue Doppler imaging in patients with chronic congestive heart failure. *Int J Cardiol*. 2005;103:175–181.

32. Dokainish H, Zoghbi WA, Lakkis NM, et al. Incremental predictive power of B-type natriuretic peptide and tissue Doppler echocardiography in the prognosis of patients with congestive heart failure. *J Am Coll Cardiol*. 2005;45:1223–1226.

33. Nikitin NP, Loh PH, Silva R, et al. Prognostic value of systolic mitral annular velocity measured with Doppler tissue imaging in patients with chronic heart failure caused by left ventricular systolic dysfunction. *Heart*. 2006;92:775–779.

34. Moller JE, Sondergaard E, Poulsen SH, Seward JB, Appleton CP, Egstrup K. Color M-mode and pulsed wave tissue Doppler echocardiography: powerful predictors of cardiac events after first myocardial infarction. *J Am Soc Echocardiogr*. 2001;14:757–763.

35. Moller JE, Sondergaard E, Poulsen SH, Appleton CP, Egstrup K. Serial Doppler echocardiographic assessment of left and right ventricular performance after a first myocardial infarction. *J Am Soc Echocardiogr*. 2001;14:249–255.

36. Redfield MM, Rodeheffer RJ, Jacobsen SJ, Mahoney DW, Bailey KR, Burnett JC Jr. Plasma brain natriuretic peptide to detect preclinical ventricular systolic or diastolic dysfunction: a community-based study. *Circulation*. 2004;109:3176–3181.

37. Hansen A, Haass M, Zugck C, et al. Prognostic value of Doppler echocardiographic mitral inflow patterns: implications for risk stratification in patients with chronic congestive heart failure. *J Am Coll Cardiol*. 2001;37:1049–1055.

38. Traversi E, Pozzoli M, Cioffi G, et al. Mitral flow velocity changes after 6 months of optimized therapy provide important hemodynamic and prognostic information in patients with chronic heart failure. *Am Heart J*. 1996;132:809–819.

39. Xie GY, Berk MR, Smith MD, Gurley JC, DeMaria AN. Prognostic value of Doppler transmitral flow patterns in patients with congestive heart failure. *J Am Coll Cardiol*. 1994;24:132–139.

40. Bruch C, Gotzmann M, Stypmann J, et al. Electrocardiography and Doppler echocardiography for risk stratification in patients with chronic heart failure: incremental prognostic value of QRS duration and a restrictive mitral filling pattern. *J Am Coll Cardiol*. 2005;45: 1072–1075.

41. Klein AL, Hatle LK, Taliercio CP, et al. Prognostic significance of Doppler measures of diastolic function in cardiac amyloidosis. A Doppler echocardiography study. *Circulation*. 1991;83:808–816.

42. Whalley GA, Doughty RN, Gamble GD, et al. Pseudonormal mitral filling pattern predicts hospital re-admission in patients with congestive heart failure. *J Am Coll Cardiol*. 2002;39:1787–1795.

43. Tei C, Ling LH, Hodge DO, et al. New index of combined systolic and diastolic myocardial performance: a simple and reproducible measure of cardiac function – a study in normals and dilated cardiomyopathy. *J Cardiol*. 1995;26:357–366.

44. Spencer KT, Kirkpatrick JN, Mor-Avi V, Decara JM, Lang RM. Age dependency of the Tei index of myocardial performance. *J Am Soc Echocardiogr*. 2004;17:350–352.

45. Tei C, Nishimura RA, Seward JB, Tajik AJ. Noninvasive Doppler-derived myocardial performance index: correlation with simultaneous measurements of cardiac catheterization measurements. *J Am Soc Echocardiogr*. 1997;10:169–178.

46. Yeo TC, Dujardin KS, Tei C, Mahoney DW, McGoon MD, Seward JB. Value of a Doppler-derived index combining systolic and diastolic time intervals in predicting outcome in primary pulmonary hypertension. *Am J Cardiol*. 1998;81:1157–1161.

47. Dujardin KS, Tei C, Yeo TC, Hodge DO, Rossi A, Seward JB. Prognostic value of a Doppler index combining systolic and diastolic performance in idiopathic-dilated cardiomyopathy. *Am J Cardiol*. 1998;82:1071–1076.

48. Arnlov J, Ingelsson E, Riserus U, Andren B, Lind L. Myocardial performance index, a Doppler-derived index of global left ventricular function, predicts congestive heart failure in elderly men. *Eur Heart J*. 2004;25:2220–2225.

49. Mikkelsen KV, Möller JE, Bie P, Ryde H, Videbaek L, Haghfelt T. Tei index and neurohormonal activation in patients with incident heart failure: serial changes and prognostic value. *Eur J Heart Fail*. 2006;8:599–608.

50. Lang RM, Bierig M, Devereux RB, et al. Recommendations for chamber quantification: a report from the American Society of Echocardiography's Guidelines and Standards Committee and the Chamber Quantification Writing Group, developed in conjunction with the European Association of Echocardiography, a branch of the European Society of Cardiology. *J Am Soc Echocardiogr*. 2005;18:1440–1463.

51. Malm S, Frigstad S, Sagberg E, Larsson H, Skjaerpe T. Accurate and reproducible measurement of left ventricular volume and ejection fraction by contrast echocardiography: a comparison with magnetic resonance imaging. *J Am Coll Cardiol*. 2004;44:1030–1035.

52. Hundley WG, Kizilbash AM, Afridi I, Franco F, Peshock RM, Grayburn PA. Administration of an intravenous perfluorocarbon contrast agent improves echocardiographic determination of left ventricular volumes and ejection fraction: comparison with cine magnetic resonance imaging. *J Am Coll Cardiol*. 1998;32:1426–1432.

53. Yu EH, Sloggett CE, Iwanochko RM, Rakowski H, Siu SC. Feasibility and accuracy of left ventricular volumes and ejection fraction determination by fundamental, tissue harmonic, and intravenous contrast imaging in difficult-to-image patients. *J Am Soc Echocardiogr*. 2000;13:216–224.

54. Spencer KT, Bednarz J, Rafter PG, Korcarz C, Lang RM. Use of harmonic imaging without echocardiographic contrast to improve two-dimensional image quality. *Am J Cardiol*. 1998,82:794–799.

55. Lang RM, Mor-Avi V, Zoghbi WA, Senior R, Klein AL, Pearlman AS. The role of contrast enhancement in echocardiographic assessment of left ventricular function. *Am J Cardiol*. 2002;90:28 J–34 J.

56. Bellenger NG, Burgess MI, Ray SG, et al. Comparison of left ventricular ejection fraction and volumes in heart failure by echocardiography, radionuclide ventriculography and cardiovascular magnetic resonance; are they interchangeable? *Eur Heart J*. 2000;21: 1387–1396.

57. Jacobs LD, Salgo IS, Goonewardena S, et al. Rapid online quantification of left ventricular volume from real-time three-dimensional echocardiographic data. *Eur Heart J*. 2006;27:460–468.

58. Cohen-Solal A, Tabet JY, Logeart D, Bourgoin P, Tokmakova M, Dahan M. A non-invasively determined surrogate of cardiac power ('circulatory power') at peak exercise is a powerful prognostic factor in chronic heart failure. *Eur Heart J*. 2002;23:806–814.

59. Smart N, Haluska B, Leano R, Case C, Mottram PM, Marwick TH. Determinants of functional capacity in patients with chronic heart failure: role of filling pressure and systolic and diastolic function. *Am Heart J*. 2005;149:152–158.

60. Vasan RS, Larson MG, Benjamin EJ, Evans JC, Reiss CK, Levy D. Congestive heart failure in subjects with normal versus reduced left ventricular ejection fraction: prevalence and mortality in a population-based cohort. *J Am Coll Cardiol*. 1999;33:1948–1955.

61. Wong M, Staszewsky L, Latini R, et al. Severity of left ventricular remodeling defines outcomes and response to therapy in heart failure: Valsartan heart failure trial (Val-HeFT) echocardiographic data. *J Am Coll Cardiol*. 2004;43:2022–2027.

62. Grayburn PA, Appleton CP, DeMaria AN, et al. Echocardiographic predictors of morbidity and mortality in patients with advanced heart failure: the Beta-blocker Evaluation of Survival Trial (BEST). *J Am Coll Cardiol*. 2005;45:1064–1071.

63. Sanz G, Castaner A, Betriu A, et al. Determinants of prognosis in survivors of myocardial infarction: a prospective clinical angiographic study. *N Engl J Med.* 1982;306:1065–1070.

64. Risk stratification and survival after myocardial infarction. *N Engl J Med.* 1983;309:331–336

65. Ahnve S, Gilpin E, Henning H, Curtis G, Collins D, Ross J Jr. Limitations and advantages of the ejection fraction for defining high risk after acute myocardial infarction. *Am J Cardiol.* 1986;58:872–878.

66. White HD, Norris RM, Brown MA, Brandt PW, Whitlock RM, Wild CJ. Left ventricular end-systolic volume as the major determinant of survival after recovery from myocardial infarction. *Circulation.* 1987;76:44–51.

67. St John Sutton M, Pfeffer MA, Plappert T, et al. Quantitative two-dimensional echocardiographic measurements are major predictors of adverse cardiovascular events after acute myocardial infarction. The protective effects of captopril. *Circulation.* 1994;89:68–75.

68. Cleland JG, Torabi A, Khan NK. Epidemiology and management of heart failure and left ventricular systolic dysfunction in the aftermath of a myocardial infarction. *Heart.* 2005;91(suppl 2):ii7–ii13; discussion ii31, ii43–ii48.

69. Burns RJ, Gibbons RJ, Yi Q, et al. The relationships of left ventricular ejection fraction, end-systolic volume index and infarct size to six-month mortality after hospital discharge following myocardial infarction treated by thrombolysis. *J Am Coll Cardiol.* 2002;39: 30–36.

70. Marchioli R, Avanzini F, Barzi F, et al. Assessment of absolute risk of death after myocardial infarction by use of multiple-risk-factor assessment equations: GISSI-Prevenzione mortality risk chart. *Eur Heart J.* 2001;22:2085–2103.

71. Cooper RS, Simmons BE, Castaner A, Santhanam V, Ghali J, Mar M. Left ventricular hypertrophy is associated with worse survival independent of ventricular function and number of coronary arteries severely narrowed. *Am J Cardiol.* 1990;65:441–445.

72. Quinones MA, Greenberg BH, Kopelen HA, et al. Echocardiographic predictors of clinical outcome in patients with left ventricular dysfunction enrolled in the SOLVD registry and trials: significance of left ventricular hypertrophy. Studies of Left Ventricular Dysfunction. *J Am Coll Cardiol.* 2000;35:1237–1244.

73. Yancy CW. Heart failure in African Americans. *Am J Cardiol.* 2005;96:3i–12i.

74. Park SH, Shub C, Nobrega TP, Bailey KR, Seward JB. Two-dimensional echocardiographic calculation of left ventricular mass as recommended by the American Society of Echocardiography: correlation with autopsy and M-mode echocardiography. *J Am Soc Echocardiogr.* 1996;9:119–128.

75. Devereux RB, de Simone G, Ganau A, Roman MJ. Left ventricular hypertrophy and geometric remodeling in hypertension: stimuli, functional consequences and prognostic implications. *J Hypertens Suppl.* 1994;12:S117–S127.

76. Chaudhry FA, Tauke JT, Alessandrini RS, Vardi G, Parker MA, Bonow RO. Prognostic implications of myocardial contractile reserve in patients with coronary artery disease and left ventricular dysfunction. *J Am Coll Cardiol.* 1999;34:730–738.

77. Galatro K, Chaudhry FA. Prognostic implications of myocardial contractile reserve in patients with ischemic cardiomyopathy. *Echocardiography.* 2000;17:61–67.

78. Chaudhry FA, Singh B, Galatro K. Reversible left ventricular dysfunction. *Echocardiography.* 2000;17:495–506.

79. Edner M, Bonarjee VV, Nilsen DW, Berning J, Carstensen S, Caidahl K. Effect of enalapril initiated early after acute myocardial infarction on heart failure parameters, with reference to clinical class and echocardiographic determinants. CONSENSUS II Multi-Echo Study Group. *Clin Cardiol.* 1996;19:543–548.

80. Vantrimpont P, Rouleau JL, Wun CC, et al. Additive beneficial effects of beta-blockers to angiotensin-converting enzyme inhibitors in the Survival and Ventricular Enlargement (SAVE) Study. SAVE Investigators. *J Am Coll Cardiol.* 1997;29:229–236.

81. MERIT-HF Study Group. Effect of metoprolol CR/XL in chronic heart failure: Metoprolol CR/XL Randomised Intervention Trial in Congestive Heart Failure (MERIT-HF). *Lancet.* 1999;353:2001–2007

82. Pitt B, Zannad F, Remme WJ, et al. The effect of spironolactone on morbidity and mortality in patients with severe heart failure. Randomized Aldactone Evaluation Study Investigators. *N Engl J Med.* 1999;341:709–717.

83. Pitt B, Remme W, Zannad F, et al. Eplerenone, a selective aldosterone blocker, in patients with left ventricular dysfunction after myocardial infarction. *N Engl J Med.* 2003;348: 1309–1321.

84. Australia/New Zealand Heart Failure Research Collaborative Group. Randomised, placebo-controlled trial of carvedilol in patients with congestive heart failure due to ischaemic heart disease. *Lancet.* 1997;349:375–380

85. Youssef G, Links M. The prevention and management of cardiovascular complications of chemotherapy in patients with cancer. *Am J Cardiovasc Drugs.* 2005;5:233–243.

86. Tassan-Mangina S, Codorean D, Metivier M, et al. Tissue Doppler imaging and conventional echocardiography after anthracycline treatment in adults: early and late alterations of left ventricular function during a prospective study. *Eur J Echocardiogr.* 2006;7:141–146.

87. Moss AJ, Zareba W, Hall WJ, et al. Prophylactic implantation of a defibrillator in patients with myocardial infarction and reduced ejection fraction. *N Engl J Med.* 2002;346: 877–883.

88. Bardy GH, Lee KL, Mark DB, et al. Amiodarone or an implantable cardioverter-defibrillator for congestive heart failure. *N Engl J Med.* 2005;352:225–237.

89. Hohnloser SH, Kuck KH, Dorian P, et al. Prophylactic use of an implantable cardioverter-defibrillator after acute myocardial infarction. *N Engl J Med.* 2004;351:2481–2488.

90. Bristow MR, Saxon LA, Boehmer J, et al. Cardiac-resynchronization therapy with or without an implantable defibrillator in advanced chronic heart failure. *N Engl J Med.* 2004;350: 2140–2150.

91. Achilli A, Sassara M, Ficili S, et al. Long-term effectiveness of cardiac resynchronization therapy in patients with refractory heart failure and "narrow" QRS. *J Am Coll Cardiol.* 2003;42:2117–2124.

92. Pitzalis MV, Iacoviello M, Romito R, et al. Cardiac resynchronization therapy tailored by echocardiographic evaluation of ventricular asynchrony. *J Am Coll Cardiol.* 2002;40: 1615–1622.

93. Stellbrink C, Breithardt OA, Franke A, et al. Impact of cardiac resynchronization therapy using hemodynamically optimized pacing on left ventricular remodeling in patients with congestive heart failure and ventricular conduction disturbances. *J Am Coll Cardiol.* 2001;38:1957–1965.

94. Yu CM, Bleeker GB, Fung JW, et al. Left ventricular reverse remodeling but not clinical improvement predicts long-term survival after cardiac resynchronization therapy. *Circulation.* 2005;112:1580–1586.

95. Bax JJ, Ansalone G, Breithardt OA, et al. Echocardiographic evaluation of cardiac resynchronization therapy: ready for routine clinical use? A critical appraisal. *J Am Coll Cardiol.* 2004;44:1–9.

96. Yu CM, Abraham WT, Bax J, et al. Predictors of response to cardiac resynchronization therapy (PROSPECT) study design. *Am Heart J.* 2005;149:600–605.

97. Nesta F, Otsuji Y, Handschumacher MD, et al. Leaflet concavity: a rapid visual clue to the presence and mechanism of functional mitral regurgitation. *J Am Soc Echocardiogr.* 2003;16:1301–1308.

98. Kwan J, Shiota T, Agler DA, et al. Geometric differences of the mitral apparatus between ischemic and dilated cardiomyopathy with significant mitral regurgitation: real-time three-dimensional echocardiography study. *Circulation.* 2003;107:1135–1140.

99. Bolling SF, Pagani FD, Deeb GM, Bach DS. Intermediate-term outcome of mitral reconstruction in cardiomyopathy. *J Thorac Cardiovasc Surg.* 1998;115:381–386.; discussion 387–388.

100. Breithardt OA, Sinha AM, Schwammenthal E, et al. Acute effects of cardiac resynchronization therapy on functional mitral regurgitation in advanced systolic heart failure. *J Am Coll Cardiol.* 2003;41:765–770.

101. Jimenez JH, Soerensen DD, He Z, He S, Yoganathan AP. Effects of a saddle shaped annulus on mitral valve function and chordal force distribution: an in vitro study. *Ann Biomed Eng*. 2003;31:1171–1181.

102. Khanna D, Miller AP, Nanda NC, Ahmed S, Lloyd SG. Transthoracic and transesophageal echocardiographic assessment of mitral regurgitation severity: usefulness of qualitative and semiquantitative techniques. *Echocardiography*. 2005;22:748–769.

103. Quere JP, Tribouilloy C, Enriquez-Sarano M. Vena contracta width measurement: theoretic basis and usefulness in the assessment of valvular regurgitation severity. *Curr Cardiol Rep*. 2003;5:110–115.

104. Athanasuleas CL, Stanley AW, Buckberg GD, Dor V, Di Donato M, Siler W. Surgical anterior ventricular endocardial restoration (SAVER) for dilated ischemic cardiomyopathy. *Semin Thorac Cardiovasc Surg*. 2001;13:448–458.

105. Suma H, Isomura T, Horii T, et al. Nontransplant cardiac surgery for end-stage cardiomyopathy. *J Thorac Cardiovasc Surg*. 2000;119:1233–1244.

106. Wilhelm MJ, Hammel D, Schmid C, et al. Partial left ventriculectomy and mitral valve repair: favorable short-term results in carefully selected patients with advanced heart failure due to dilated cardiomyopathy. *J Heart Lung Transplant*. 2005;24:1957–1964.

107. McGee EC Jr, Grady KL, McCarthy PM. Nontransplant surgical alternatives for heart failure. *Curr Treat Options Cardiovasc Med*. 2005;7:491–501.

108. Jones R, Lee K, Mark D, Bonw R. STICH trial. TS. Available at: http://www.stichtrial.org

109. Athanasuleas CL, Buckberg GD, Stanley AW, et al. Surgical ventricular restoration in the treatment of congestive heart failure due to post-infarction ventricular dilation. *J Am Coll Cardiol*. 2004;44:1439–1445.

110. Yotsumoto G, Sakata R, Ueno T, et al. Late development of mitral regurgitation after left ventricular reconstruction surgery. *Ann Thorac Cardiovasc Surg*. 2005;11:159–163.

111. Dor V. The endoventricular circular patch plasty ("Dor procedure") in ischemic akinetic dilated ventricles. *Heart Fail Rev*. 2001;6:187–193.

112. Cherniavsky AM, Karaskov AM, Marchenko AV, Mikova NV. Preoperative modeling of an optimal left ventricle volume for surgical treatment of ventricular aneurysms. *Eur J Cardiothorac Surg*. 2001;20:777–782.

113. Rose EA, Gelijns AC, Moskowitz AJ, et al. Long-term mechanical left ventricular assistance for end-stage heart failure. *N Engl J Med*. 2001;345:1435–1443.

114. Shapiro GC, Leibowitz DW, Oz MC, Weslow RG, Di Tullio MR, Homma S. Diagnosis of patent foramen ovale with transesophageal echocardiography in a patient supported with a left ventricular assist device. *J Heart Lung Transplant*. 1995;14:594–597.

115. Reilly MP, Wiegers SE, Cucchiara AJ, et al. Frequency, risk factors, and clinical outcomes of left ventricular assist device-associated ventricular thrombus. *Am J Cardiol*. 2000;86:1156–1159, A10.

116. Horton SC, Khodaverdian R, Chatelain P, et al. Left ventricular assist device malfunction: an approach to diagnosis by echocardiography. *J Am Coll Cardiol*. 2005;45:1435–1440.

117. Gulati VK, Katz WE, Follansbee WP, Gorcsan J, 3rd. Mitral annular descent velocity by tissue Doppler echocardiography as an index of global left ventricular function. *Am J Cardiol*. 1996;77:979–984.

118. Yip G, Wang M, Zhang Y, Fung JW, Ho PY, Sanderson JE. Left ventricular long axis function in diastolic heart failure is reduced in both diastole and systole: time for a redefinition? *Heart*. 2002;87:121–125.

119. Yu CM, Lin H, Yang H, Kong SL, Zhang Q, Lee SW. Progression of systolic abnormalities in patients with "isolated" diastolic heart failure and diastolic dysfunction. *Circulation*. 2002;105:1195–1201.

120. Wang M, Yip GW, Wang AY, et al. Peak early diastolic mitral annulus velocity by tissue Doppler imaging adds independent and incremental prognostic value. *J Am Coll Cardiol*. 2003;41:820–826.

121. Troughton RW, Prior DL, Frampton CM, et al. Usefulness of tissue Doppler and color M-mode indexes of left ventricular diastolic function in predicting outcomes in systolic left ventricular heart failure (from the ADEPT study). *Am J Cardiol.* 2005;96:257–262.
122. Okura H, Takada Y, Kubo T, et al. Tissue Doppler-derived index of left ventricular filling pressure, E/E', predicts survival of patients with non-valvular atrial fibrillation. *Heart.* 2006;92:1248–1252.
123. Sun JP, Popovic ZB, Greenberg NL, et al. Noninvasive quantification of regional myocardial function using Doppler-derived velocity, displacement, strain rate, and strain in healthy volunteers: effects of aging. *J Am Soc Echocardiogr.* 2004;17:132–138.
124. Koyama J, Ray-Sequin PA, Falk RH. Longitudinal myocardial function assessed by tissue velocity, strain, and strain rate tissue Doppler echocardiography in patients with AL (primary) cardiac amyloidosis. *Circulation.* 2003;107:2446–2452.
125. Palka P, Lange A, Donnelly JE, Nihoyannopoulos P. Differentiation between restrictive cardiomyopathy and constrictive pericarditis by early diastolic Doppler myocardial velocity gradient at the posterior wall. *Circulation.* 2000;102:655–662.
126. Bax JJ, Bleeker GB, Marwick TH, et al. Left ventricular dyssynchrony predicts response and prognosis after cardiac resynchronization therapy. *J Am Coll Cardiol.* 2004;44:1834–1840.
127. Bax JJ, Abraham T, Barold SS, et al. Cardiac resynchronization therapy: part 1 – issues before device implantation. *J Am Coll Cardiol.* 2005;46:2153–2167.
128. Sogaard P, Egeblad H, Pedersen AK, et al. Sequential versus simultaneous biventricular resynchronization for severe heart failure: evaluation by tissue Doppler imaging. *Circulation.* 2002;106:2078–2084.
129. Helle-Valle T, Crosby J, Edvardsen T, et al. New noninvasive method for assessment of left ventricular rotation: speckle tracking echocardiography. *Circulation.* 2005;112:3149–3156.
130. Notomi Y, Lysyansky P, Setser RM, et al. Measurement of ventricular torsion by two-dimensional ultrasound speckle tracking imaging. *J Am Coll Cardiol.* 2005;45:2034–2041.
131. Knudtson ML, Galbraith PD, Hildebrand KL, Tyberg JV, Beyar R. Dynamics of left ventricular apex rotation during angioplasty: a sensitive index of ischemic dysfunction. *Circulation.* 1997;96:801–808.
132. Stuber M, Scheidegger MB, Fischer SE, et al. Alterations in the local myocardial motion pattern in patients suffering from pressure overload due to aortic stenosis. *Circulation.* 1999;100:361–368.
133. Vannan MA, Pedrizzetti G, Li P, et al. Effect of cardiac resynchronization therapy on longitudinal and circumferential left ventricular mechanics by velocity vector imaging: description and initial clinical application of a novel method using high-frame rate B-mode echocardiographic images. *Echocardiography.* 2005;22:826–830.
134. Fuchs E, Muller MF, Oswald H, Thony H, Mohacsi P, Hess OM. Cardiac rotation and relaxation in patients with chronic heart failure. *Eur J Heart Fail.* 2004;6:715–722.
135. Sugeng L, Weinert L, Lang RM. Left ventricular assessment using real time three dimensional echocardiography. *Heart.* 2003;89(suppl 3):iii29–iii36.
136. Jenkins C, Bricknell K, Hanekom L, Marwick TH. Reproducibility and accuracy of echocardiographic measurements of left ventricular parameters using real-time three-dimensional echocardiography. *J Am Coll Cardiol.* 2004;44:878–886.
137. Sugeng L, Mor-Avi V, Weinert L, et al. Quantitative assessment of left ventricular size and function: side-by-side comparison of real-time three-dimensional echocardiography and computed tomography with magnetic resonance reference. *Circulation.* 2006;114:654–661.
138. Corsi C, Lang RM, Veronesi F, et al. Volumetric quantification of global and regional left ventricular function from real-time three-dimensional echocardiographic images. *Circulation.* 2005;112:1161–1170.
139. Mor-Avi V, Sugeng L, Weinert L, et al. Fast measurement of left ventricular mass with real-time three-dimensional echocardiography: comparison with magnetic resonance imaging. *Circulation.* 2004;110:1814–1818.

140. Sugeng L, Spencer KT, Mor-Avi V, et al. Dynamic three-dimensional color flow Doppler: an improved technique for the assessment of mitral regurgitation. *Echocardiography*. 2003;20:265–273.

141. Lang RM, Mor-Avi V, Sugeng L, Nieman PS, Sahn DJ. Three-dimensional echocardiography: the benefits of the additional dimension. *J Am Coll Cardiol*. 2006;48:2053–2069.

142. Senni M, Rodeheffer RJ, Tribouilloy CM, et al. Use of echocardiography in the management of congestive heart failure in the community. *J Am Coll Cardiol*. 1999;33:164–170.

143. Kermani M, Dua A, Gradman AH. Underutilization and clinical benefits of angiotensin-converting enzyme inhibitors in patients with asymptomatic left ventricular dysfunction. *Am J Cardiol*. 2000;86:644–648.

144. Get with the Guidelines AHA. Available at: http://www.americanheart.org/presenter.jhtml?identifier=3027533

145. Guidelines Applied in Practice ACoC. Available at: http://www.acc.org/qualityandscience/gap/or/oregon_gap.htm

146. Nagueh SF, Zoghbi WA. Clinical assessment of LV diastolic filling by Doppler echocardiography. *ACC Curr J Rev*. July/August 2001;10:45–49.

# Chapter 27
# Future Applications of Echocardiography in Acute Coronary Syndrome

P. Tung, P. Kee, H. Kim, S.L. Huang, M. Klegerman, and D. McPherson

## Case Presentation

RJ is a 55-year-old male who presents to your clinic due to his concern for cardiovascular disease. His past medical history is notable for hypertension and hyperlipidemia, both of which are controlled with medications. He has no history of alcohol, tobacco, or drug use. His medications include atenolol 25 mg daily, lipitor 40 mg daily, and aspirin 81 mg daily. He is an avid runner and is currently training for an upcoming marathon. Currently, he has no cardiovascular symptoms. He is seeking care from you because he has a strong family history of heart disease and is concerned about his cardiovascular risk. His father, grandfather, and older brother all died suddenly before age 50 from myocardial infarction. RJ is afraid that he will "drop dead like the rest of his family."

His physical examination is essentially unremarkable. His blood pressure is 125/80 mmHg, heart rate 64 bpm, respiratory rate 12/min, body mass index 23. His carotids are normal with brisk upstrokes and without bruit. His lung fields are clear to auscultation, and heart sounds are regular and without murmurs. His distal pulses are symmetric and normal.

An electrocardiogram performed in clinic shows normal sinus rhythm with no evidence of accelerated conduction and normal QRS, ST, and T segments. His laboratory results are notable for total cholesterol 160 mg/dL, low-density lipoprotein cholesterol 110 mg/dL, high-density lipoprotein cholesterol 38 mg/dL, high-sensitivity C-reactive protein 2.2 mg/L, homocysteine 8 μmol/L. The rest of his complete blood count and chemistry panels are unremarkable.

You discuss with RJ that according to the Framingham's risk score, his cardiovascular risk for the next 10 years is low – estimated at 7%. However, you recognize the Framingham's risk score does not account for family history. You are also

P. Tung (✉)

Department of Internal Medicine, University of Texas Health Science Center,
Houston, TX, USA
e-mail: poyee.p.tung@uth.tmc.edu

E. Herzog, F.A. Chaudhry (eds.), *Echocardiography in Acute Coronary Syndrome*,
DOI 10.1007/978-1-84882-027-2_27, © Springer-Verlag London Limited 2009

wary of the mildly elevated high-sensitivity C-reactive protein level, which may convey a higher risk of future heart attack. You recommend RJ undergo an exercise echocardiogram which would offer further information regarding risk stratification and prognosis.

The patient exercises on the Bruce protocol for 14 min 30 s, achieving 90% of his maximum predicted heart rate. He has no ischemic symptoms. His blood pressure goes from 130/80 mmHg at rest to 160/85 mmHg with peak exercise. His echocardiogram at rest is unremarkable showing normal biventricular size, systolic and diastolic function, and no significant valvular abnormalities. At peak exercise, his left ventricle augments appropriately and all myocardial segments thicken normally.

You are confident that the normal stress echocardiogram has high negative predictive value in excluding obstructive coronary artery disease. In addition, you know from the literature that having a completely normal stress echocardiogram confers low, although not zero, risk of cardiac event in the next 3–5 years.[1–5] Now, RJ wants to know if it is okay to conclude he does not have coronary artery disease.

## Introduction

Currently available imaging modalities including stress echocardiography, single-photon emission computed tomography, and coronary angiography are used for detecting advanced stages of atherosclerosis when significant luminal narrowing has occurred. Detection of early stages of atherosclerosis is prudent because it allows opportunities for aggressive medical intervention. More importantly, previous studies have shown that coronary occlusion resulting in infarction does not correlate with site of high-grade stenosis.[6–8] This highlights the importance of identifying the vulnerable patient rather than the obstructive lesion. We now recognize that inflammation and neovascularization in the arterial wall are pathological changes in early atherosclerosis. With the aid of acoustically active ultrasound contrast agents, we now have the opportunities to image earlier markers of disease and explore potential applications of these agents for targeted drug delivery.

## Acoustically Active Contrast Agents for Ultrasound Imaging

Acoustically active contrast agents are intravascular tracers that can be engineered to target and enhance detection of endothelial and adventitial markers present in early stages of atherosclerosis. Entrapped air or gas within the contrast agents makes them good acoustic reflectors. Their outer shells can be modified, so ligands such as peptides or antibodies against endothelial markers, or drugs can be attached. A number of formulations including commercial formulations (i.e., Optison[TM], Definity[TM]) are available. Our group pioneered liposome-based acoustically active contrast agents with air entrapped in the phospholipid bilayers.[9] These agents can be used to target and highlight early atheroma components.

## Imaging of Inflammation

Acoustically active contrast agents can detect arterial inflammation via passive or active targeting. Basalyga et al. demonstrated albumin in the microbubble shell was able to bind passively to denuded aorta via electrostatic interactions,[10] presumably mediated through adherence of leukocytes to the inflamed endothelium.[11] In active targeting, the surface components of acoustically active contrast agents are modified to interact with and highlight the markers of inflammation. Villanueva et al. used anti-human anti-ICAM-1 (intercellular adhesion molecule expressed in the membranes of leukocytes and endothelial cells)-conjugated microbubbles to attach to activated coronary artery endothelial cells in vitro.[12] We have demonstrated that our echogenic liposomes were able to highlight both endothelial and adventitial components of atheroma in vivo. Using Yucatan miniswines as a model, we showed anti-ICAM-1- and anti-VCAM-1-conjugated liposomes bound to atherosclerotic arterial wall (Figs. 27.1 and 27.2).[13,14] Furthermore, we demonstrated improved characterization of the binding of anti-ICAM echogenic liposomes to atheroma using 3-D intravascular ultrasound (Fig. 27.3, unpublished data).

## Imaging of Thrombus

Thrombus formation and arterial occlusion are important features of inflammation and atherosclerosis. Noninvasive imaging of thrombus formation using thrombus-targeted microbubbles and echogenic liposomes has been studied. Lanza et al. demonstrated feasibility of highlighting arterial thrombi in vivo using microbubbles targeted with antifibrin antibodies.[15]

## Potential Therapeutic Applications of Ultrasound in Coronary Artery Disease

By coupling drugs or small molecules to acoustically active contrast agents, they can potentially be delivered to sites of interest which would enhance their therapeutic effects. Preliminary data suggested in vivo binding of thrombus to MRX-408, a peptide coupled to the lipid shell, may enhance thrombolysis when activated by ultrasound.[16] Another potential strategy to achieve targeted thrombolysis is by coupling tissue plasminogen activator to ultrasound contrast agents.

Our group has demonstrated the feasibility of loading nitric oxide, a biologically active agent, onto echogenic liposomes for delivery to vascular smooth muscle cells (Fig. 27.4, unpublished data). Administration of these nitric oxide-containing contrast agents to balloon-injured carotid arteries results in the inhibition of intimal thickening when compared with controls (Fig. 27.5, unpublished data). This provides a new approach for delivering a variety of bioactive agents to target tissues.

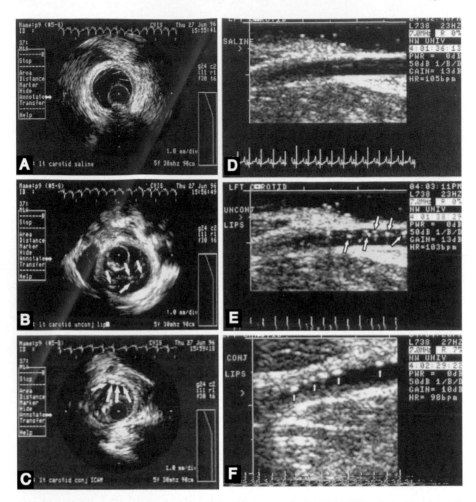

**Fig. 27.1** In vivo data demonstrating the attachment of anti-ICAM-1-conjugated echogenic immunoliposomes to the atherosclerotic arterial wall. Intravascular ultrasound imaging of the atherosclerotic left carotid artery of a Yucatan miniswine (notice the circular atheroma deposition). (**A**) Following injection of saline (*arrows* point to early atheroma). (**B**) Following injection of unconjugated liposomes (*arrows* point to liposomes within lumen). (**C**) Following injection of anti-ICAM-1-labeled liposomes (*arrows* point to liposomes attached to the atherosclerotic plaque). Transvascular ultrasound images of the atherosclerotic left carotid artery of a Yucatan miniswine. (**D**) Following saline injection. (**E**) Following injection of unconjugated liposomes (*arrows* point to liposomes within the lumen). (**F**) Following injection of anti-ICAM-1-labeled liposomes (*arrows* point to liposomes attached to the atherosclerotic plaque)

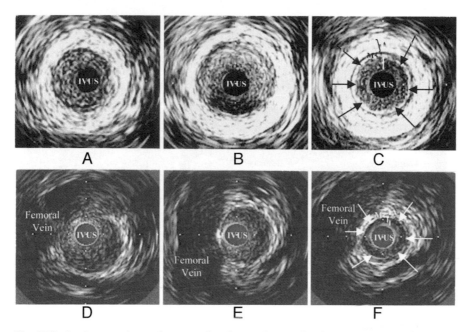

**Fig. 27.2** In vivo experiment demonstrating the attachment of anti-ICAM-1 and anti-VCAM-1-conjugated echogenic immunoliposomes to atherosclerotic arterial wall. Intravascular ultrasound imaging of the atherosclerotic left carotid artery of a Yucatan miniswine. (**A**) Following saline injection. (**B**) Five minutes after injection of unconjugated liposomes. (**C**) Following injection of anti-ICAM-1-labeled liposomes. There is enhancement of the atheroma (*arrows*) as well as adventitia (**A**). Intravascular ultrasound imaging of the atherosclerotic femoral artery of a Yucatan miniswine. (**D**) Following saline injection. (**E**) Five minutes after injection of unconjugated liposomes. (**F**) Postinjection of anti-VCAM-1-labeled liposomes (*arrows* point to enhanced atheroma)

We have also demonstrated it is possible to deliver a small molecule (in this case, calcein was used as a surrogate) to vascular smooth muscle cells by conjugating anti-smooth muscle cell actin antibody to the liposomes (Fig. 27.6, unpublished data). The ability to regulate or manipulate vascular SMC function is an important step in the treatment of atherosclerosis.

## Case Presentation (Year 2020)

In year 2020, our patient RJ will have more diagnostic and therapeutic options. Despite a normal exercise echocardiogram, you feel that RJ is at risk of vascular disease because of his strong family history and abnormal C-reactive protein levels. The patient undergoes ultrasound-based molecular imaging of his coronary arteries using anti-ICAM and anti-VCAM-loaded liposomes as contrast agents. The test reveals he does indeed have diffuse inflammation of his vessels, which is a sign of subclinical atherosclerosis. You prescribe RJ with more potent anti-lipid and

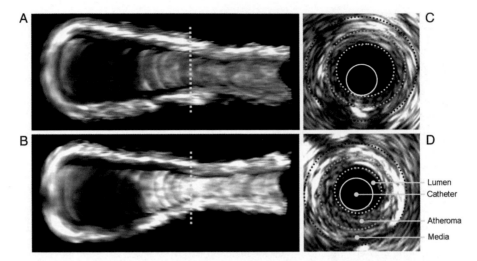

**Fig. 27.3** 2-D and 3-D volumetric intravascular ultrasound images of an atheroma of the common carotid artery. A longitudinal section of the artery is displayed to better demonstrate the extent and distribution of plaque to the endothelial surface and across the arterial wall. The *dark* luminal region indicates the bifurcation of the common carotid artery and is used as a landmark ensuring the same arterial segment has been selected at baseline and after treatment with anti-ICAM-1-conjugated immunoliposomes. Acoustic enhancement by anti-ICAM-1 immunoliposomes was observed across the arterial wall and over the endothelial surface, especially beyond the bifurcation point. (**A**) Baseline before anti-ICAM-1 liposomes injection. (**B**) Five minutes after anti-ICAM-1 liposomes injection. (**C** and **D**) 2-D intravascular ultrasound images detailing enhancement of endothelium and atheroma by anti-ICAM-1 immunoliposomes on the cross-sectional view along the *yellow line* in the 3-D image

anti-inflammatory drugs and plan to follow his clinical response with a repeat imaging study. If RJ fails to respond with regression of disease in 6 months, you plan to administer small molecule-loaded echogenic liposomes to modify his vascular smooth muscle function directly. Your patient RJ is very satisfied with your plan, and he remains your loyal patient for the next 40 years!

## Conclusion

The ability to use targeted acoustically active tracers to detect inflammation within the vessel wall and thrombus formation is an important step in identifying vulnerable patients at risk for vascular disease. This technique is a promising future tool for identifying patients with early disease, monitoring their response to therapies and potentially as a therapeutic treatment option through targeted drug delivery.

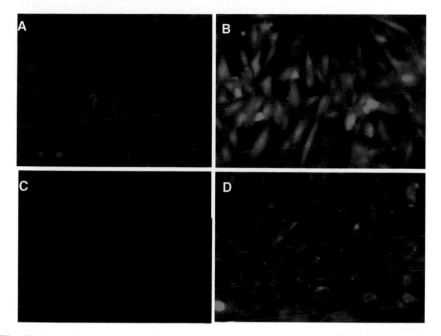

**Fig. 27.4** In vitro experiment demonstrating loading of NO onto echogenic liposomes allows delivery of NO onto vascular smooth muscle cells. Hemoglobin normally sequesters NO. However, NO-loaded liposomes are not sequestered by hemoglobin and can be delivered onto smooth muscle cells. (**A**) Nitric oxide saturated solution in the absence of hemoglobin. (**B**) Nitric oxide saturated solution in the presence of hemoglobin. (**C**) Liposomes containing nitric oxide in the absence of hemoglobin. (**D**) Liposomes containing nitric oxide in the presence of hemoglobin

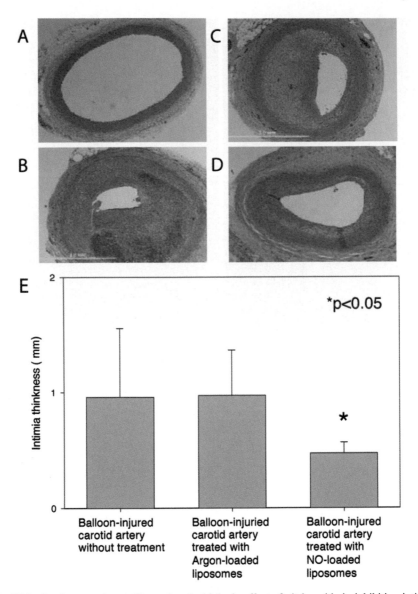

**Fig. 27.5** In vivo experiment illustrating the biologic effect of nitric oxide in inhibiting intimal hyperplasia in balloon-injured carotid arteries in a rabbit model. (**A**) Histology of a controlled carotid artery showing normal intima. (**B**) Histology of a balloon-injured carotid artery showing intimal hyperplasia. (**C**) Histology of a balloon-injured carotid artery treated with argon, which has no biologic effect. (**D**) Histology of a balloon-injured carotid artery treated with nitric oxide, which is effective in inhibiting intimal hyperplasia. (**E**) Nitric oxide-loaded liposomes inhibit intimal thickness by $51 \pm 6\%$

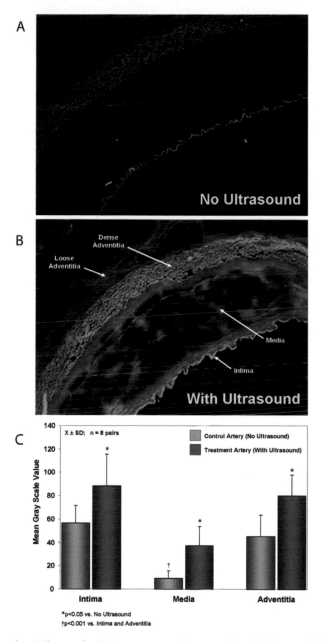

**Fig. 27.6** In vivo delivery of calcein, a surrogate for a small molecule, to all three layers of the arterial wall in Yucatan miniswines using ultrasound and smooth muscle cell actin-targeted liposomes. (**A**) Without ultrasound, very little uptake in the arterial media was noted. (**B**) With ultrasound treatment, greater uptake in the media is seen. (**C**) The bar graph demonstrates uptake of calcein in all three arterial layers following ultrasound treatment

# References

1. Cortigiani L, Dodi C, Paolini E, Bernardi D, Bruno G, Nannini E. Prognostic value of pharmacological stress echocardiography in women with chest pain and unknown coronary artery disease. *J Am Coll Cardiol*. 1998;32(7):1975–1981.
2. Cortigiani L, Lombardi M, Landi P, Paolini EA, Nannini E. Risk stratification by pharmacological stress echocardiography in a primary care cardiology centre. Experience in 1082 patients. *Eur Heart J*. 1998;19(11):1673–1680.
3. Cortigiani L, Picano E, Coletta C, et al. Safety, feasibility, and prognostic implications of pharmacologic stress echocardiography in 1482 patients evaluated in an ambulatory setting. *Am Heart J*. 2001;141(4):621–629.
4. Steinberg EH, Madmon L, Patel CP, Sedlis SP, Kronzon I, Cohen JL. Long-term prognostic significance of dobutamine echocardiography in patients with suspected coronary artery disease: results of a 5-year follow-up study. *J Am Coll Cardiol*. 1997;29(5):969–973.
5. Yao S, Qureshi E, Sherrid MV, Chaudhry FA. Practical applications in stress echocardiography: risk stratification and prognosis in patients with known or suspected ischemic heart disease. *J Am Coll Cardiol*. 2003;42(6):1084–1090.
6. Ambrose J, Hjemdahl-Monsen C, Borrico S, Gorlin R, Fuster V. Angiographic demonstration of a common link between unstable angina pectoris and non-Q-wave acute myocardial infarction. *Am J Cardiol*. 1988;61(4):244–247.
7. Ambrose J, Tannenbaum M, Alexopoulos D, et al. Angiographic progression of coronary artery disease and the development of myocardial infarction. *J Am Coll Cardiol*. 1988;12(1):56–62.
8. Little W, Constantinescu M, Applegate R, et al. Can coronary angiography predict the site of a subsequent myocardial infarction in patients with mild-to-moderate coronary artery disease? *Circulation*. 1988;78(5 Pt 1):1157–1166.
9. Huang S, Hamilton A, Nagaraj A, et al. Improving ultrasound reflectivity and stability of echogenic liposomal dispersions for use as targeted ultrasound contrast agents. *J Pharm Sci*. 2001;90(12):1917–1926.
10. Basalyga DM, Wagner WR, Beer-Stolz D, Fenyus ML, Villanueva FS. Albumin microbubbles adhere to exposed extracellular matrix of perfused whole vessels. *Circulation*. 1998;98:I-290.
11. Yasu T, Greener Y, Jablonski E, et al. Activated leukocytes and endothelial cells enhance retention of ultrasound contrast microspheres containing perfluoropropane in inflamed venules. *Int J Cardiol*. 2005;98(2):245–252.
12. Villanueva F, Jankowski R, Klibanov S, et al. Microbubbles targeted to intercellular adhesion molecule-1 bind to activated coronary artery endothelial cells. *Circulation*. 1998;98(1):1–5.
13. Demos SM, Alkan-Onyuksel H, Kane BJ, et al. In vivo targeting of acoustically reflective liposomes for intravascular and transvascular ultrasonic enhancement. *J Am Coll Cardiol*. 1999;33(3):867–875.
14. Hamilton A, Huang S, Warnick D, et al. Intravascular ultrasound molecular imaging of atheroma components in vivo. *J Am Coll Cardiol*. 2004;43(3):453–460.
15. Lanza GM, Wallace KD, Scott MJ, et al. A novel site-targeted ultrasonic contrast agent with broad biomedical application. *Circulation*. 1996;94(12):3334–3340.
16. Wu Y, Unger EC, McCreery TP, et al. Binding and lysing of blood clots using MRX-408. *Invest Radiol*. 1998;33(12):880–885.

# Chapter 28
# Myocardial Contrast Echocardiography in the Emergency Department

**J. Todd Belcik and Jonathan R. Lindner**

## Diagnostic Algorithms for Chest Pain in the Emergency Room

Emergency departments across the United States annually treat close to 6 million patients who present with chest pain (CP).[1] Only a minority of these patients (10–30%) are ultimately diagnosed as having an acute myocardial infarction or acute coronary syndrome (ACS).[2,3] Yet, many patients with noncardiac CP are admitted to the hospital or to observation units incurring enormous burden to the health-care system. It has been estimated that the majority of patients admitted to the hospital with CP have a noncardiac etiology.[1] Of those who do have ACS, the standard diagnostic algorithms that are currently employed are frequently nondiagnostic, leading to a delayed or even missed diagnosis.[2–4] These standard practices include detailed history, physical examination, 12-lead electrocardiogram (ECG), and circulating biomarkers for myocardial cell injury. Although the ECG can rapidly identify patients with ST-elevation MI, its overall sensitivity is relatively low and is diagnostic in roughly 30–50% of patients who have acute myocardial infarction (MI) other than acute ST-elevation MI.[5,6] One of the most important diagnostic advances over the last two decades has been cardiac-specific troponin assays that can be used to identify high-risk patients. However, these assays may remain negative for a period of time depending on the timing of presentation and the degree of necrosis, are somewhat limited in their ability to detect ischemia without necrosis, and can also be falsely elevated by other comorbid conditions.[7–9] Because of the limitations in current evaluation methods, approximately 4–5% of patients with evolving myocardial infarctions are mistakenly discharged from the emergency department.[2,4,10] These patients have a particularly high mortality risk.[2]

To address limitations of the current state-of-the-art practice, protocols for rapid imaging of myocardial function and perfusion have been developed and have been

J.T. Belcik (✉)
Division of Cardiovascular Medicine, Oregon Health and Science University,
Portland, Oregon, USA
e-mail: lindnerj@ohsu.edu

E. Herzog, F.A. Chaudhry (eds.), *Echocardiography in Acute Coronary Syndrome*,
DOI 10.1007/978-1-84882-027-2_28, © Springer-Verlag London Limited 2009

tested for incremental value. The widespread availability, low cost, and portable bedside capabilities of ultrasound make echocardiography the most practical imaging technique for rapid evaluation of patients presenting to the emergency department with chest pain. A critical component of the echocardiographic examination in this setting is the use of ultrasound contrast agents. These agents are comprised of acoustically active microbubbles that are generally encapsulated with a shell composed of protein, lipid, or biocompatible polymers and contain either air (nitrogen) or high-molecular weight gases (perfluorocarbons, sulfur hexafluoride) that have low solubility and diffusivity.[11] The use of these agents to enhance wall motion assessment and to detect perfusion abnormalities in patients presenting with CP will be discussed.

## Left Ventricular Opacification

Assessment of regional wall motion by echocardiography in the acute setting can provide powerful prognostic information in patients with CP, particularly in those without prior MI who do not have preexisting wall motion abnormalities.[12,13] In particular, the negative predictive value of the technique is high. In other words, the presence of completely normal wall motion can exclude ischemia, provided that imaging is performed during CP or very soon after resolution of symptoms. This approach hinges on adequate visualization of all myocardial segments. Despite advances in imaging technology, such as harmonic filtering, adequate evaluation of the endocardial border is still not possible in 5–15% of patients due to factors such as obesity and lung disease. Microbubble-based ultrasound contrast agents improve endocardial border delineation of the left ventricle in these technically suboptimal studies (Fig. 28.1).[14-17] This issue is of particular importance in the evaluation of patients who present to the emergency department with CP since (1) every segment needs to be visualized, (2) a high level of reader confidence is needed, and (3) the imaging environment in the emergency department is often suboptimal.

Several clinical studies have demonstrated that ultrasound contrast agents used in technically suboptimal studies can substantially increase the number of interpretable

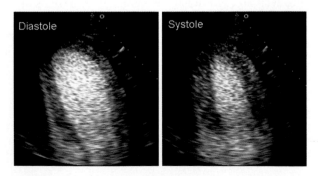

**Fig. 28.1** End-diastolic and end-systolic frames during left ventricular opacification from a patient with technically difficult baseline windows. Endocardial borders are defined by the change in contrast intensity between the cavity and the myocardium

segments and decrease interobserver variability.[14–16] Improvement in endocardial definition and an increase in the number of segments that can be adequately visualized with contrast administration have led to greater diagnostic accuracy.[14,18] Physician confidence also increases with contrast administration, particularly in those with less experience in echocardiographic interpretation.[19] The issue of reader confidence is not inconsequential since often rapid decisions must be made in the emergency department on the basis of bedside interpretation.

The additional diagnostic value of left ventricular opacification with contrast echocardiography has recently been demonstrated in emergency room patients presenting with chest pain.[20] Regional wall motion information with contrast echocardiography performed in patients without ST-segment elevation on initial ECG provided substantial incremental diagnostic for diagnosis of ACS. It also provided prognostic information for short- and long-term risk for adverse

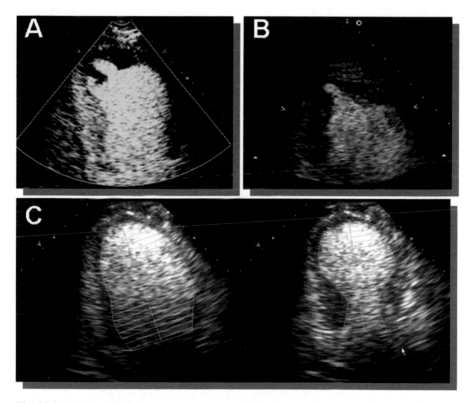

**Fig. 28.2** Ancillary findings on contrast echocardiography in patients presenting with chest pain. (**A**) Left ventricular apical thrombus in a patient presenting with acute MI and a wall motion abnormality in the LAD distribution. (**B**) Left ventricular apical pseudoaneurysm which was not visualized on the baseline noncontrast study in patients with recurrence of chest pain several weeks after MI. (**C**) End-diastolic (*left*) and end-systolic (*right*) frames in a patient with apical ballooning syndrome and normal coronary artery anatomy. The wall motion abnormality from the end-systolic frames is atypical for coronary artery distribution pattern

cardiovascular events and for mortality. In patients who are confirmed to have an ischemic cause of their CP, contrast echocardiography can also reveal other important manifestations of disease such as the presence of ventricular pseudoaneurysms or ventricular thrombus (Fig. 28.2). Several case studies have also shown that other miscellaneous disease states that can manifest as chest pain, such as apical variant hypertrophic cardiomyopathy and idiopathic apical ballooning (Takotsubo cardiomyopathy), are easily identifiable with the use of ultrasound contrast agents for left ventricular opacification.[21,22]

## Evaluation of Regional Myocardial Blood Flow

The ability to rapidly assess myocardial perfusion at the patient bedside provides additional diagnostic potential for myocardial contrast echocardiography (MCE). Most of the microbubble ultrasound contrast agents that have been approved for use in patients are smaller than the average capillary diameter and have a similar rheology to erythrocytes.[23,24] Hence, they act as a pure intravascular blood pool agent and can be used to evaluate regional perfusion by measuring contrast enhancement within the myocardium.[25] Appropriate use of MCE in patients with possible or known ACS relies on user knowledge of the technical components of perfusion imaging.

The degree of acoustic signal enhancement generated by microbubbles, measured as a video intensity (VI), reflects the concentration of microbubbles in tissues. Hence, regional VI reflects relative myocardial blood volume, provided imaging is being performed with a method that does not compromise microbubble integrity. Since the vast majority of the intramyocardial blood volume resides in the capillary compartment,[26] the VI from contrast administration reflects capillary blood volume. Information on capillary blood volume alone can be useful in patients presenting with CP. Perfusion abnormalities at rest are generally characterized by reduced myocardial blood volume due to either capillary loss (prior infarction), complete lack of capillary filling (acute infarction), or capillary derecruitment in the face of reduced perfusion pressure (flow-limiting stenosis at rest). All of these pathophysiologic processes can be detected by imaging blood volume with nondestructive, low-mechanical index imaging (Fig. 28.3). Imaging blood volume alone in this manner should be used with caution though for several reasons. First, attenuation defects can appear identical to blood volume abnormalities. Second, if microbubble concentration is too high, then system saturation (signal enhancement that is beyond the upper limit of the dynamic range) may obfuscate a defect that is due to resting hypoperfusion.[11] Finally, flow information rather than volume information is necessary in certain circumstances such as when evaluating the adequacy of collateral flow or antegrade flow in the infarct-related artery.

For evaluation of blood flow, microbubbles within the imaging sector volume must be destroyed and the rate of their replenishment measured.[25] The rate of microbubble replenishment is assessed by the rate constant of video intensity

**Fig. 28.3** Perfusion defect at the left ventricular apex and the distal lateral wall where there is complete absence of contrast enhancement during continuous low-power myocardial contrast echocardiography. There is an underlying mural apical thrombus that also does not opacify

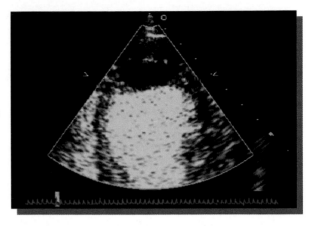

recovery. This parameter can be quantified by fitting postdestructive imaging data to a one-exponential function. Data for such curve fitting can be obtained by one of two methods: (1) continuous low-power imaging after several frames of high-power destructive imaging or (2) progressive prolongation of the pulsing interval (time interval between frames) during high-power imaging that destroys microbubbles with each imaging pulse.[11] Blood flow can then be calculated by the product of the rate constant (capillary blood velocity) and relative blood volume, which is measured by the relative plateau intensity once refill is complete.[25]

In the setting of ACS, assessment of flow is often needed immediately at the patient bedside without recourse to quantitative regional analysis from curve fitting. In this setting, visual evaluation of reduced microvascular velocity must suffice. This can be accomplished by either visually detecting regional heterogeneity in the time or pulsing interval required to reach plateau intensity, or identification of a territory that requires more than five cardiac cycles to fill (in the absence of bradycardia or tachycardia). Evaluation of regional capillary blood velocity provides the most accurate depiction of the perfusion territory of the culprit vessel since it can detect regions that are supplied by collateral perfusion that can have relatively normal blood volume despite reduced blood flow.[27]

## Perfusion Imaging for Diagnosis of ACS

The incremental value of perfusion imaging in patients presenting to the emergency department with CP has been evaluated in several studies that used the visual inspection techniques described above.[20,28,29] The premise of these studies was that perfusion imaging could provide additive diagnostic and/or prognostic information to wall motion assessment for several reasons. First, not all global or regional ventricular dysfunction is secondary to ischemia. Second, wall motion can be difficult to assess in certain patient populations, such as those with left bundle branch block.

Finally, in those with ACS, the finding of abnormal function but normal perfusion often denotes a "myocardial stunning" physiology, which is likely to convey a different prognosis than persistent hypoperfusion.

Studies comparing MCE and radionuclide imaging have demonstrated equivalent diagnostic performance for the two techniques in patients presenting with chest pain.[29] In a series of almost 1,000 patients who presented to the emergency department with prolonged CP, MCE performed within 12 h was shown to provide incremental diagnostic and prognostic information.[20,28] For diagnostic purposes, the combination of regional function and perfusion was found to be superior to standard clinical assessment. In particular, perfusion and wall motion with MCE was superior to the TIMI risk score, particularly when taking into account only the initial troponin value. These findings indicate that MCE at the patient bedside provides the ability to rapidly risk stratify patients with CP very early after presentation. It should be noted, however, that the incremental *diagnostic* value of perfusion imaging to regional function was very small. However, perfusion imaging data were particularly helpful in determining long-term *prognosis*. Those patients with abnormal regional function but preserved perfusion (stunning or nonischemic etiologies) had

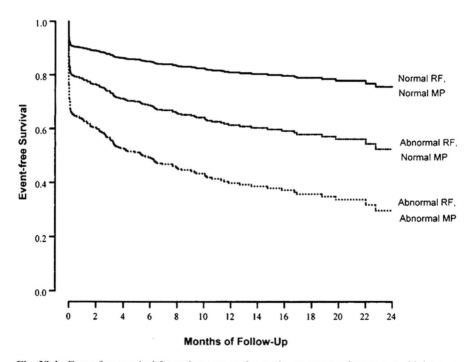

**Fig. 28.4** Event-free survival for patients presenting to the emergency department with intermediate TIMI risk score according to regional function (RF) and myocardial perfusion (MP) status. Events were defined as death, myocardial infarction, unstable angina, or coronary revascularization. Reproduced with permission[28]

a significantly better event-free survival than those with abnormal function and perfusion (Fig. 28.4).[20,28]

## MCE in Patients with Known MI

Myocardial contrast echocardiography may provide important information even in those patients in whom the diagnosis of ACS or ST-elevation MI has been made. One such application is the measurement of the risk area. The myocardial risk area is the region that is destined to undergo necrosis unless adequate perfusion is restored. In the setting of acute coronary occlusion, the risk area is the territory supplied by the infarct-related artery minus the territory that is supplied by sufficient collateral flow to maintain viability (approximately 0.20–0.25 ml/min/g tissue).[30] These territorial patterns can be assessed with MCE perfusion imaging (Fig. 28.5). In canine models of occlusion, it has been demonstrated that central territories that lack perfusion are the regions that are destined to undergo necrosis, which occurs in a time-dependent fashion.[27,31] Surrounding regions that have delayed contrast replenishment compared to remote territories are ischemic but receive sufficient collateral flow to maintain viability even if occlusion is prolonged.[27,31] Wall motion cannot differentiate between collateralized zones and regions that are destined to necrosis since both will produce severe hypokinesis to akinesis.[32]

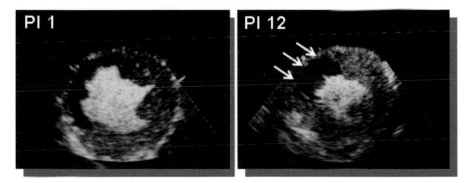

**Fig. 28.5** Illustration of true risk area and collateralized regions during occlusion of the LAD in a canine model. The perfusion defect at a short pulsing interval (PI) illustrates the ischemic region subtended by the LAD. With prolongation of the PI, there is gradual filling of the borders due to collateral blood flow, thereby revealing the true risk area at the center of the perfusion bed (*arrows*)

The use of MCE for evaluating risk area in patients has been confirmed whereby perfusion imaging was performed immediately before primary percutaneous coronary intervention (PCI) for acute ST-elevation MI.[33] Regions with severe wall motion abnormality but the presence of some degree of perfusion during coronary occlusion almost always demonstrated recovery of resting function at follow-up echocardiography several months later. Therefore, the presence of perfusion within the territory of an infarct-related artery, whether from antegrade or collateral flow, can give reassurance that viability will be maintained. On the other hand, the lack of perfusion at the time of presentation does not necessarily imply that wall motion or contractile reserve will not recover since prompt revascularization may still result in complete salvage.

Although MCE can measure the true risk area with excellent spatial resolution, the clinical utility of this information and whether it should be used to make treatment decisions is not clear at the present time. This approach has instead been used to evaluate new treatment strategies aimed at improving microvascular reflow. The best measure of any therapy aimed at improving myocardial salvage is to evaluate eventual infarct size as a proportion to the true risk area rather than measurement of infarct size alone. The ability of MCE to provide this information on percent salvage has been demonstrated in trials where the therapeutic effect of adenosine given as an adjunct to primary PCI was studied.[34]

In those with recognized MI, MCE can also be used to assess the adequacy of reperfusion therapy. Since the technique evaluates perfusion at the capillary level, lack of perfusion after thrombolysis or PCI can also occur from microvascular no-reflow that occurs in 20–30% of instances when epicardial artery patency with TIMI-3 flow has been achieved.[35–37] The complete lack of myocardial reflow in the territory of the infarct-related artery detected by MCE predicts with lack of functional recovery and a high risk for adverse remodeling.[38–41] Partial or non-transmural perfusion defects, which tend to match well with regions with delayed enhancement on Gd-DTPA magnetic resonance imaging,[42] may or may not recover resting function depending on their extent.[33,40] Even if resting function does not recover, the presence of residual perfusion does denote the presence of viability confirmed by the presence of contractile reserve during low-dose dobutamine.[33,43] It should be cautioned that although MCE can provide information on acute reflow patterns in patients in the emergency department, assessment of microvascular integrity is most accurate for predicting long-term outcome when performed several days after revascularization therapy, since reactive hyperemia and temporal heterogeneity of microvascular flow occur in the first few days after epicardial artery recanalization.[44,45]

# References

1. Nawar EW, Niska RW, Xu J. National Hospital Ambulatory Medical Care Survey: 2005 Emergency Department Summary. Advance Data from Vital and Health Statistics; no. 386. Centers for Disease Control and Prevention, and the National Center for Health Statistics. Available at: http://www.cdc.gov/nchs
2. Pope JH, Aufderheide TP, Ruthazer R, et al. Missed diagnoses of acute cardiac ischemia in the emergency department. *N Engl J Med*. 2000;342:1163–1170.
3. Hamm CW, Goldmann BU, Heeschen C, Kreymann G, Berger J, Meinertz T. Emergency room triage of patients with acute chest pain by means of rapid testing for cardiac troponin T or troponin I. *N Engl J Med*. 1997;337:1648–1653.
4. Mehta RH, Eagle KA. Missed diagnoses of acute coronary syndromes in the emergency room – continuing challenges. *N Engl J Med*. 2000;342:1207–1210.

5. Lee TH, Rouan GW, Weisberg MC et al. Sensitivity of routine clinical criteria for diagnosing myocardial infarction within 24 hours of hospitalization. *Ann Intern Med*. 1987;106:181–186.

6. Gibler WB, Young GP, Hedges JR, et al. Acute myocardial infarction in chest pain patients with nondiagnostic ECGs: serial CK-MB sampling in the emergency department. *Ann Emerg Med*. 1992;21:504–512.

7. Malasky BR, Alpert JS. Diagnosis of myocardial injury by biochemical markers: problems and promises. *Cardiol Rev*. 2002;10:306–317.

8. Babuin L, Vasile VC, Rio Perez JA, et al. Elevated cardiac troponin is an independent risk factor for short- and long-term mortality in medical intensive care unit patients. *Crit Care Med*. 2008;36:759–765.

9. Maeder M, Fehr T, Rickli H, Ammann P. Sepsis-associated myocardial dysfunction: diagnostic and prognostic impact of cardiac troponins and natriuretic peptides. *Chest*. 2006;129: 1349–1366.

10. Rude RE, Poole WK, Muller JE, et al. Electrocardiographic and clinical criteria for recognition of acute myocardial infarction based on analysis of 3,697 patients. *Am J Cardiol*. 1983;52:936–942.

11. Kaufmann B, Wei K, Lindner JR. Contrast echocardiography. *Curr Prob Cardiol*. 2007;32: 45–96.

12. Sabia P, Afrookteh A, Touchstone DA, Keller MW, Esquivel L, Kaul S. Value of regional wall motion abnormality in the emergency room diagnosis of acute myocardial infarction: a prospective study using 2-dimensional echocardiography. *Circulation*. 1991;84:I85–I92.

13. Sabia P, Abbott RD, Afrookteh A, Keller MW, Touchstone DA, Kaul S. The importance of two-dimensional echocardiographic assessment of left ventricular systolic function in patients presenting to the emergency room with cardiac-related symptoms. *Circulation*. 1997;96: 785–792.

14. Reilly JP, Tunick PA, Timmermans RJ, Stein B, Rosenzweig BP, Kronzon I. Contrast echocardiography clarifies uninterpretable wall motion in intensive care unit patients. *J Am Coll Cardiol*. 2000;35:485–490.

15. Crouse LJ, Cheirif J, Hanly DE, et al. Opacification and border delineation improvement in patients with suboptimal endocardial border definition in routine echocardiography: results of the Phase III Albunex Multicenter Trial. *J Am Coll Cardiol*. 1993;22:1494–1500.

16. Rainbird AJ, Mulvagh SL, Oh JK, et al. Contrast dobutamine stress echocardiography: clinical practice assessment in 300 consecutive patients. *J Am Soc Echocardiogr*. 2001;5:378–385.

17. Hoffmann R, von BS, ten CF et al. Assessment of systolic left ventricular function: a multicentre comparison of cineventriculography, cardiac magnetic resonance imaging, unenhanced and contrast-enhanced echocardiography. *Eur Heart J*. 2005;6:607–616.

18. Dolan MS, Riad K, El-Shafei A, et al. Effect of intravenous contrast for left ventricular opacification and border definition on sensitivity and specificity of dobutamine stress echocardiography compared with coronary angiography in technically difficult patients. *Am Heart J*. 2001;5:908–915.

19. Lindner JR, Dent JM, Moos SP, Jayaweera AR, Kaul S. Enhancement of left ventricular cavity opacification by harmonic imaging after venous injection of Albunex. *Am J Cardiol*. 1997;79:1657–1662.

20. Rinkevich D, Kaul S, Wang XQ, et al. Regional left ventricular perfusion and function in patients presenting to the emergency department with chest pain and no ST-segment elevation. *Eur Heart J*. 2005;26:1606–1611.

21. Ward RP, Weinert L, Spencer KT, et al. Quantitative diagnosis of apical cardiomyopathy using contrast echocardiography. *J Am Soc Echocardiogr*. 2002;15:316–322.

22. Abe Y, Kondo M, Matsuoka R, Araki M, Dohyama K, Tanio H. Assessment of clinical features in transient left ventricular apical ballooning. *J Am Coll Cardiol*. 2003;41:737–742.

23. Jayaweera AR, Edwards N, Glasheen WP, Villanueva FS, Abbott RD, Kaul S. In vivo myocardial kinetics of air-filled albumin microbubbles during myocardial contrast echocardiography. Comparison with radiolabeled red blood cells. *Circ Res*. 1994;74:1157–1165.

24. Lindner JR, Song J, Jayaweera AR, Sklenar J, Kaul S. Microvascular rheology of definity microbubbles after intra-arterial and intravenous administration. *J Am Soc Echocardiogr*. 2002;5:396–403.

25. Wei K, Jayaweera AR, Firoozan S, Linka A, Skyba DM, Kaul S. Quantification of myocardial blood flow with ultrasound-induced destruction of microbubbles administered as a constant venous infusion. *Circulation*. 1998;97:473–483.

26. Kassab GS, Lin DH, Fung YC. Morphometry of pig coronary venous system. *Am J Physiol*. 1994;7(6 Pt 2):H2100–H2113.

27. Coggins MP, Sklenar J, Le DE, Wei K, Lindner JR, Kaul S. Noninvasive prediction of ultimate infarct size at the time of acute coronary occlusion based on the extent and magnitude of collateral-derived myocardial blood flow. *Circulation*. 2001;104:2471–2477.

28. Tong KL, Kaul S, Wang X, et al. Myocardial contrast echocardiography versus thrombolysis in myocardial infarction score in patients presenting to the emergency department with chest pain and a nondiagnostic electrocardiogram. *J Am Coll Cardiol*. 2005;46:920–927.

29. Kaul S, Senior R, Firschke C, et al. Incremental value of cardiac imaging in patients presenting to the emergency department with chest pain and without ST-segment elevation: a multicenter study. *Am Heart J*. 2004;148:129–136.

30. Gewirtz H, Fischman AJ, Abraham S, Gilson M, Strauss HW, Alpert NM. Positron emission tomographic measurements of absolute regional myocardial blood flow permits identification of nonviable myocardium in patients with chronic myocardial infarction. *J Am Coll Cardiol*. 1994;23:851–859.

31. Lafitte S, Higashiyama A, Masugata H, et al. Contrast echocardiography can assess risk area and infarct size during coronary occlusion and reperfusion: experimental validation. *J Am Coll Cardiol*. 2002;39:1546–1554.

32. Leong-Poi H, Coggins MP, Sklenar J, Jayaweera AR, Wang XQ, Kaul S. Role of collateral blood flow in the apparent disparity between the extent of abnormal wall thickening and perfusion defect size during acute myocardial infarction and demand ischemia. *J Am Coll Cardiol*. 2005;45:565–572.

33. Balcells E, Powers ER, Lepper W, et al. Detection of myocardial viability by contrast echocardiography in acute infarction predicts recovery of resting function and contractile reserve. *J Am Coll Cardiol*. 2003;41:827–833.

34. Micari A, Belcik TA, Balcells EA, et al. Improvement in microvascular reflow and reduction of infarct size with adenosine in patients undergoing primary coronary stenting. *Am J Cardiol*. 2005;96:1410–1415.

35. Ito H, Okamura A, Iwakura K et al. Myocardial perfusion patterns related to thrombolysis in myocardial infarction perfusion grades after coronary angioplasty in patients with acute anterior wall myocardial infarction. *Circulation*. 1996;93:1993–1999.

36. Iwakura K, Ito H, Takiuchi S, et al. Alternation in the coronary blood flow velocity pattern in patients with no reflow and reperfused acute myocardial infarction. *Circulation*. 1996;94:1269–1275.

37. Kamp O, Lepper W, Vanoverschelde JL, et al. Serial evaluation of perfusion defects in patients with a first acute myocardial infarction referred for primary PTCA using intravenous myocardial contrast echocardiography. *Eur Heart J*. 2001;22:1485–1495.

38. Porter TR, Li S, Oster R, Deligonul U. The clinical implications of no reflow demonstrated with intravenous perfluorocarbon containing microbubbles following restoration of thrombolysis in myocardial infarction (TIMI) 3 flow in patients with acute myocardial infarction. *Am J Cardiol*. 1998;82:1173–1177.

39. Ito H, Maruyama A, Iwakura K, et al. Clinical implications of the 'no reflow' phenomenon. A predictor of complications and left ventricular remodeling in reperfused anterior wall myocardial infarction. *Circulation*. 1996;93:223–228.

40. Janardhanan R, Moon JC, Pennell DJ, Senior R. Myocardial contrast echocardiography accurately reflects transmurality of myocardial necrosis and predicts contractile reserve after acute myocardial infarction. *Am Heart J*. 2005;149:355–362.

41. Main ML, Magalski A, Chee NK, Coen MM, Skolnick DG, Good TH. Full-motion pulse inversion power Doppler contrast echocardiography differentiates stunning from necrosis and predicts recovery of left ventricular function after acute myocardial infarction. *J Am Coll Cardiol.* 2001;38:1390–1394.
42. Janardhanan R, Moon JC, Pennell DJ, Senior R. Myocardial contrast echocardiography accurately reflects transmurality of myocardial necrosis and predicts contractile reserve after acute myocardial infarction. *Am Heart J.* 2005;149:355–362.
43. Andrassy P, Zielinska M, Busch R, Schomig A, Firschke C. Myocardial blood volume and the amount of viable myocardium early after mechanical reperfusion of acute myocardial infarction: prospective study using venous contrast echocardiography. *Heart.* 2002;87:350–355.
44. Villanueva FS, Glasheen WP, Sklenar J, Kaul S. Assessment of risk area during coronary occlusion and infarct size after reperfusion with myocardial contrast echocardiography using left and right atrial injections of contrast. *Circulation.* 1993;88:596–604.
45. Sakuma T, Okada T, Hayashi Y, Otsuka M, Hirai Y. Optimal time for predicting left ventricular remodeling after successful primary coronary angioplasty in acute myocardial infarction using serial myocardial contrast echocardiography and magnetic resonance imaging. *Circ J.* 2002;66:685–690.

# Index

Printed in the United States of America